Novel Anticancer Drug Protocols

METHODS IN MOLECULAR MEDICINE™

John M. Walker, SERIES EDITOR

METHODS IN MOLECULAR MEDICINE™

Novel Anticancer Drug Protocols

Edited by

John K. Buolamwini, PhD

University of Tennessee Health Science Center, Memphis, TN

and

Alex A. Adjei, MD, PhD

Mayo Clinic and Foundation, Rochester, MN

Humana Press ✳ Totowa, New Jersey

Production Editor: Mark J. Breaugh.

Cover illustration: Microphotographs obtained from dorsal skinfold chamber in 6 wk nu/nu mouse. (*See* Fig. 1, p. 67.) Background: Second column, bottom frame. Inset: Fourth column, bottom frame.

Cover design by Patricia F. Cleary.

For additional copies, pricing for bulk purchases, and/or information about other Humana titles, contact Humana at the above address or at any of the following numbers: Tel.: 973-256-1699; Fax: 973-256-8341; E-mail: humana@humanapr.com; Website: humanapress.com

Printed in the United States of America. 10 9 8 7 6 5 4 3 2 1

Library of Congress Cataloging in Publication Data

Novel anticancer drug protocols / edited by John K. Buolamwini and Alex A. Adjei.
    p. cm. -- (Methods in molecular medicine)
    Includes bibliographical references and index.
    ISBN 0-89603-963-3 (alk. paper)   e-ISBN 1-59259-380-1
    1. Antineoplastic agents--Research--Methodology. I. Buolamwini, John K. II. Adjei, Alex A. III. Series

    RC271.C5 N476 2003
    616.99'4061--dc21

                                                                      2002038702

Preface

We are in an exciting era in the war against cancer, with real prospects for novel anticancer drugs that are cancer cell-specific without the toxicities that have been the hallmark of conventional cytotoxic cancer chemotherapy. Advances in cancer cell biology fueled by the molecular biology revolution have resulted in the uncovering of many novel potential molecular targets for cancer therapy. New anticancer drug discovery and development is now largely focused on exploiting these new molecular targets, which encompass oncogenes, tumor suppressor genes, and their gene products, as well as targets involved in tumor angiogenesis, metastasis, survival, and longevity mechanisms. Exploitation of some of these targets has already yielded fruits and introduced new paradigms of molecularly targeted cancer therapy into the clinic, namely, protein kinase inhibition by antibodies or small molecules, exemplified by Herceptin® (trastuzumab), a humanized antibody targeted against the HER-2 growth factor receptor tyrosine kinase for the treatment of metastatic breast cancer; and Gleevec, a small molecule bcr-abl kinase inhibitor for the treatment of chronic myelogenous leukemia.

With many potential molecular targets having already been identified, and many more yet to be discovered, we face challenges in their validation, the use of relevant assays for successful drug discovery, and efficient preclinical and clinical development strategies to enable the translation of the discoveries into effective clinical regimens for cancer patients. To meet these challenges, novel tools in the form of basic and clinical research and testing protocols are required. In this volume on *Novel Anticancer Drug Protocols,* we have provided not only a broad overview of the whole arena of novel anticancer drug targets, but also a wide-ranging selection of cutting-edge techniques that are being applied to novel anticancer drug discovery and development. These comprise protocols involving, or applied to, growth factors, receptor/nonreceptor tyrosine kinases and their downstream signal transduction targets, serine/threonine kinases, angiogenesis, metastasis, apoptosis, cell longevity, protein chaperoning and degradation, functional genomics, antibody methods, antisense oligonucleotide strategies, protein–protein and protein–DNA interactions, and miscellaneous pertinent methods. With the exception of the introductory chapter on novel anticancer drug targets and a

v

review chapter on assays for in vitro and in vivo synergy, each methodological-cal chapter begins with background information, followed by a detailed description of the experimental protocols in easy-to-follow reproducible reci-pes, and notes to ensure their successful use by other investigators.

We hope that *Novel Anticancer Drug Protocols* will serve its purpose of making available, in a user-friendly format, a broad range of the cutting-edge methodologies now being used in the discovery and development of novel anticancer drugs, to basic scientists and clinical researchers in academia, in-dustry, and government laboratories, as well as cancer research institutions. Our gratitude goes to all the authors who have contributed chapters to the book.

John K. Buolamwini, PhD
Alex A. Adjei, MD, PhD

Contents

Contributors

JULIAN ADAMS • *Millennium Pharmaceuticals Inc., Cambridge, MA*

ALEX A. ADJEI • *Department of Oncology, Mayo Clinic and Foundation, Rochester, MN*

WYNNE AHERNE • *CRC Centre for Cancer Therapeutics, Institute of Cancer Research, Surrey, UK*

GREGORY J. AHMANN • *Department of Hematology and Internal Medicine, Mayo Clinic, Rochester, MN*

MARGARET-MARY AMEYAW • *Washington University School of Medicine, St. Louis, MO*

HAREGEWEIN ASSEFA • *Department of Pharmaceutical Sciences, College of Pharmacy, University of Tennessee Health Science Center, Memphis, TN*

ROBLE G. BEDOLLA • *Department of Surgery, University of Texas Health Science Center, San Antonio, TX*

PER BORGSTRÖM • *Sidney Kimmel Cancer Center, San Diego, CA*

KATHERINE BOXALL • *CRC Centre for Cancer Therapeutics, Institute of Cancer Research, Surrey, UK*

MICHAEL G. BRATTAIN • *Department of Pharmacology and Therapeutic, Roswell Park Cancer Institute, Buffalo, NY*

JOHN K. BUOLAMWINI • *Department of Pharmaceutical Sciences, College of Pharmacy, University of Tennessee Health Science Center, Memphis, TN*

PAUL CLARKE • *CRC Centre for Cancer Therapeutics, Institute of Cancer Research, Surrey, UK*

MEGHAN CUNNINGHAM • *Department of Biology, Georgetown University, Washington, DC*

PETER J. ELLIOTT • *CombinatorRx Inc., Boston, MA*

RAFAEL FONSECA • *Department of Hematology and Internal Medicine, Mayo Clinic, Rochester, MN*

ANNA FREDRIKSSON • *Karolinska Pharmacy, Karolinska Hospital, Stockholm, Sweden*

GREGORY I. FROST • *Sidney Kimmel Cancer Center, San Diego, CA*

MICHIKO N. FUKUDA • *Glycobiology Program, The Burnham Institute, La Jolla, CA*

xi

JACEK GAN • *Comprehensive Cancer Center and Department of Human Oncology, The University of Wisconsin, Madison, WI*

STEPHEN D. GILLIES • *Lexigen Pharmaceuticals Inc., Lexington, MA*

RONALD S. GO • *Sections of Hematology and Medical Oncology, Gundersen-Lutheran Medical Center, La Crosse, WI*

PAUL H. GUMERLOCK • *Division of Hematology and Oncology, Department of Internal Medicine, University of California Davis Cancer Center, Sacramento, CA*

JACQUELYN A. HANK • *Comprehensive Cancer Center and Department of Human Oncology, The University of Wisconsin, Madison, WI*

ANTHEA HARDCASTLE • *CRC Centre for Cancer Therapeutics, Institute of Cancer Research, Surrey, UK*

ROMAN HERRERA • *Cancer Molecular Sciences Department, Pfizer Global Research and Development, Ann Arbor, MI*

MANUEL HIDALGO • *Sidney Kimmel Comprehensive Cancer Center, Johns Hopkins University School of Medicine, Baltimore, MD*

WILL S. HOLLAND • *Division of Hematology and Oncology, Department of Internal Medicine, University of California Davis Cancer Center, Sacramento, CA*

KENNETH HOOK • *Cancer Pharmacology Department, Pfizer Global Research and Development, Ann Arbor, MI*

ELZBIETA IZBICKA • *Institute for Drug Development Cancer Therapy and Research Center, San Antonio, TX*

TOMOYA KAWAGUCHI • *Division of Hematoloya and Oncology, Department of Internal Medicine, University of California Davis Cancer Center, Sacramento, CA*

MERIUM KHAN • *Department of Biology, Georgetown University, Washington, DC*

KAY KLAUSING • *Molecular and Cell Biology, Ligand Pharmaceuticals Inc., San Diego, CA*

CHRISTOPHER P. KOLBERT • *Microarray Shared Resource, Mayo Clinic Cancer Center, Rochester, MN*

KELLY L. KRAJNIK • *Microarray Shared Resource, Mayo Clinic Cancer Center, Rochester, MN*

JEFFREY I. KREISBERG • *Department of Surgery, University of Texas Health Science Center; Audie Murphy Veterans Administration Hospital, San Antonio, TX*

TYLER LAHUSEN • *Molecular Therapeutics Unit, Oral and Pharyngeal Cancer Branch, National Institute of Dental and Craniofacial Research, National Institutes of Health, Bethesda, MD*

ERIC S. LIGHTCAP • *Millennium Pharmaceuticals Inc., Cambridge, MA*

SHAZLI N. MALIK • *Departments of Surgery, University of Texas Health Science Center, San Antonio, TX*

ALISON MALONEY • *CRC Centre for Cancer Therapeutics, Institute of Cancer Research, Surrey, UK*

VANESSA MARCELL • *Department of Biology, Georgetown University, Washington, DC*

SHARON MARSH • *Washington University School of Medicine, St. Louis, MO*

HOWARD L. McLEOD • *Washington University School of Medicine, St. Louis, MO*

LOREA MENDOZA • *PharmaKine Ltd., Zamudio Technology Park, Bizkaia, Spain*

MANISHA MURTHY • *Department of Pharmaceutical Sciences, University of Southern California, School of Pharmacy, Los Angeles, CA*

NOURI NEAMATI • *Department of Pharmaceutical Sciences, University of Southern California, School of Pharmacy, Los Angeles, CA*

DAVID NISHIOKA • *Department of Biology, Georgetown University, Washington, DC*

DENNIS J. O'KANE • *Microarray Shared Resource, Mayo Clinic Cancer Center, Rochester, MN*

ELVIRA OLASO • *Department of Cell Biology, Basque Country University School of Medicine and Dentistry, Leioa, Spain*

AMY OSTENDORF • *Comprehensive Cancer Center and Department of Human Oncology, The University of Wisconsin, Madison, WI*

WHYTE G. OWEN • *Departments of Physiology, Biophysics, Biochemistry, and Molecular Biology, Mayo Clinic and Foundation, Rochester, MN*

LAURENCE PEARL • *Section of Structural Biology, Institute of Cancer Research, Chester Beatty Laboratories, London, UK*

CHRISTINE S. PIEN • *Toler Rx Inc., Cambridge, MA*

CHRIS PRODROMOU • *Section of Structural Biology, Institute of Cancer Research, Chester Beatty Laboratories, London, UK*

ELIZABETH QUACKENBUSH • *Merck Research Laboratories, Rahway, NJ*

CHRISTINE M. ROSE • *Washington University School of Medicine, St. Louis, MO*

MARTIN G. ROWLANDS • *CRC Centre for Cancer Therapeutics, Institute of Cancer Research, Surrey, UK*

RAVI SALGIA • *Department of Medical Oncology, Dana-Farber Cancer Institute; Department of Medicine, Brigham and Women's Hospital and Harvard Medical Schoxol, Boston, MA*

JANN N. SARKARIA • *Department of Oncology, Mayo Foundation, Rochester, MN*

MARTIN SATTLER • *Department of Medical Oncology, Dana-Farber Cancer Institute, Brigham and Women's Hospital and Harvard Medical School, Boston, MA*

JUDITH S. SEBOLT-LEOPOLD • *Cancer Molecular Sciences Department, Pfizer Global Research and Development, Ann Arbor, MI*

ADRIAN M. SENDEROWICZ • *Molecular Therapeutics Unit, Oral and Pharyngeal Cancer Branch, National Institute of Dental and Craniofacial Research, National Institutes of Health, Bethesda, MD*

PAUL M. SONDEL • *Comprehensive Cancer Center and Departments of Human Oncology and Pediatrics and Medical Genetics, The University of Wisconsin, Madison, WI*

TERESA A. SOUCY • *Millennium Pharmaceuticals Inc., Cambridge, MA*

DAVID P. STEENSMA • *Division of Hematology, Department of Internal Medicine, Mayo Clinic and Mayo Foundation, Rochester, MN*

SHARON STONE-ELANDER • *Karolinska Pharmacy, Karolinska Hospital, Stockholm, Sweden*

JEAN E. SURFUS • *Comprehensive Cancer Center and Department of Human Oncology, The University of Wisconsin, Madison, WI*

WILLIAM R. TAYLOR • *Microarray Shared Resource, Mayo Clinic Cancer Center, Rochester, MN*

BEVERLY A. TEICHER • *Genzyme Corporation, Framingham, MA*

MICHAEL TIMM • *Department of Laboratory Medicine and Pathology, Mayo Clinic and Mayo Foundation, Rochester, MN*

CURTIS M. TYREE • *Neurogenetics Inc., La Jolla, CA*

KERI VAN BECELAERE • *Cancer Molecular Sciences Department, Pfizer Global Research and Development, Ann Arbor, MI*

FERNANDO VIDAL-VANACLOCHA • *Department of Cell Biology, Basque Country University School of Medicine and Dentistry, Leioa, Spain*

DANIEL D. VON HOFF • *Institute for Drug Development, Cancer Therapy and Research Center, San Antonio, TX*

MICHAEL I. WALTON • *CRC Centre for Cancer Therapeutics, Institute of Cancer Research, Surrey, UK*

HUI WANG • *Division of Clinical Pharmacology, Department of Pharmacology and Toxicology, and Comprehensive Cancer Center, University of Alabama at Birmingham, Birmingham, AL*

YUN-XING WANG • *Program in Structural Biology, National Cancer Institute Frederick, Frederick, MD*

THOMAS E. WITZIG • *Division of Hematology, Department of Internal Medicine, Mayo Clinic and Mayo Foundation, Rochester, MN*

PAUL WORKMAN • *CRC Centre for Cancer Therapeutics, Institute of Cancer Research, Surrey, UK*

JIANING ZHANG • *Glycobiology Program, The Burnham Institute, La Jolla, CA*

RUIWEN ZHANG • *Division of Clinical Pharmacology, Department of Pharmacology and Toxicology, and Comprehensive Cancer Center, University of Alabama at Birmingham, Birmingham, AL*

I

INTRODUCTION

1

Overview of Novel Anticancer Drug Targets

John K. Buolamwini and Haregewein Assefa

1. Introduction

There has been an explosion in the number of potential molecular targets
that can be explored for selective cancer treatment. The stage is now set
to translate years of productive cancer research into more patient-friendly
anticancer therapeutics. At present, the challenge is how to identify bonafide
and viable targets and efficiently exploit these for the development of selective
nontoxic cancer therapies, to overcome the major drawbacks of conventional
cytotoxic cancer chemotherapy. To this end, it is gratifying that the selective
inhibition of some of these novel targets, especially those in mitogenic signal
transduction pathways like HER-2 and bcr-abl tyrosine kinases, has resulted
in successful treatments of cancer patients. HER-2 is targeted by the antibody
traszumamab (Herceptin®), approved for the treatment of metastatic breast
cancer *(1)*, while bcr-abl tyrosine kinase is targeted by the small molecule drug
STI571 (Imatinib, Gleevec), for the treatment of chronic myelogenous leukemia
(CML) *(2)*. Other promising therapies targeted to other signal transduction
targets are in the pipeline, the most advanced probably being small molecules
targeted to the epidermal growth factor receptor (EGFR) tyrosine kinase *(3)*.
This chapter will provide a broad overview of a wide range of emerging
molecular targets, highlighting some of the strategies used to exploit them for
molecularly-targeted cancer therapy, such as small molecules, antibodies, and
antisense oligonucleotides.

The application of molecular biology technologies to cancer research has
resulted in the identification of many potential anticancer molecular targets that
can be considered 'cancer selective'. These targets span the gamut of proteins

From: *Methods in Molecular Medicine, vol. 85: Novel Anticancer Drug Protocols*
Edited by: J. K. Buolamwini and A. A. Adjei © Humana Press Inc., Totowa, NJ

and genes involved in cancer cell proliferation, differentiation, malignant transformation, survival, replicative longevity, angiogenesis, and metastasis. They include growth factors and their receptor tyrosine kinases, non-receptor tyrosine kinases, serine/threonine kinases, protein phosphatases, regulatory proteins, transcription factors, and proteins involved in shuttling, sequestration, and/or degradation of other proteins, as well as proteins involved in extracellular matrix modeling and interactions *(4–11)*. Cancer results from processes involving genetic changes that activate oncogene *(12)* and/or deactivate tumor suppressor gene function *(13,14)*. Oncogenes, activated by mutation, amplification, and/or overexpression, cause neoplastic transformation and promote tumor progression. On the other hand, deactivating mutations in tumor suppressor genes or deactivating events involving their transcription or gene products result in loss of function and give way to tumor formation. The ability of cancer cells to resist apoptosis (i.e., programmed cell death by which cells commit suicide), in large part, allows cancer establishment and progression, as well as drug resistance *(15)*.

In this chapter, the targets are considered under the following general pathways: (1) mitogenic signal transduction, (2) cell-cycle, (3) apoptosis/survival, (4) angiogenesis and metastasis, and (5) cell replicative lifespan/longevity. This classification should not be considered rigid, as overlaps do occur. Approaches to exploit these targets are varied, including small molecule drug development *(9,11)*, antibodies *(16)*, antisense oligonucleotides *(17)*, and gene therapy *(18,19)*.

2. Mitogenic Signal Transduction Pathway Targets

Targeting signal transduction pathways was the first approach to the current paradigms of molecularly-targeted cancer therapeutics *(4,20)*. The most studied targets in the group are the growth factor receptor tyrosine kinases, non-receptor tyrosine kinases, adaptor proteins, GTP-binding proteins, and serine/threonine kinases, which comprise members of mitogenic signaling cascades and networks spanning the cell surface and the cytoplasm. Binding of growth factors to their cognate receptor tyrosine kinases (RTKs) causes receptor homo- or heterodimerization, resulting in autophosphorylation of the receptors to begin signal transduction cascades *(21,22)*. The tyrosine phosphorylation creates a binding sites in the cytoplasmic domain of the RTKs for adapter proteins such as Grb2, which binds to the RTK via its SH2 domain. This binding activates Grb2, enabling it to bind to the guanine nucleotide exchange factor, the sos (son of sevenless) protein via the Grb2 SH3 domain. Grb2 binding to sos causes the latter to translocate to the cell membrane where it interacts with the GTP-binding protein ras, causing a molecular switch in ras that results in release of bound GDP from ras, to be replaced by GTP instead, resulting in the activation of ras. Ras is a signaling hub that has several other upstream regulators and downstream effectors *(23–26)*. In the most studied ras signaling cascade, activated ras binds to and activates raf-1 kinase, to initiate the mitogen activated protein (MAP) kinase cascade. Activated raf-1 phosphorylates MEK kinase, which in turn phosphorylates the last member in the cascade, extracellular regulated kinase, ERK. Phosphorylated ERK then translocates to the cell nucleus to propagate the mitogenic signal by phosphorylating transcription factors which induce the expression of cell division cycle genes *(21,27)*.

RTKs have been implicated in many human cancers, especially breast, ovarian, and non-small cell lung cancers *(21,28)*, and are being pursued intensely for cancer therapy *(11,29–31)*. Notable among these kinases are EGFR, HER-2 (c-erbB-2), platelet-derived growth factor receptor (PDGFR), vascular endothelial growth factor receptor (VEGFR) and basic fibroblast growth factor receptor (bFGFR). Many reviews have appeared on drug discovery efforts targeting the RTKs *(3,32–36)*. Strategies for the discovery of tyrosine kinase inhibitors with anticancer activity have also been presented by Fry et al. *(37)*; these include the production of the target kinases, primary screening for potency and specificity, investigation of cellular effects, and in vivo evaluation for anticancer activity.

2.1. The ErbB/HER Growth Factor Receptor Tyrosine Kinases

The EGFR (erbB-1, HER-1), HER-2 (erbB-2, neu), HER-3 (erbB-3) and HER-4 (erbB-4) are members of the type 1 growth factor receptor tyrosine kinase (RTK) family, also known as the erbB or HER family *(27,38)*. Specific ligands have been identified for EGFR (EGF and TGFα, HER-3 and HER-4 (heregulin, neu differentiation factor or neuregulin 1), but none has yet been identified for HER-2 *(39)*. EGFR and HER-2 have emerged as the most viable anticancer molecular targets in this family, and their overexpression or mutational activation is frequently encountered in breast, ovarian, and non-small cell lung cancers *(21,28,38)*. Numerous small organic compounds have been synthesized and evaluated as inhibitors of EGFR and/or c-erbB-2 tyrosine kinases *(3,32,36,40)*. The most successful compounds to date are the anilinoquinazolines, some of which are in clinical trials, including the orally active ZD1839 (Iressa®) *(3)*. Antibodies are also being pursued as therapeutic agents against EGFR and HER2 *(3)*. In this regard, trastzumamab (Herceptin®, Genentech, South San Franscisco, CA), a humanized monoclonal antibody is already in the clinic for the treatment of HER-2-overexpressing metastatic breast cancer *(41)*. Cetuximab (IMC-C225, ImClone, New York, NY) is a monoclonal antibody targeted against EGFR that is in clinical trials *(42)*. Interestingly, HER-2 has also been shown to be depleted by inhibitors of the heat shock protein HSP90, such as geldanamycin, making this class of compounds indirect inhibitors of HER-2 function as well *(43,44)*.

2.2. Other Receptor Tyrosine Kinases

Platelet-derived growth factor (PDGF) signaling affects proliferation, actin rearrangement, chemotaxis and angiogenesis, and provides protection against apoptosis *(45)*. This signaling is frequently deregulated in gliomas *(28)*. The platelet-derived growth factor receptor (PDGFR) is also being targeted for novel anticancer drug discovery, albeit less so than the EGFR family. Small molecule selective inhibitors of PDGFR include 2-phenylaminopyrimidines such as CGP57148 (STI571), 3-arylsubstituted quinoxalines, and quinolines *(34)*. The vascular endothelial growth factor receptors, VEGFR-1 (flt-1) and VEGFR-2, are implicated in tumor angiogenesis *(46–48)*, while VEGFR-3 has been demonstrated to be involved in maintaining the integrity of the endothelial lining during angiogenesis *(49)*. The most prominent angiogenic growth factor receptor tyrosine kinases are VEGFR-2 (flk-1), basic fibroblast growth factor receptor (bFGFR) and PDGFRβ *(28,50)*. It is interesting that in addition to its angiogenic function, the bFGFR ligand, bFGF, has been shown to induce MDM2 protein expression by a p53-independent mechanism to prolong cell survival and resistance to cisplatin *(51)*. Suramin and its analogs, such as FCE 27266, have been found to block the growth stimulatory activities of the growth factors VEGF, PDGF, and bFGF by inhibiting their binding to cognate receptors *(48)*.

Clinically promising small molecule drugs are those that inhibit the kinase activities of these growth factor receptors. The clinical development of inhibitors targeted to VEGF and its receptors has been reviewed recently *(52)*. SU5416, a VEGFR-2 (flk-1)-selective kinase inhibitor *(53)*, is in advanced clinical development as an anti-angiogenic agent (SUGEN/Pharmacia, South San Francisco, CA). PD145709 and SU5402, selective bFGF receptor kinase inhibitors *(54,55)*. Leflunomide (SU 101), a PDGFβ receptor kinase inhibitor, has been shown to be an effective inhibitor of PDGFβ-promoted glioma tumor growth in vivo *(56)*. SCH 13929 has been shown to interact with, and competitively inhibit the binding of PDGF to its receptors, and to inhibit its biological functions in vitro and in vivo *(57)*. PTK787 is a new potent kinase inhibitor of both VEGFR-1 and VEGFR-2 receptors, with IC_{50} values of 0.077 and 0.037 μM, respectively *(52)*. Another potential receptor tyrosine kinase target is c-kit, which has been shown to harbor gain-of-function mutations in some human gastrointestinal stromal tumors *(58)*. C-kit together with its ligand, stem cell factor, is expressed in about 75% of small cell lung cancers (SCLC), and is being targeted for the treatment of SCLC using STI571 (Gleevec™) *(59)*, discussed in the next section.

2.3. Non-Receptor Tyrosine Kinases

In addition to the receptor tyrosine kinases, non-receptor tyrosine kinases are also involved in mitogenic signal transduction. Notable oncogenic non-receptor protein tyrosine kinases involved in human cancer are the src gene product pp60^{src}, which is deregulated in colon *(28)* and pancreatic *(60)* cancers; the src family member lck gene product p56^{lck} *(61)*, which is deregulated in T-cell lymphomas *(62)*; and the bcr-abl gene product p210$^{bcr-abl}$, which is deregulated in most chronic myelogenous leukemias *(28)*. 2-Substituted aminopyrido[2,3-*d*]pyrimidinones *(63)* have been found to have selective inhibitory activity against pp60^{src}. Other small molecule pp60^{src}-selective inhibitors include 5,10-dihydropyrimidino[4,5-*b*]quinolin-4(1*H*)-ones and 3-(N-phenyl)carboxamide-2-iminochromene derivatives *(34)*. The 3-(N-phenyl) carboxamide-2-iminochromene derivatives also inhibit the kinase activity of p56^{lck}. X-ray crystal structure-based design of novel small molecule inhibitors has also been undertaken *(64)*. The 2-phenylaminopyrimidine derivative, CGP 57148 (STI571, Gleevec™) is a potent inhibitor of the bcr-abl gene product p210$^{bcr-abl}$ tyrosine kinase in vitro and in vivo *(65)*, and has recently been approved for the treatment of CML *(2)*. This drug, as mentioned in the previous section, also inhibits c-kit tyrosine kinase *(58,66)*, as well as PDGFR kinase *(34)*. Key small molecule inhibitors have also been identified for p56^{lck}, including dihydroxystyrene salicylic acid, a dihydroxyisoquinoline derivative, and a pyrazolo[3,4-*d*]pyrimidine derivative *(34)*.

2.4. Cytoplasmic Serine/Threonine Kinases

Several cytoplasmic oncogenic serine/threonine kinases have also been identified, including some members of the protein kinase C (PKC) family, protein kinase A (PKA), and the MAP kinases, all of which are being investigated as novel targets for cancer therapy.

2.4.1. Protein Kinases C, A, and B

The development of specific inhibitors targeting serine/threonine kinases, including protein kinase A (PKA), PKC, mitogen-activated protein (MAP) kinases and cell-cycle related kinases, as probes and potential drugs, has been reviewed *(67)*. PKC isozymes are very much involved in cell growth regulation and tumor promotion, being the major molecular targets of tumor promoting phorbol esters *(68,69)*. Endogenously, they are activated by diacylglycerol *(70)*. PKC effects are mediated, at least in part by ERK via Raf-1 and ras

(25). Some isozymes are calcium-dependent, while others are not *(71)*. It has been demonstrated that the PKC family is a potential target for cancer therapy *(72–78)*. PKC overexpression has been observed in estrogen receptor-negative breast cancer, thyroid cancer, gliomas, and melanoma *(76)*. PKC overexpression has also been implicated in angiogenesis *(76)*. The PKCα isoform has been shown to be especially overexpressed in multidrug resistant cancers *(73,76,79,80)*. The antiproliferative effect of PKC inhibitors is cell context dependent *(73)*. Several PKC inhibitors, albeit not isozyme specific, have been identified, including 7-hydroxystaurosporin (UCN-01) and safingol *(72,73,75,81)*. CGP 53506 is a selective inhibitor of PKCα, and has been shown to inhibit tumor growth *(82)*. Computer-aided drug design has been applied to the discovery of novel PKC modulators exploiting the 3D structure of PKCδ in complex with a phorbol ester *(83–85)*. The lack of specificity of current PKC modulators makes it questionable whether their effects are really due to modulation of PKC, since many also inhibit other serine/threonine kinases, especially cyclin-dependent kinases. Antisense approaches to the inhibition of PKCα have advanced into clinical trials *(17)*.

Considerable effort has also been put into targeting PKA for anticancer therapy. A cyclic AMP analog, 8-chloro-cyclic AMP, has been shown to inhibit tumor growth by targeting PKA *(86)*. The antisense oligonucleotide approach has been applied more extensively in this regard *(17)*.

Protein kinase B, also known as AKT, is involved in oncogenic signaling through PI3 kinase pathways involved in cancers such as breast, prostate, colon, and brain *(87)*, and is negatively regulated by the PTEN tumor suppressor gene *(88,89)*. Anticancer targeting of this pathway has not advanced as much as the targeting of PKC and PKA.

2.4.2. MAP Kinases

The ERK cascade comprising MAP kinases downstream of ras *(90)*, is the most characterized MAP kinase cascade *(91–93)* in signal transduction. Two proteins in the pathway, Raf-1 and MEK, are the important oncogenic members in this cascade *(12)*, and have emerged as potential novel anticancer drug targets *(94–96)*. The cascade starts with raf-1, which is activated by ras, and in turn activates MEK. MEK then activates the last MAP kinase in the cascade, ERK, which enters into the cell nucleus to propagate the mitogenic signal for cell division. Raf-1 is also involved in anti-apoptotic signaling via MEK-dependent and MEK-independent pathways. In the former pathway, MEK activation by raf-1 is followed by MEK activation of ERK, which activates Rsk1, which in turn phosphorylates and inactivates the pro-apoptotic protein BAD *(97)*, and/or activates the cell survival promoting transcription factor CREB *(98)*. The MEK-independent cell survival signaling of raf-1 is associated with its being targeted to mitochondria, and the possible involvement of the Bcl-2 family of proteins *(99–101)*. In addition to its kinase-dependent effects, raf-1 has also been shown to promote cell survival in a kinase-independent fashion by antagonizing the activity of apoptosis signal-regulating kinase 1 (ASK-1) through protein-protein interactions *(102)*. Antisense oligonucleotide strategies have being pursued for raf-1 modulation in cancer, some of which are being evaluated in advanced clinical trials *(17,103)*. As well, a small molecule raf-1 kinase inhibitor, BAY-43-9006, is in clinical trials *(104)*. Selective small molecule inhibitors of MEK have also been discovered, such as PD 98059, which inhibits cell growth and reverses ras transformation *(105)*, and CI-1040, which suppresses colon tumor growth in vivo *(96)*.

2.5. Cyclin-Dependent Kinases

In mitogenic signaling, activated terminal MAP kinases such as ERK translocate to the cell nucleus to activate transcription factors that induce cell division cycle gene expression to initiate the cell cycle. Serine/threonine kinases, termed cyclin-dependent kinases (CDKs), work in concert with their activating cyclins (regulatory units) to drive progression through the different phases of the cell division cycle *(106–108)*. CDKs are kept under control by nuclear proteins termed cyclin-dependent kinase inhibitors (CKIs), exemplified by p21, p27, p57 and p16 *(109–113)*. Phosphorylation substrates of activated CDKs include the retinoblastoma (Rb) tumor suppressor gene product and related proteins, as well as the E2F transcription factor family *(114–116)*. CDKs have emerged as potential targets for novel anticancer drug discovery *(117–121)*. Several small molecule ATP-site competitive CDK inhibitors are under anticancer drug development *(67,108,122)*. Notable CDK inhibitors are flavopiridol, olumoucine, and its analog roscovitine. Flavopiridol is a broad-spectrum CDK inhibitor that inhibits CDK1, CDK2, CDK4, CDK6, and CDK9 *(120)* and causes cell cycle arrest in G1 independent of functional p53 or Rb *(123)*, as well as cell cycle arrest at G2, attributed to the alteration of the phosphorylation state of CDK1, and/or inhibition of the kinase activity of cyclin B-CDK1. The CDK-selectivity among these molecules, both within the CDK family and relative to non-CDK enzymes has been reviewed *(120,122)*. Flavopiridol inhibits the growth of human tumor xenografts originating from lung, colon, stomach, breast, and brain, and has been under clinical development *(75,124)*. The ability to induce p53-independent apoptosis is an attractive property of the CDK inhibitors. This property in flavopiridol is now being attributed to the ability of CDK inhibitors to antagonize the effects of non-cell cycle CDKs like CDK9/cyclin T involved in RNA polymerase regulation *(125)*. The inhibition of CDK9/cyclin T has been shown to be the mechanism for the newly discovered anti-HIV activity of CDK inhibitors like flavopiridol

(126). The purine-derivative CDK inhibitors olumoucine and analog roscovitine are more selective than flavopyridol, and have also emerged as clinical trials candidates *(127)*. Other important small molecule CDK inhibitors are new purine derivatives like the purvalanols *(128)*, the paulones *(129)*, and the the indigoids *(130)*, as well as CDK4-selective compounds like the aminothiazoles *(131)*.

2.5.1. Other Cell Cycle Oncogenic Kinases

Emerging cell-cycle related non-cyclin-depdendent serine/threonine kinase anticancer targets include polo-like *(132)* and aurora *(133)* kinases, which have been shown to be aberrantly expressed in non-small cell lung cancer and colorectal cancers, respectively. No small molecule inhibitors of these have been reported. Chk1 is an important mediator of cell cycle arrest in G2 following DNA damage, and has become a potential anticancer target as well *(134)*. The G2 checkpoint abrogation achieved with the staurosporine derivative UCN-01 results from its inhibition of Chk1 kinase *(135)*. A 1.7 Å resolution X-ray crystal structure of human Chk1 kinase domain in complex with an ATP analog has been reported *(102)*, making this target amenable to structure-based design for small molecule inhibitor discovery.

2.6. Protein Phosphatases

Unlike protein kinases, protein phosphatases have not been shown to be very extensively involved in oncogenesis. However, a few oncogenic protein phosphatases have been identified such as the Cdc25 proteins *(136)*. Overexpression of Cdc25B has been demonstrated in 32% of human primary breast cancers *(136)*. Specific Cdc25B protein phosphatase inhibitors that inhibit tumor growth have been reported recently *(137)*.

2.7. The Grb2 Adapter Protein

The Grb2 adapter protein *(138)*, which is involved in both receptor and non-receptor tyrosine kinase signaling, provides an attractive target for simultaneously abrogating mitogenic signals from various protein tyrosine kinases *(139,140)*. There are two types of domains on the Grb2 protein, which it uses to perform its adapter functions: the SH2 (src homology 2) and SH3 (src homology 3) domains *(141)*. Small molecule inhibitors of the Grb-2 SH2 domain have been discovered *(139)*.

2.8. Ras Oncogene

The 21 kDa ras gene product is a GTP-binding protein that acts as a key hub in cellular proliferation and differentiation signal transduction *(142)*. In humans, the ras family is made up of three members, K-ras, H-ras, and N-ras *(143,144)*. Mutated ras genes are oncogenic, and are found in about 30%

of human cancers, being highly prevalent in pancreatic (90%), lung (40%), colorectal (50%) cancers and myeloid leukemias (30%), but rarely present (<5%) in breast, ovarian, or cervical cancers *(145)*. Activation of ras occurs by the binding of a GTP molecule that replaces a GDP molecule. This GTP binding is caused by the binding of sos protein to ras. The three-dimensional (3D) structure of the ras-sos complex has been reported *(146)*. Anticancer drug discovery targeting ras has taken two main routes: (1) antisense *(17)*, and (2) ras farnesyl transferase inhibitors *(147,148)*. Ras farnesylation is required to anchor newly translated ras protein to the cell membrane before it can perform its signal transduction functions *(149,150)*. A farnesyl moiety is coupled to the cysteine in the CAAX amino acid sequence at the C-terminus (where C is cysteine, A is any aliphatic amino acid and X is any amino acid), by farnesyl transferase (Fiase) using farnesyl pyrophosphate as substrate *(147,151)*. An undersirable effect of some farnesyl transferase inhibitors is their inhibition of geranylgeranyl transferase as well. Many FTase-selective inhibitors have been discovered, and constitute the most popular agents for targeting ras for cancer chemotherapy *(151–153)*. Representative ras FTase inhibitors in clinical trials are SCH66336 and R115777 *(148,154)*. The ras-related GTP-binding proteins Rac and Rho, have also been proposed as potential drug discovery targets for ras-mediated cancers *(155)*. These proteins are key players in cytoskeletal reorganization. Rho suppresses the p21^{WAF1} gene product to allow ras to drive cells into S phase *(26)*.

2.9. Oncogenic Transcription Factors

Several transcription factors involved in cell proliferation and differentiation, such as myc, ets, fos, jun, rel/NF-κB and myb, are known oncogenes *(12, 156,157)*. Cyclin D1 overexpression has been shown to promote malignancy in B-cell lymphoma in cooperation with myc *(158,159)*. The Bcl-2 anti-apototic protein has also been shown to cooperate with myc to cause oncogenic transformation *(160)*. Myc has also been shown to activate telomerase in human mammary epithelial cells and normal human diploid fibroblasts *(161)*. It has been suggested that inhibiting *c-myc* expression may induce differentiation and reverse transformation *(162)*. Antisense oligonucleotides against *c-myc* are being pursued for cancer therapy *(17)*. NF-κB is another transcription factor that is emerging as a potential anticancer target *(163,164)*. It is implicated in both carcinogenesis and tumor progression, playing a role in cell survival and proliferation. Recently, the transcription factor hypoxia-inducible factor 1 (HIF-1) has also been shown to be important in cancer progression and angiogenesis. Its overexpression has been correlated with treatment failure and mortality in brain, breast, cervical, esophageal, oropharyneal and ovarian cancers *(165)*.

3. p53 and Apoptosis Targets

The p53 tumor suppressor protein was chosen as *Science* Magazine's molecule of the year in 1993 *(166)*. p53 has been dubbed as the 'guardian of the genome' *(167)*. p53 functions as a transcription factor causing cell cycle arrest or apoptosis, in response to DNA damage *(135,168)*. It is also a player in DNA repair *(169)*. Cell cycle arrest and apoptosis, as well as DNA repair, are the mechanisms by which p53 performs its tumor suppressor functions. The cell cycle arrest function of p53 is achieved primarily through the transcriptional induction of the cyclin-dependent kinase inhibitor p21 and/or GADD45 gene product *(170)*. p53 induces apoptosis by transcriptional induction of the Bax gene product *(171)*, or by transcription-independent mechanisms *(15,169,172)*. p53 mutations, which occur in more than 50% of human cancers *(173)*, cause loss of function *(174,175)*. Loss of p53 function correlates with drug resistance and aggressiveness in many cancers, including ovarian *(176)* and breast cancers *(177)*. Although some questions remain, many anticancer agents are thought to act by induction of apoptosis in the context of functional p53 *(174,175,178)*. Inducing or maintaining p53 function appears to be an attractive cancer therapeutic modality. A variety of anticancer therapeutic approaches devised to manipulate the p53 pathway are currently being pursued, including gene therapy, exploitation of lack of p53 function for selective oncolytic viral replication, reactivation of mutant p53 through conformational changes, and the inhibition of p53 binding to MDM2 which results in its degradation *(173,179,180)*. It has been observed that the tumor suppressor function of p53 can be inhibited even in the absence of inactivating mutations. The major player in this respect is the MDM2 gene product *(181)*. MDM2 protein is transcriptionally induced by p53 in a negative feedback control loop that regulates p53 function *(182–184)*. The overexpression of MDM2 *(185)* is thought to suppress normal p53 function *(186)* by both protein-protein interaction and by direct interference with the basal transcriptional machinery *(187)*. The overexpression of MDM2 occurs in many human cancers, including sarcomas, esophageal carcinomas, brain tumors, breast cancer, ovarian cancer, cervical cancer, lung cancer, colon cancer, bronchogenic carcinoma, nasopharyngeal carcinoma, neuroblastomas, testicular germ-cell tumor, urothelial cancers, and pediatric solid tumors *(185,188,189)*. Polypeptides that bind to MDM2 protein *(190,191)*, antibodies against MDM2 protein *(192)*, small molecule MDM2 inhibitors *(193,194)*, as well as anti-MDM2 antisense oligonucleotides *(195–197)* are strategies that have been used to cause disruption of p53-MDM2 interaction and to increase the cellular function of wild-type p53. These approaches could be developed as cancer therapeutics in their own right, or could be combined with other cancer treatment modalities *(197)*.

The anti-apoptotic oncogene, Bcl-2 *(198)* is also a potential anticancer target. As mentioned above, Bcl-2 cooperates with myc to cause oncogenic transformation *(160)*. It is especially important in B-cell lymphomas *(199)*. Overexpression of Bcl-2 has been observed in prostate, breast, colorectal, small cell lung, and non-small cell lung cancers *(200)*. There are other Bcl-2 family proteins that also have anti-apoptotic effects, such as Bcl-xL, that may also serve as potential chemotherapy targets *(200)*. Peptidyl blockers of the dimerization of the Bcl-2 family proteins have been designed *(201)*, as well as small molecule inhibitors, which were reported recently *(202)*. One concern to keep in mind in attempts to use Bcl-2 inhibitors in cancer therapy is their potential adverse effects in patients with ischemic cardiac disease, where the anti-apoptotic effects of Bcl-2 are beneficial *(200)*.

Another anti-apoptosis molecular target is survivin *(203)*. Survivin is expressed in the most common human cancers but not in normal adult tissues *(203)*. In one study, it was shown that survivin mRNA was overexpressed in 85% of non-small cell lung tumors *(204)*. Inhibition of melanoma tumor growth in vivo by survivin targeting has been demonstrated *(205)*. No small molecule inhibitors of this target are yet available.

4. Cell Lifespan Targets

The enzyme telomerase is a ribonucleoprotein DNA polymerase that lenghtens telomeres, which are specialized nucleotide sequences at the ends of chromosomes consisting of long tandem repeats of the sequence TTAGGG *(206)*. This function is known to prolong the proliferative lifespan in cells *(207)*. Telomerase maintains telomere length by using its integral RNA as a template to add TTAGGG tracks to telomeres, and is induced in actively dividing cells and cancer cells, but not in otherwise normal cells *(207,208)*. Telomerase activity is said to be elevated in 86% of all cancers studied *(209)*. Telomerase may serve as a viable cancer target for selective cancer chemotherapy *(209–212)*. The telomerase repeat amplification protocol (TRAP) assay *(207)* has been used to identify telomerase inhibitors *(209,213,214)*, including porphyrins, anthraquinones, and 7-deaza-nucleotide analogs. The occurrence of telomerase in renewable tissues, such as the liver, may pose toxicity problems in the use of telomerase inhibitors as anticancer agents *(208)*.

5. Tumor Angiogenesis and Metastasis Targets

Angiogenesis is critical for cancer establishment and metastasis *(215–217)*. Tumor angiogenesis is a complex process involving differential expansion and coalescence of endothelial cell precursors into a network of vessels, as well as the recruitment of supporting cells to feed the incipient tumor *(46,47)*. Several angiogenesis pathways targets for cancer therapy have been identified and many small molecule inhibitors of these have been discovered *(48,218)*. The growth factors and their receptor tyrosine kinases shown to be involved in angiogenesis, as well as the small molecule inhibitors targeting them have already been considered under receptor tyrosine kinases (*see* **Subheading 2.2.**). Another important tumor angiogenic factor is angiogenin, a non-mitogenic polypeptide that can both induce or suppress angiogenesis *(50)*. It has been shown that the peptidyl agents angiostatin and endostatin antagonize the angiogenic effects of angiogenin, and are highly effective in eliminating tumors in mice, which has led to human clinical trials of the agents *(219)*. Thalidomide and the fumagilins such as AG-1470, are also important antiangiogenic agents, but their mechanism of action is not well understood as yet *(48)*. Recently, a new thalidomide analog, *S*-3-[3-aminophthalimido]-glutarimide (S-3APG) was shown to inhibit angiogenesis and the growth of B-cell neoplasias in mice *(220)*. Indirect induction of angiogenesis through other pathways has also been demonstrated, the HIF-1 signaling pathway being one of such *(165)*, and may be targeted also for antiangionesis cancer therapy.

Matrix metalloproteinases (MMPs) have been studied extensively as anti-cancer molecular targets, and many small molecule inhibitors have been discovered in their wake, some of which are selective while others are not. MMPs constitute a large family of zinc-binding proteins that degrade the extracellular matrix, allowing cancer invasion *(221,222)*, and can be divided into five classes based on substrate preference as follows: (1) type 1 col-lagenases, comprising MMP-1, MMP-8, and MMP-13, (2) type IV col-lagenases, MMP-2 and MMP-9, (3) stromelysins, MMP-3, MMP-7, MMP-10 and MMP-11, (4) elastases, MMP-12, and (5) membrane type matrix metal-loproteases, MT-MMPs *(223)*. Several MMP inhibitors have been advanced into clinical trials *(222)*. The results of the clinical trials conducted with MMP inhibitors so far have been disappointing *(224)*. The reasons for this may have to do with the clinical trials design, and therefore new trials are being initiated based on the lessons learned from the failed trials *(222)*.

Urokinase (uPA), a serine protease formed initially as high molecular weight uPA (HMWuPA) that is cleaved into an amino terminal fragment (ATF) and low molecular weight uPA (LMWuPA), has been shown to be involved in tumor metastasis and angiogenesis *(223,225)*. LMWuPA causes proteolytic degradation and activation of TGF-β. In addition, it also converts plasminogen to plasmin, the active product with proteolytic activity that affects various extracellular matrix components. Binding of ATF to the uPA receptor (uPAR), results in cell migration and osteoblast proliferation *(223)*. uPA and uPAR have been shown to cooperate with MMPs, especially MMP-9 to cause tumor cell intravasation *(226)*. The uPA/uPAR system has also been a target for novel anticancer drug discovery *(227)*. The potential role of urokinase receptor antagonists in metastatic disease has been summarized *(225)*. Amiloride-analog potent uPA enzyme inhibitors, such as B623, have been shown to block tumor invasion in vivo *(48)*.

Another category of extracellular matrix interacting molecules relevant to cancer invasion, is the cell adhesion molecules (CAMs) class. These molecules mediate cell-matrix and cell-cell interactions, appear to be involved in cancer invasion and organ-specific metastasis *(228,229)*, and are potential anticancer molecular targets *(230)*. The integrins constitute the largest group of CAMs. They are transmembrane heterodimeric proteins, composed of α and β subunits, which function as receptors for matrix proteins such as fibronectin, vitronectin, laminin, and collagen *(231)*. Other groups of cell adhesion molecules of importance are the cadherins, selectins, mucins, hyaluronan (CD44), the major histocompatibility (MHC) antigens, CD2, CD4, and CD8, and other Igs such as ICAM-1, ICAM-2, VCAM-1, CEA, C-CAMs, and DCC *(228,230)*, and gangliosides *(232)*. Synthetic peptides designed to antagonize cell adhesion interactions, incorporating an RGD (Arg-Gly-Asp) motif, have been shown to prevent metastasis *(48,228,230)*.

6. Conclusion

The cure for cancer may yet be a dream, but the future may see a situation where many cancers can be controlled like many other diseases, so that a diagnosis of cancer will no longer be a death sentence as it has been for most patients with disseminated malignant tumors. Many potential novel anticancer molecular targets have been identified and validated. There are other emerging targets, such as protein lipid kinases like phosphoinositide 3-OH kinase *(87)*, proteasomes, chaperone proteins, as well as chromatin associated and hypoxia associated targets *(233)*. Early successes have been achieved with a few targets, and the paradigms of their successful development are being applied to many other potential targets. Some of the clinical results have been disappointing, like the case of the MMP inhibitors, but even then, it is thought that better clinical trial designs may bring success. The novel drugs are acting primarily as cytostatic rather than cytocidal agents, and therefore clinical end points and markers, as well as the tumor stage for clinical trial entry, have to be chosen expediently. Furthermore, different cancers harbor different molecular targets and therefore therapies will have to be tailored to individual molecular target profiles. The challenges we face in translating target information into clinical agents call for novel anticancer drug protocols to expedite the validation of targets, the discovery agents to exploit the targets, and the correlation of drug effects on targets with clinical response.

References

1. Shak, S. (1999) Overview of the trastuzumab (Herceptin) anti-HER-2 monoclonal antibody clinical programme in HER-2 overexpressing metastatic breast cancer. Herceptin Multinational Investigator Study Group. *Semin. Oncol.* **26,** 71–77.
2. Druker, B. J. (2002) STI571 (Gleevec™) as a paradigm for cancer therapy. *Trend. Mol. Med.* **8** (Issue 4 Suppl), S14–S18.
3. de Bono, J. S. and Rowinsky, E. K. (2002) The ErbB receptor family: a therapeutic target for cancer. *Trend. Mol. Med.* **8** (Issue 4 Suppl), S19–S26.
4. Workman, P. (1994) The Potential for molecular oncology to define new drug targets, in *New Molecular Targets for Cancer Chemotherapy* (Kerr, D. J. and Workman, P., eds.), CRC Press, Boca Raton, FL, pp. 1–44.
5. Karp, J. E. and Broder, S. (1995) Molecular foundations of cancer: new targets for intervention. *Nat. Med.* **1,** 309–320.
6. Oliff, A., Gibbs, J. B., and McCormick, F. (1996) New molecular targets for cancer therapy. *Sci. Am.* **275,** 144–149.
7. Kuwano, N. (1997) Novel molecular targets for anticancer drugs. *Jpn. J. Cancer Chemother.* **24,** 2187–2189.
8. Aszalos, A. and Eckhardt, S. (1997) Molecular events as targets of anticancer drug therapy. *Path. Oncol. Res.* **3,** 147–158.
9. Seymore, L. (1999) Novel anti-cancer agents in development: exciting prospects and new challenges. *Cancer Treat. Rev.* **25,** 301–312.
10. Buolamwini, J. K. (1999) Novel anticancer drug discovery. *Curr. Opin. Chem. Biol.* **3,** 500–509.
11. Buolamwini, J. K. (2002) Novel molecular targets for cancer drug discovery. In *The Molecular Basis of Human Cancer* (Coleman, W. B. and Tsongalis, G. J., eds.), Humana Press, Totowa, NJ, pp. 521–540.
12. Hunter, T. (1997) Oncoprotein networks. *Cell* **88,** 573–582.
13. Weinberg, R. A. (1991) Tumor suppressor genes. *Science* **254,** 1138–1146.
14. Hanahan, D. and Weinberg, A. (2000) The hallmarks of cancer. *Cell* **100,** 57–70.
15. White, E. (1996) Life, death and the pursuit of apoptosis. *Genes Dev.* **10,** 1–15.
16. Jurcic, J. G., Scheinberg, D. A., and Houghton, A. N. (1997) Monoclonal antibody therapy of cancer. *Cancer Chemother. Biol. Response Modif.* **17,** 195–216.
17. Wang, H., Prasad, G., Buolamwini, J. K., and Zhang, R. (2001) Antisense anticancer oligonucleotide therapeutics. *Curr. Cancer Drug Targets* **1,** 177–196.
18. Chong, C. and Vile, R. (1997) Gene therapy for cancer. *Drugs Future* **22,** 857–874.
19. Gomez-Navarro, J., Bilbao, G., and Curiel, D. T. (2002) Gene therapy in the treatment of human cancer. In *The Molecular Basis of Human Cancer* (Coleman, W. B. and Tsongalis, G. J., eds.), Humana Press, Totowa, NJ, pp. 541–565.
20. Adjei, A. A. (2000) Signal transduction pathway targets for anticancer drug discovery. *Curr. Pharm. Des.* **6,** 361–378.

21. Ullrich, A. and Schlessinger, J. (1991) Signal transduction by receptors with tyrosine kinase activity. *Cell* **61,** 203–212.
22. Sauseville, E. A. and Longo, D. L. (1994) Growth factors and growth factor inhibitors. In *Cancer Therapeutics: Experimental and Clinical Agents* (Teicher, B., ed.), Humana Press, Totowa, NJ, pp. 337–370.
23. Gishizky, M. L. (1995) Tyrosine kinase induced mitogenesis. Breaking the link with cancer. *Ann. Rep. Med. Chem.* **30,** 247–253.
24. Katz, M. E. and McCormick, F. (1997) Signal transduction from multiple ras effectors. *Curr. Opin. Genet. Dev.* **7,** 75–79.
25. Marais, R., Light, Y., Mason, C., Paterson, H., Olson, M. F., and Marshall, C. J. (1998) Requirement of Ras-GTP-Raf complexes for activation of Raf-1 by protein kinase C. *Science* **280,** 109–112.
26. Olson, M. F., Paterson, H. F., and Marshall, C. J. (1998) Signals from Ras and Rho GTPases interact to regulate expression of p21[Waf1/Cip1]. *Nature* **394,** 295–299.
27. Fantl, W. J., Johnson, D. E., and Williams, L. T. (1993) Signalling by receptor tyrosine kinases. *Ann. Rev. Biochem.* **62,** 453–481.
28. Kolibaba, K. S. and Druker, B. J. (1997) Protein tyrosine kinases and cancer. *Biochim. Biophys. Acta* **1333,** F217–F248.
29. Lofts, F. J. and Gullick, W. J. (1994) Growth factor receptors as targets. In *New Molecular Targets for Cancer Chemotherapy* (Kerr, D. J. and Workman, P., eds.), CRC Press, Boca Raton, FL, pp. 45–66.
30. Levitzki, A. (1994) Protein tyrosine kinase inhibitors. In *New Molecular Targets for Cancer Chemotherapy* (Kerr, D. J. and Workman, P., eds.), CRC Press, Boca Raton, FL, pp. 67–79.
31. Levitzki, A. and Gazit A. (1995) Tyrosine kinase inhibition: an approach to drug development. *Science* **267,** 1782–1788.
32. Burke, T. R. (1992) Protein tyrosine kinase inhibitors. *Drugs Future* **17,** 119–131.
33. Zwick, E., Bange, J., and Ullrich, A. (2002) Receptor tyrosine kinases as targets for anticancer drugs. *Trends Mol. Med.* **8,** 17–23.
34. Fry, D. W. (1996) Recent advances in tyrosine kinase inhibitors. *Ann. Rep. Med. Chem.* **31,** 151–160.
35. Traxler, P. and Lydon, N. (1995) Recent advances in protein tyrosine kinase inhibitors. *Drugs Future* **20,** 1261–1274.
36. Traxler, P., Furet, P., Met, H., Buchdunger, E., Meyer, T., and Lydon, N. (1997) Design and synthesis of novel tyrosine kinase inhibitors using a pharmacophore model of the ATP-binding site of the EGF-R. *J. Pharm. Belg.* **52,** 88–96.
37. Fry, D. W., Kraker, A. J., Connors, R. C., et al. (1994) Strategies for the discovery of novel tyrosine kinase inhibitors with anticancer activity. *Anti-Cancer Drug Design* **9,** 331–351.
38. Aaronson, S. A. (1991) Growth factors and cancer. *Science* **254,** 1146–1152.
39. Tzahar, E. and Yarden, Y. (1998) The ErbB-2/HER2 oncogenic receptor of adenocarcinomas: from orphanhood to multiple stromal ligands. *Biochim. Biophys. Acta* **1377,** M25–M37.

40. Yaish, P., Gazit, A., Gilom, C., and Levitzki, A. (1988) Blocking of EGF-dependent cell proliferation by EGF receptor kinase inhibitors. *Science* **242,** 933–935.
41. Slamon, D. J., Leyland-Jones, B., Shak, S., et al. (2001) Use of chemotherapy plus a monoclonal antibody against HER2 for metastatic breast cancer that overexpresses HER2. *N. Engl. J. Med.* **344,** 783–792.
42. Baselga, J. (2001). The EGFR as a target for anticancer therapy: focus on Cetuxumab. *Eur. J. Cancer* **37,** S16–S22.
43. Miller, P., DiOrio, C., Moyer, M., et al. (1994) Depletion of the erbB-2 gene product p185 by the benzoquinone ansamycins. *Cancer Res.* **54,** 2724–2730.
44. Neckers, L. (2002) Hsp90 inhibitors as novel cancer chemotherapeutic agents. *Trend. Mol. Med.* **8** (Issue 4 Suppl), S55–S61.
45. Heldin, C.-H., Ostman, A., and Ronnstrand, L. (1998) Signal transduction via platelet-derived growth factor receptors. *Biochim. Biophys. Acta* **1378,** F79–F113.
46. Hanahan, D. (1997) Signaling vascular morphogenesis and maintenance. *Science* **277,** 48–50.
47. Risau, W. (1997) Mechanisms of angiogenesis. *Nature* **386,** 671–674.
48. Powell, D., Skotnicki, J., and Upeslacis, J. (1997) Angiogenesis inhibitors. *Ann. Rep. Med. Chem.* **32,** 161–170.
49. Kubo, H., Fujiwara, T., Jussila, L., et al. (2000) Involvement of vascular endothelial growth factor receptor-3 in maintenance of integrity of endothelial cell lining during tumor angiogenesis. *Blood* **96,** 546–553.
50. Folkman, J. and Klagsbrun, M. (1987) Angiogenic factors. *Science* **235,** 442–447.
51. Shaulian, E., Resnitzky, D., Shifman, O., et al. (1997) Induction of Mdm2 and enhancement of cell survival by bFGF. *Oncogene* **15,** 2717–2725.
52. Zhu, Z., Bohlen, P., and Witte, L. (2002) Clinical development of angiogenesis inhibitors to vascular endothelial growth factor and its receptors as cancer therapeutics. *Curr. Cancer Drug Targets* **2,** 135–156.
53. Fong, T. A., Shawver, L. K., Sun, L., et al. (1999) SU5416 is a potent and selective inhibitor of the vascular endothelial growth factor receptor (Flk-1/KDR) that inhibits tyrosine kinase catalysis, tumor vascularization, and growth of multiple tumor types. *Cancer Res.* **59,** 99–106.
54. Fry, D. W. and Nelson, J. M. (1995) Inhibition of fibroblast growth factor-mediated tyrosine phosphorylation and protein synthesis by PD 145709, a member of the 2-thioindole class of tyrosine kinase inhibitors. *Anti-Cancer Drug Design* **10,** 604–622.
55. Mohammadi, M., McMahon, G., Sun, L., et al. (1997) Structures of the tyrosine kinase domain of fibroblast growth factor receptor in complex with inhibitors. *Science* **276,** 955–960.
56. Shawver, L. K., Schwartz, D. P., Mann, E., et al. (1997) Inhibition of platelet-derived growth factor-mediated signal transduction and tumor growth by *N*-[4-(trifluoromethyl)phenyl]-5-methylisoxazole-4-carboxamide. *Clin. Cancer Res.* **3,** 1167–1177.

57. Mullins, D. E., Hamud, F., Reim, R., and Davis, H. R. (1994) Inhibition of PDGF receptor binding and PDGF-stimulated biological activity in vitro and of intimal lesion formation in vivo by 2-bromomethyl-5-chlorobenzene sulfonylphthalimide. *Arterioscler. Thromb.* **14,** 1047–1055.
58. Hirota, S., Isozaki, K., Moriyama, Y., et al. (1998) Gain-of-function mutations of c-kit in human gastrointestinal stromal tumors. *Science* **279,** 577–580.
59. O'Dwyer, M. E. and Druker, B. J. (2001) The role of the tyrosine kinase inhibitor STI571 in the treatment of cancer. *Curr. Cancer Drug Targets* **1,** 49–57.
60. Lutz, M.P., Eber, I. B. S., Flossmann-Kast, B. B. M., et al. (1998) Overexpression and activation of the tyrosine kinase Src in human pancreatic carcinoma. *Biochem. Biophys. Res. Commun.* **243,** 503–508.
61. Bolen, J. B. and Veillet A. A. (1989) Function for the *lck* proto-oncogene. *Trends Biochem. Sci.* **14,** 404–407.
62. Cheung, R. K. and Dosch, H. M. (1991) The tyrosine kinase lck is critically involved in the growth transformation of human B lymphocytes. *J. Biol. Chem.* **266,** 8667–8670.
63. Klutchko, S. R., Hamby, J. M., Boschelli, D. H., et al. (1998) 2-Substituted aminopyrido[2,3-*d*]pyrimidin-7(8H)-ones. Structure-activity relationships against selected tyrosine kinases and in vitro and in vivo anticancer activity. *J. Med. Chem.* **41,** 3276–3292.
64. Lunney, E. A., Para, K. S., Rubin, J. R., et al. (1997) Structure-based design of a novel series of ligands that bind to the pp60^{src} SH2 domain. *J. Am. Chem. Soc.* **119,** 12,471–12,476.
65. Buchdunger, E., Zimmerman, J., Mett, H., et al. (1996) Inhibition of the Abl protein-tyrosine kinase in vitro and in vivo by a 2-phenylaminopyrimidine derivative. *Cancer Res.* **56,** 100–104.
66. Heinrich, M. C., Griffith, D. J., Druker, B. J., Wait, C. K., Ott, K. A., and Zigler, A. J. (2000) Inhibition of c-kit receptor tyrosine kinase activity by STI 571, a selective tyrosine kinase inhibitor. *Blood* **96,** 925–932.
67. Lee, J. C. and Adams, J. L. (1995) Inhibitors of serine/threonine kinases. *Curr. Opin. Biotech.* **6,** 657–661.
68. Castagna, M., Takai, Y., Kaibuchi, K., Sano, K., Kikkawa, U., and Nishizuka, Y. (1982) Direct activation of calcium-activated phospholipid-dependent protein kinase by tumor-promoting phorbol esters. *J. Biol. Chem.* **257,** 7847–7851.
69. Niedel, J. E., Kuhn, L. J., and Vandenbank, G. R. (1983) Phorbol diester receptor copurifies with protein kinase C. *Proc. Natl. Acad. Sci. USA* **80,** 36–40.
70. Exton, J. H. (1997) Cell signalling through guanine-nucleotide-binding regulatory proteins (G proteins) and phospholipases. *Eur. J. Biochem.* **243,** 10–20.
71. Dekker, L. V. and Parker, P. J. (1994) Protein kinase C. A question of specificity. *Trends Biochem. Sci.* **19,** 73–77.
72. Grescher, A. and Dale, I. L. (1989) Protein kinase C—a novel target for rational anticancer drug design? *Anti-Cancer Drug Design* **4,** 93–105.
73. Basu, A. (1993) The potential of protein kinase C as a target for anticancer treatment. *Pharmac. Ther.* **59,** 257–280.

74. Philip, P. A. and Harris A. L. (1995) Potential for protein kinase C inhibitors in cancer therapy. *Cancer Treat. Res.* **178,** 3–27.
75. Schwartz, G. K. (1996) Protein kinase C inhibitors as inducers of apoptosis for cancer treatment. *Exp. Opin. Invest. Drugs* **5,** 1601–1615.
76. Capronigro, F., French, R. C., and Kaye, S. B. (1997) Protein kinase C: a worthwhile target for anticancer drugs? *Anti-Cancer Drugs* **8,** 26–33.
77. Goekjian, P. G. and Jirousek, M. R. (2001) Protein kinase C inhibitors as novel anticancer drugs. *Expert Opin. Investig. Drugs* **10,** 2117–2140.
78. Hofmann, J. (2002) Modulation of protein kinase C in antitumor treatment. *Rev. Physiol. Biochem. Pharmacol.* **142,** 1–96.
79. Blobe, G. C., Sachs, C. W., Khan, W. A., et al. (1993) Selective regulation of expression of protein kinase C (PKC) isozymes in multidrug-resistant MCF-7 cells. Functional significance of enhanced expression of PKCα. *J. Biol. Chem.* **268,** 658–664.
80. Gill, P. K., Gescher, A., and Gant, T. W. (2001) Regulation of MDR1 promoter activity in human breast carcinoma cells by protein kinase C isozymes alpha and theta. *Eur. J. Biochem.* **268,** 4151–4157.
81. Harris, W., Hill, C. H., Lewis, E. J., Nixon, J. S., and Wilkinson, S. E. (1993) Protein kinase C inhibitors. *Drugs Future* **18,** 727–735.
82. Zimmermann, J., Caravatti, G., Mett, H., et al. (1996) Phenylamino-pyrimidine (PAP) derivatives: a new class of potent and selective inhibitors of protein kinase C (PKC). *Arch. Pharm.* **329,** 371–376.
83. Wang, S., Milne, G. W. A., Nicklaus, M. C., Marquez, V. E., Lee, J., and Blumberg, P. M. (1994) Protein kinase C. Modeling of the binding site and prediction of binding constants. *J. Med. Chem.* **37,** 1326–1338.
84. Wang, S., Zaharevitz, D. W., Sharma, R., et al. (1994) Discovery of novel, structurally diverse protein kinase C agonists through computer 3D-database pharmacophore search. Molecular modeling studies. *J. Med. Chem.* **37,** 4479–4489.
85. Qiao, L., Wang, S., George, C., Lewin, L. E., Blumberg, P. M., and Kozikowski, A. P. (1998) Structure-based design of a new class of protein kinase C modulators. *J. Am. Chem. Soc.* **120,** 6629–6630.
86. Ramage, A. D., Langdon, S. P., Ritchie, A. A., Urns, D. J., and Miller, W. R. (1995) Growth inhibition by 8-chloro-cyclic AMP of human HT29 colorectal and ZR-75-1 breast carcinoma xenografts is associated with selective modulation of protein kinase A isoenzymes. *Eur. J. Cancer* **31A,** 969–973.
87. Blume-Jensen, P. and Hunter, T. (2001) Oncogenic kinase signalling. *Nature* **411,** 355–356.
88. Zhong, H., Chiles, K, Feldser, D., et al. (2000) Modulation of hypoxia-inducible factor 1-alpha expression by the epidermal growth factor/phosphoinositide-3 kinase/PTEN/AKT/FRAP pathway in human protrate cancer cells: implications for tumor angiogenesis and therapeutics. *Cancer Res.* **60,** 1541–1545.
89. Leslie, L. R. and Downes, P. C. (2002) PTEN: the down side of PI 3-kinase signalling. *Cell. Signalling* **14,** 285–295.

90. Stein, B. and Anderson, D. (1996) The MAP kinase family: new "MAPs" for signal transduction pathways targets. *Ann. Rep. Med Chem.* **31,** 289–298.
91. Lewis, T. S., Shapiro, P. S., and Ahn, N. G. (1998) Signal transduction through MAP kinase cascades. *Adv. Cancer Res.* **74,** 49–139.
92. Cobb, M. H. (1999) MAP kinase pathways. *Prog. Biophys. Mol. Biol.* **71,** 479–500.
93. Kolch, W. (2000) Meaningful relationships: the regulation of the Ras/Raf/MEK/ ERK pathway by protein interactions. *Biochem. J.* **351,** 289–305.
94. Kumar, C. C. and Madison, V. (2001) Drugs targeted against protein kinases. *Expert Opin. Emerging Drugs* **6,** 308–315.
95. Herrera R. and Sebolt-Leopold J. S. (2002) Unraveling the complexities of the Raf/MAP kinase pathway for pharmacological intervention. *Trends Mol. Med.* **8(4),** S27–S31.
96. Sebolt-Leopold, J. S., Dudley, D. T., Herrera, R., et al. (1999) Blockade of the MAP kinase pathway suppresses growth of colon tumors in vivo. *Nat. Med.* **5,** 810–816.
97. Shimamura, A, Ballif, B. A., Richards, S. A., and Blenis, J. (2000) Rsk1 mediates a MEK-MAP kinase cell survival signal. *Curr. Biol.* **10,** 127–135.
98. Bonni, A., Brunet, A., West, A. E., Datta, S. R., Takasu, M. A., and Greenberg, M. E. (1999) Cell survival promoted by the Ras-MAPK signalling pathway by transcription-dependent and -independent mechanisms. *Science* **286,** 1358–1362.
99. Wang, H. G., Miyashita, T., Takayama, S., et al. (1994) Apoptosis regulation by interaction of Bcl-2 protein and Raf-1 kinase. *Oncogene* **9,** 2751–2756.
100. Pardo, O. E., Arcaro, A., Salerno, G., Raguz, S., Downward, J., and Seckl, M. J. (2002) Fibroblast and growth factor-2 induces translational regulation of Bcl-X_L and Bcl-2 via a MEK-dependent pathway. Correlation with resistance to etoposide-induced apoptosis. *J. Biol. Chem.* **277,** 12,040–12,046.
101. Zhong, J., Troppmair, J., and Rapp, U. R. (2001) Independent control of cell survival by Raf-1 and Bcl-2 at the mitochondria. *Oncogene* **20,** 4807–4816.
102. Chen, J., Fujii, K., Zhang, L., Roberts, T., and Fu, H. (2001) Raf-1 promotes cell survival by antagonizing signal-regulating kinase 1 through a MEK-ERK independent mechanism. *Proc. Natl. Acad. Sci. USA* **98,** 7783–7788.
103. Monia, B. P. (1997) First- and second-generation antisense inhibitors targeted to human c-*raf* kinase: in vitro and in vivo studies. *Anti-Cancer Drug Design* **12,** 327–339.
104. Chow, S., Patel, H., and Hedley, D. W. (2001) Measurement of MAP kinase activation by flow cytometry using phospho-specific antibodies to MEK and ERK: potential for pharmacodynamic monitoring of signal transduction inhibitors. *Cytometry* **46,** 72–78.
105. Dudley, D. T., Pang, L., Decker, S. J., Bridges, A. J., and Saltiel, A. R. (1995) A synthetic inhibitor of the mitogen-activated protein kinase cascade. *Proc. Natl. Acad. Sci. USA* **92,** 7686–7689.
106. Draetta, G. (1990) Cell cycle control in eukaryotes: molecular mechanisms of cdc2 activation. *Trends Biol. Sci.* **15,** 378–383.

107. Sherr. C. J. (1993) Mammalian G1 cyclins. *Cell* **73,** 1059–1065.
108. Coleman, K. G., Lyssikatos, J. P., and Yang, B. V. (1997) Chemical inhibitors of cyclin-dependent kinases. *Ann. Rep. Med. Chem.* **32,** 171–179.
109. Hunter, T. and Pines, J. (1994) Cyclins and cancer II: cyclin D and CDK inhibitors come of age. *Cell* **79,** 573–582.
110. Morgan, D. O. (1995) Principles of CDK regulation. *Nature* **374,** 131–134.
111. Lee, M. H., Renisdottir, I., and Massague, J. (1995) Cloning of p57KIP2, a cyclin-dependent kinase inhibitor with unique domain structure and tissue distribution. *Genes Dev.* **9,** 639–649.
112. Sherr, C. J. and Roberts, J. M. (1999) CDK inhibitors, positive and negative regulators of G1-phase progression. *Genes Dev.* **13,** 1505–1512.
113. Ortega, S., Malumbres, M., and Barbacid, M. (2002) Cyclin-dependent kinases, INK4 inhibitors and cancer. *Biochim. Biophys. Acta* **1602,** 73–87.
114. Lees, E. M. and Harlow, E. (1995). Cancer and the cell cycle. In *Cell Cycle Control* (Hutchison, C. and Glover, D. M., eds.), IRL Press, New York, pp. 228–263.
115. Weinberg, R. A. (1995) The retinoblastoma protein and cell cycle control. *Cell* **81,** 323–330.
116. Draetta, G. and Pagano, M. (1996) Cell cycle control and cancer. *Ann. Rep. Med. Chem.* **31,** 241–248.
117. Imoto, M. (1998) Molecular target therapy of cancer: a. cell cycle. *Kagaku Ryo no Ryoiki* **14,** 13–19.
118. Buolamwini, J. K. (2000) Cell cycle molecular targets in novel anticancer drug discovery. *Curr. Pharm. Design* **6,** 379–392.
119. Buolamwini, J. K. (2001) Cell cycle molecular targets and drug discovery. In *Cell Cycle Checkpoints and Cancer* (Blagosklonny, M. V., ed.), Landes Bioscience, Georgetown, TX, pp. 235–246.
120. Sausville, E. A. (2002) Complexities in the development of cyclin-dependent kinase inhibitor drugs. *Trends Mol. Med.* **8** (Issue 4 Suppl), S32–S37.
121. Hardcastle, I. R., Golding, B. T., and Griffin, R. J. (2002) Designing inhibitors of cyclin-dependent kinases. *Annu. Rev. Pharmacol. Toxicol.* **42,** 325–348.
122. Meijer, L. (1996) Chemical inhibitors of cyclin-dependent kinases. *Trends Cell Biol.* **6,** 393–397.
123. Carlson, B. A., Dubay, M. M., Sausville, E. A., Brizuella, L., and Worland, P. J. (1996) Flavopiridol induces G1 arrest with inhibition of cyclin-dependent kinase (CDK) 2 and CDK4 in human breast carcinoma cells. *Cancer Res.* **56,** 2973–2978.
124. Christain, M. C., Puda, J. M., Ho, P. T. C., Arbuck, S. G., Murgo, A. J., and Sausville E. A. (1997) Promising new agents under development by the division of cancer treatment, diagnosis, and centers of the National Cancer Institute. *Semin. Oncol.* **24,** 219–240.
125. Chao, S.-H. and Price, D. H. (2001) Flavopyridol inactivates P-TEFb and blocks most RNA polymerase II transcription in vivo. *J. Biol. Chem.* **276,** 31,793–31,799.

126. Wang, D., de la Fuente, C., Deng, L., et al. (2001) Inhibition of human immunodeficiency virus type-1 transcription by chemical cyclin-dependent kinase inhibitors. *J. Virol.* **75,** 7266–7279.

127. Iseki, H., Ko, T. C., Xue, X. Y., Seapan, A., Hellmich, M. R., and Townsend, C. W. (1997) Cyclin-dependent kinase inhibitors block proliferation of human gastric cancer cells. *Surgery* **122,** 187–194.

128. Gray, N. S., Wodika, L., Thunnissen, A.-M. W. H., et al. (1998) Exploiting chemical libraries, structure, and genomics in the search for kinase inhibitors. *Science* **281,** 533–538.

129. Sauseville, E. A., Zaharevitz, D., Gussio, R., et al. (1999) Cyclin-dependent kinases: initial approaches to exploit a novel therapeutic target. *Pharmacol. Ther.* **82,** 285–292.

130. Hoessel, R., Leclerc, S., Endicott, J. A., et al. (1999) Indirubin, the active constituent of a Chinese antileukemia medicine, inhibits cyclin-dependent kinases. *Nat. Cell Biol.* **1,** 60–67.

131. Toogood, P. (2001) Cyclin-depenent kinase inhibitors for treating cancer. *Med. Res. Revs.* **21,** 487–498.

132. Wolf, G., Elez, R., Doermer, A., et al. (1997) Prognostic significance of polo-like kinase (PLK) expression in non-small cell lung cancer. *Oncogene* **14,** 543–549.

133. Bischoff, J. R., Anderson, L., Zhu, Y., et al. (1998) A homologue of *Drosophila* aurora kinase is oncogenic and amplified in human colorectal cancers. *EMBO J.* **17,** 3052–3065.

134. Graves, P. R., Yu, L., Schwarz, J. K., et al. (2000) The Chk1 protein kinase and the Cdc25C regulatory pathways are targets of the anticancer agent UCN-01. *J. Biol. Chem.* **275,** 5600–5605.

135. Bates, S. and Vousden, K. H. (1996) p53 in signaling checkpoint arrest or apoptosis. *Curr. Opin. Genet. Dev.* **6,** 12–19.

136. Galaktionov, K., Lee, A. K., Eckstein, J., et al. (1995) CDC25 phosphatases as potential human oncogenes. *Science* **269,** 1575–1577.

137. Ducruet, A. P., Rice, R. L., Tamura, K., et al. (2000) Identification of new Cdc25 dual specificity phosphatase inhibitors in a targeted small molecule array. *Bioorg. Med. Chem.* **8,** 1451–1466.

138. Lowenstein, E. J., Daly, R. J., Batzer, A. G., et al. (1992) The SH2 and SH3 domain-containing protein GRB2 links receptor tyrosine kinases to ras signaling. *Cell* **70,** 431–442.

139. Botfield, M. C. and Green, J. (1995) SH2 and SH3 domains: choreographers of multiple signaling pathways. *Ann. Rep. Med. Chem.* **30,** 227–237.

140. Gishizky, M. L. (1995) Tyrosine kinase induced mitogenesis. Breaking the link with cancer. *Ann. Rep. Med. Chem.* **30,** 247–253.

141. Mayer, B. J. and Gupta, R (1998) Functions of SH2 and SH3 domains. *Curr. Top. Microb. Immunol.* **228,** 1–22.

142. Bourne, H. R., Sanders, D. A., and McCormic, F. (1990) The GTPase superfamily: a conserved switch for diverse cell functions. *Nature* **348,** 125–132.

143. Mulcahy, L. S., Smith, M. R., and Stacey, D. (1985) Requirement for ras proto-oncogene function during serum-stimulated growth in NIH 3T3 cells. *Nature* **313,** 241–243.
144. Barbacid, M. (1987) Ras genes. *Ann. Rev. Biochem.* **56,** 779–827.
145. Bos, J. L. (1989) Ras oncogenes in human cancer: a review. *Cancer Res.* **49,** 4682–4689.
146. Boriack-Sjodin, P. A., Margait, S. M., Bar-Sagi, D., and Kuriyan, J. (1998) The structural basis of the activation of ras by Sos. *Nature* **394,** 337–343.
147. Sebolt-Leopold, J. S. (1994) A case for ras targeted agents as antineoplastics. In *Cancer Therapeutics: Experimental and Clinical Agents* (Teicher, B., ed.), Humana Press, Totowa, NJ, pp. 395–415.
148. Herrera, R. and Sebolt-Leopold, J. S. (2002) Unraveling the complexities of the Raf/MAP kinase pathway for pharmacological intervention. *Trends Mol. Med.* **8** (Issue 4 Suppl), S27–S31.
149. Jackson, J. H., Cochrane, C. G., Bourne, J. R., Solski, P.A., Buss, J. E., and Der, C. J. (1990) Farnesyl modification of Kirsten-ras Exon 4B protein is essential for transformation. *Proc. Natl. Acad. Sci. USA* **87,** 3042–3046.
150. Kato, K., Cox, A. D., Hisaka, M. M., Graham, S. M., Buss, J. E., and Der, C. J. (1992) Isoprenoid addition to ras protein is the critical modification for its membrane association and transformation activity. *Proc. Natl. Acad. Sci. USA* **89,** 6403–6407.
151. Cox, A. D. and Der, C. J. (1997) Farnesyl transferase inhibitors and cancer treatment: targeting simply ras? *Biochim. Biophys. Acta* **1333,** F51–F71.
152. Bolton, G. L., Sebolt-Leopold, J. S., and Hodges, J. C. (1994) Ras oncogene directed approaches in cancer chemotherapy. *Ann. Rep. Med. Chem.* **29,** 165–174.
153. Leonard, D.M. (1997) Ras farnesyltransferase: a new therapeutic target. *J. Med. Chem.* **40,** 2971–2990.
154. Zujewski, J. (1998) *NCI Cancernet Web Site.* http://cancernet.nci.gov/cgi-bin/cancer-phy
155. Symons, M. (1995) The Rac and Rho pathway as a source of drug targets for ras-mediated malignancies. *Curr. Opin. Biotech.* **6,** 668–674.
156. Latchman, D. S. (1996) Transcription-factor mutations in disease. *N. Engl. J. Med.* **334,** 28–33.
157. Papavassiliou, A. G. (1997) Transcription factor-based drug design in anticancer drug development. *Mol. Med.* **3,** 99–810.
158. Lovec, H., Grzeschiczek, A., Kowalski, M.-B., and Moroy, T. (1994) Cyclin D1/*bcl-2* cooperates with myc genes in the generation of B-Cell lymphoma in transgenic mice. *EMBO J.* **13,** 3487–3495.
159. Bodrug, S. E., Warner, B. J., Bath, M. L., Linderman, D. J., Harris, A. W., and Adams, J. M. (1994) Cyclin D1 transgene impedes lymphocyte maturation and collaborates in lymphomagenesis with the myc Gene. *EMBO J.* **13,** 2124–2130.
160. Gauwerky, C. E., Haluska, F. G., Tsujimoto, Y., Nowell, P. C., and Croce, C. M. (1988) Evolution of B-Cell malignancy: pre-B-cell leukemia resulting from MYC

activation in a B-cell neoplasm with a rearranged *BCL2* gene. *Proc. Natl. Acad. Sci. USA* **85**, 8548–8552.

161. Wang, J., Xie, L. Y., Allan, S., Beach, D., and Hannon, G. J. (1998) Myc activates telomerase. *Genes Dev.* **12**, 1769–1774.

162. Wickstrom, E. L., Bacon, T. A., Gonzalez, A., Freeman, D. L., Lyman, G. H., and Wickstrom, E. (1988) Human promyelocytic leukemia HL-60 cell proliferation and c-myc protein expression are inhibited by an antisense pentadecadeoxynucleotide targeted against c-myc mRNA. *Proc Natl. Acad. Sci. USA* **85**, 1028–1032.

163. Hideshima, T., Chauhan, D., Richardson, P., et al. (2002) NF-kappa B as a therapeutic target in multiple myeloma. *J. Biol. Chem.* **277**, 16,639–16,647.

164. Haefner, B. (2002) NF-κB: arresting a major culprit in cancer. *Drug Discovery Today* **7**, 653–663.

165. Semenza, G. L. (2002) HIF-1 and tumor progression: pathophysiology and therapeutics. *Trends Mol. Med.* **8** (Issue 4 Suppl), S62–S67.

166. Culotta, E. and Koshland, D. E. (1993) Molecule of the year: p53 sweeps cancer research. *Science* **262**, 1958–1961.

167. Lane, D. P. (1992) p53 guardian of the genome. *Nature* **358**, 15–16.

168. Levine, A. J. (1997) p53, the cellular gate keeper for growth and division. *Cell* **88**, 323–331.

169. Harris, C. C. (1996) Structure and function of the p53 tumor suppressor gene: clues for rational cancer therapeutic strategies. *J. Natl. Cancer Inst.* **88**, 1442–1455.

170. Kastan, M. B., Zhan, Q., El-Deiry, W. S., et al. (1992) A mammalian cell cycle checkpoint pathway utilizing p53 and GADD45 is defective in Ataxia-Telagiectasia. *Cell* **71**, 587–597.

171. Miyashita, T and Reed, J. C. (1995) Tumor suppressor p53 is a direct transcriptional activator of the bax gene. *Cell* **80**, 293–299.

172. Caelles, C., Helmberg, A. and Karin, M. (1994) p53-dependent apoptosis in the absence of transcriptional activation of p53-targeted genes. *Nature* **370**, 220–223.

173. Lane, D. P. and Lain, S. (2002) Therapeutic exploitation of the p53 pathway. *Trends Mol. Med.* **8(4)**, S38–S42.

174. Lowe, S. W., Ruley, H. E., Jacks, T., and Housman, D. E. (1993) p53-dependent apoptosis modulates the cytotoxicity of anticancer agents. *Cell* **74**, 957–968.

175. Kerr, D. J. and Workman, P., eds. (1994) *New Molecular Targets for Cancer Chemotherapy*, CRC Press, Boca Raton, FL.

176. Buttitta, F., Marchetti, A., Gadducci, A., et al. (1997) p53 alterations are predictive of chemoresistance and aggressiveness in ovarian carcinomas: a molecular and immunohistochemical study. *Br. J. Cancer* **75**, 230–235.

177. Aas., T, Borressen, A.-L., Geisler, S., et al. (1996) Specific p53 mutations are associated with *de novo* resistance to doxorubicin in breast cancer patients. *Nat. Med.* **2**, 811–814.

178. Herr, I. and Debatin, K.-M. (2001) Cellular stress response and apoptosis in cancer therapy. *Blood* **98,** 2603–2614.

179. Foster, B. A., Coffey, H. A., Morin, M. J., and Rastinejsd, F. (1999) Pharmacological rescue of mutant p53 conformation and function. *Science* **286,** 2507–2510.

180. Hupp, T. R., Lane, D. P., and Ball, K. L. (2000) Strategies for manipulating the p53 pathway in the treatment of human cancer. *Biochem. J.* **352,** 1–17.

181. Piette, J., Neel, H., and Marechal, V. (1997) MDM2: keeping p53 under control. *Oncogene* **15,** 1001–1010.

182. Barak, Y., Juven, T., Haffner, R., and Oren, M. (1993) MDM-2 expression is induced by wild-type p53 activity. *EMBO J.* **12,** 461–468.

183. Wu, X., Bayle, J. H., Olson, D., and Levine, J. A. (1993) The p53-mdm-2 autoregulatory feedback loop. *Genes Dev.* **7,** 1126–1132.

184. Chen, X., Bargonetti, J., and Prives, C. (1995) p53 through p21 (WAF1/CIP1), induces cyclin D1 synthesis. *Cancer Res.* **55,** 4257–4263.

185. Oliner, J. D., Kinzler, K. W., Meltzer, P. S., George, P. L., and Vogelstein, B. (1992) Amplification of a gene encoding a p53-associated protein in human sarcomas. *Nature* **358,** 80–83.

186. Finlay, C. A. (1993) The mdm-2 oncogene can overcome wild-type p53 suppression of transformed cell growth. *Mol. Cell. Biol.* **13,** 301–306.

187. Thut, C. J., Goodrich, J. A., and Tjian, R. (1997) Repression of p53-mediated transcription by MDM2: a dual mechanism. *Genes Dev.* **11,** 1974–1986.

188. Momand, J., Jung, D., Wilczynski, S., and Niland, J. (1998) The MDM2 gene amplification database. *Nucl. Acid. Res.* **26,** 3453–3459.

189. Zhang, R. and Wang, H. (2000) MDM2 oncogene as a novel target for human cancer therapy. *Curr. Pharm. Design* **6,** 393–416.

190. Bottger, A., Bottger, V., Garcia-Echeverria, C., et al. (1997) Molecular characterization of the mdm2-p53 interactions. *Mol. Biol.* **9,** 744–756.

191. Garcia-Echeverria, C., Chene, P., Blommers, M. J. J., and Furet, P. (2000) Discovery of potent antagonists of the interaction between human double minute 2 and tumor suppressor p53. *J. Med. Chem.* **43,** 3205–3208.

192. Midgley, C. A. and Lane, D. P. (1997) p53 protein stability in tumor cells is not determined by mutation but is dependent on mdm2 binding. *Oncogene* **15,** 1179–1189.

193. Arriola, E. L., Lopez, A. R., and Chresta, C. M. (1999) Differential regulation of p21/waf-1/cip-1 and mdm2 by etoposide: etoposide inhibits the p53-mdm2 autoregulatory feedback loop. *Oncogene* **18,** 1081–1091.

194. Stoll, R., Renner, C., Hansen, S., et al. (2001) Chalcone derivatives antagonize interactions between the human oncoprotein mdm2 and p53. *Biochemistry* **40,** 336–344.

195. Chen, L., Agrawal, S., Zhou, W., Zhang, R., and Chen, Z. (1998) Synergistic activation of p53 by inhibition of mdm2 expression and DNA damage. *Proc. Natl. Acad. Sci. USA* **95,** 195–200.

196. Chen, L., Lu, W., Agrawal, S., Zhou, W., Zhang, R., and Chen, J. (1999) Ubiquitous induction of p53 in tumor cells by antisense inhibition of mdm2 expression. *Mol. Med.* **5,** 21–34.

197. Wang, H., Oliver, P., Zeng, X., et al. (1999) MDM2 oncogene as a target for cancer therapy: an antisense approach. *Intl. J. Oncol.* **15,** 653–660.
198. Bissonnette, R., Echeverri, F., Mahboubi, A., and Green, D. R. (1992) Apoptotic cell death induced by c-myc is inhibited by bcl-2. *Nature* **359,** 552–554.
199. Korsmeyer, S. J. (1992) Bcl-2 initiates a new category of oncogenes: regulators of cell death. *Blood* **80,** 879–886.
200. Oltersdorf, T. and Fritz, L. C. (1998) The bcl-2 family: targets for the regulation of apoptosis. *Ann. Rep. Med. Chem.* **33,** 253–262.
201. Diaz, J.-L., Oltersdorf, T., Horne, W., et al. (1997) A common binding site mediates heterodimerization and homodimerization of bcl-2 family members. *J. Biol. Chem.* **272,** 11,350–11,355.
202. Enyedy, I. J., Ling, Y., Nacro, K., et al. (2001) Discovery of small-molecule inhibitors of Bcl-2 through structure-based computer screening. *J. Med. Chem.* **44,** 4313–4324.
203. Ambrosini, G., Adida, C., Sirugo, G., and Altieri, D. C. (1998) Induction of apoptosis and inhibition of cell proliferation by *survivin* gene targeting. *J. Biol. Chem.* **273,** 11,177–11,182.
204. Monzo, M., Rosell, R., Felip, E., et al. (1999) A novel anti-apoptosis gene: re-expression of surviving messenger RNA as a prognosis marker in non-small cell lung cancers. *J. Clin. Oncol.* **17,** 2100–2104.
205. Grossman, D., Kim, P. J., Schechner, J. S., and Altieri, D. C. (2001) Inhibition of melanoma tumor growth in vivo by survivin targeting. *Proc. Natl. Acad. Sci. USA* **98,** 635–640.
206. Blackburn, E. H. (1992) Telomerases. *Ann. Rev. Biochem.* **61,** 113–129.
207. Kim, N. W., Piatyszek, M. A., Prowse, K. R., et al. (1994) Specific association of human telomerase activity with immortal cells and cancer. *Science* **266,** 2011–2015.
208. Burger, A. M., Bibby, M. C., and Double, J. A. (1997) Telomerase activity in normal and malignant mammalian tissues: feasibility of telomerase as a target for cancer chemotherapy. *Br. J. Cancer* **75,** 516–522.
209. Sharma, S., Raymond, E., Soda, H., and Von Hoff, D. D. (1997) Telomerase and telomere inhibitors in preclinical development. *Exp. Opin. Invest. Drugs* **6,** 1179–1185.
210. Hamilton, S. E. and Corey, D. R. (1996) Telomerase: anti-cancr target or just a fascinating enzyme? *Chem. Biol.* **3,** 863–867.
211. Parkinson, E. K. (1996) Do telomerase antagonists represent a novel anti-cancer strategy? *Br. J. Cancer* **73,** 1–4.
212. Stewart, S. A. and Hahn, W. C. (2002) Prospects for anti-neoplastic therapies based on telomere biology. *Curr. Cancer Drug Targets* **2,** 1–17.
213. Aszalos, A. and Eckhardt, S. (1997) Molecular events as targets of anticancer drug therapy. *Path. Oncol. Res.* **3,** 147–158.
214. Perry, P. J., Gowan, S. M., Reszka, A. P., et al. (1998) 1,4- and 2,6-disubstituted amidoanthracene-9,10-dione derivatives as inhibitors of human telomerase. *J. Med. Chem.* **41,** 3253–3260.

215. Folkman, J. (1995) Angiogenesis in cancer, vascular rheumatoid and other diseases. *Nat. Med.* **1**, 27–31.
216. Folkman, J. (1995) Clinical applications of research on angiogenesis. *N. Engl. J. Med.* **333**, 1757–1763.
217. Folkman, J. (1996) Fighting cancer by attacking its blood supply. *Sci. Am.* **275**, 150–154.
218. Gourley, M. and Williamson, J. S. (2000) Angiogenesis: new targets for the development of anticancer chemotherapies. *Curr. Pharm. Des.* **6**, 417–439.
219. Nelson, N. J. (1998) News item: inhibitors of angiogenesis enter phase III testing. *J. Natl. Cancer Inst.* **90**, 960–963.
220. Lentzsch, S., Rogers, M. S., LeBlanc, R., et al. (2002) *S*-3-Amino-phthalimido-glutarimide inhibits angiogenesis and growth of B-cell neoplasias in mice. *Cancer Res.* **62**, 2300–2305.
221. Mazzieri, R., Masiero, L., Zanetta, L., et al. (1997) Control of type IV collagenase activity by components of the urokinase-plasmin system: a regulatory mechanism with cell-bound reactants. *EMBO J.* **16**, 2319–2332.
222. Vihinen, P. and Kahari, V.-M. (2002) Matrix metalloproteinases in cancer: prognostic markers and therapeutic targets. *Int. J. Cancer* **99**, 157–166.
223. Rabbani, S. A. (1998) Metalloproteases and urokinase in angiogenesis and tumor progression. *In Vivo* **12**, 135–142.
224. Coussens, L. M., Fingleton, B., and Matrisian, L. M. (2002) Matrix metalloproteinase inhibitors and cancer: trials and tribulations. *Science* **295**, 2387–2392.
225. Weidle, U. H. and Konig, B. (1998) Urokinase receptor antagonists: novel agents for the treatment of cancer. *Exp. Opin. Invest. Drugs* **7**, 391–404.
226. Kim, J., Wu, W., Kovalski, K., and Ossowski, L. (1998) Requirement of specific proteases in cancer cell intravasation as revealed by a novel semi-quantitative PCR-based assay. *Cell* **94**, 335–362.
227. Edwards, D. R. and Murphy, G. (1998) Proteases—invasion and more. *Nature* **394**, 527–528.
228. Huang, Y.-W., Baluna, R., and Vitetta, E. S. (1997) Adhesion molecules as targets for cnacer therapy. *Histol. Histopathol.* **12**, 467–477.
229. Shaw, L. M., Rabinovitz, I., Wang, H. H.-F., Toker, A., and Mercurio, A. M. (1997) Activation of phosphoinositol 3-OH kinase by the $\alpha6\beta4$ integrin promotes carcinoma invasion. *Cell* **91**, 949–960.
230. El-Hariry, I. and Pignatelli, M. (1997) Adhesion molecules: opportunities for modulation and a paradigm for novel therapeutic approaches in cancer. *Exp. Opin. Invest. Drugs* **6**, 1465–1478.
231. Engleman, V. W., Kellogg, M. S., and Rogers, T. E. (1996) Cell adhesion integrins as pharmaceutical targets. *Ann. Rep. Med. Chem.* **31**, 191–200.
232. Fish, R. G. (1996) Role of gangliosides in tumor progression: a molecular target for cancer therapy? *Medical Hypothesis* **46**, 140–144.
233. Workman, P. and Kaye, S. B. (2002) Translating basic cancer research into new cancer therapeutics. *Trends Mol. Med.* **8** (Issue 4 Suppl), S1–S9.

II

KINASE INHIBITOR DISCOVERY PROTOCOLS

2

Biomarker Assays for Phosphorylated MAP Kinase

Their Utility for Measurement of MEK Inhibition

Judith S. Sebolt-Leopold, Keri Van Becelaere, Kenneth Hook, and Roman Herrera

1. Introduction

Mitogen-activated protein kinase (MAP kinase) pathways are activated in response to a variety of stimuli involving receptor tyrosine kinases and G-protein coupled receptors *(1)*. Among the various families of MAP kinases, the extracellular signal-regulated kinases (ERK1 and ERK2) are the best characterized. Their involvement in proliferation-related events is highlighted by the fact that their activation is under the control of a signaling cascade of phosphorylation events downstream from the proto-oncogene Ras. Four proteins have emerged as key players in the quest to pharmacologically intervene in this pathway: Ras, Raf, MEK (MAP kinase kinase), and ERK. The reader is referred elsewhere for comprehensive reviews on the role of MAPK cascades in signal transduction *(1–3)*.

PD 184352 (CI-1040) represents the first MEK inhibitor reported to possess significant anticancer efficacy in animal models *(4)*. This agent is now undergoing Phase 1 clinical evaluation. The MAP kinase pathway is particularly amenable to pharmacodynamic evaluation, given the availability of antibodies that are specific for phosphorylated MAP kinase (pMAPK). The utility of such an assay in preclinical animal models was demonstrated for the MEK inhibitor CI-1040 *(4)*. Phosphorylated MAPK is the product of MEK activity and thus represents a direct measure of MEK inhibition. Measurement of pMAPK levels can be carried out by employing immunoblotting, flow cytometric,

From: *Methods in Molecular Medicine, vol. 85: Novel Anticancer Drug Protocols*
Edited by: J. K. Buolamwini and A. A. Adjei © Humana Press Inc., Totowa, NJ

or immunohistochemical procedures. In the following sections, we describe specific protocols that illustrate each of the above analysis methodologies.

2. Materials

1. MAPK lysis buffer: 50 mM glycerol phosphate, 10 mM Hepes, pH 7.4, 1% Triton X 100, 70 mM NaCl, 1 mM sodium vanadate, 10 μM pepstatin, 10 μM leupeptin, 100 μM phenylmethylsulfonyl fluoride (PMSF).
2. TBST: 0.9% NaCl, 10 mM Tris HCl, 0.1% Tween-20, pH 7.5.
3. pMAPK Ab: Promega pMAPK, 1:5000 in 0.5% bovine serum albumin (BSA); rabbit polyclonal.
4. Secondary Ab: BioRad Goat-anti-Rabbit HRP, 1:10,000 in 0.5% BSA.
5. Blocking solution: 1% BSA, 1% ovalbumin in TBST, filter sterilized with 0.01% sodium azide.
6. Total Erk Ab (Santa Cruz [1:2000 in 0.5% BSA; 1:1 mixture of ERK1 and ERK2 Antibodies]).
7. ECL Western blotting detection reagents (Amersham).
8. Phosphate-buffered saline (PBS).
9. Sodium vanadate.
10. Tris-glycine gels (Novex; 10%).
11. Phorbol 12-myristate 13-acetate (PMA).
12. Dimethylsulfoxide (DMSO).
13. Formaldehyde.
14. Methanol.
15. Mouse IgG (Sigma).
16. Goat anti-rabbit IgG Fab fragment (Molecular Probes; Alexa fluor 488).
17. Aqua-poly mounting media.
18. Fetal bovine serum (FBS).
19. Rabbit IgG.

3. Methods
3.1. Western Blot Analysis of pMAPK In Vitro and Ex Vivo
3.1.1. Treatment and Lysis of Cells

1. Seed 12-well plates at a cell density of 2×10^5 cells/well (1.5 mL/well) in the presence of 10% fetal bovine serum (basal conditions). Incubate at 37°C overnight.
2. Treat cells for one hour with MEK inhibitor at fixed or varying concentrations.
3. Wash cells with 1 mL of ice cold PBS containing 1 mM sodium vanadate.
4. Remove the PBS and add 100 μL of MAPK lysis buffer. Scrape the wells and transfer the lysed cells to chilled Eppendorf tubes. Spin the Eppendorf tubes at 18,000g at 4°C degrees for 5 min. Transfer the supernatants to cold eppendorf tubes and discard the pellets.

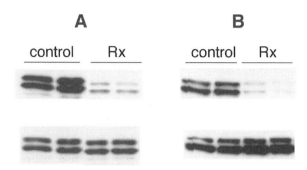

Fig. 1. Assessment of pMAPK levels by Western immunoblotting. Upper panels represent pMAPK levels and lower panels represent the same blots that have been stripped and re-blotted for total MAPK. **(A)** Mice bearing, H460 nonsmall cell lung cancer xenografts were treated with a single oral dose of CI-1040 (150 mg/kg). One hour after treatment, tumors were excised for analysis of pMAPK suppression. **(B)** Female cynomolgus monkeys were treated for 14 d with a daily oral dose of 200 mg/kg. Two hours after the day 14 dose, animals were sacrificed and their lungs were evaluated for levels of phosphorylated MAP kinase.

3.1.2. Preparation of Tissue Homogenates

1. Samples should be flash frozen in liquid nitrogen immediately upon excision and stored at –70°C. For processing, remove tissue into dry ice. Weigh out 40–100 mg of tissue, using a scalpel to slice. Add the appropriate volume of MAPK lysis buffer to give a 2.5% (w/v) tumor homogenate.
2. KEEP CELL LYSATES ON ICE AT ALL TIMES. Homogenize with a polytron homogenizer. Clean polytron with water between samples. Centrifuge samples at 1000g for 15 min at 4°C. Transfer the supernatants to cold 15-mL Falcon tubes. Determine the protein concentrations of lysates.

3.1.3. Western Blot Analysis (Fig. 1)

1. Load lysate samples (15–20 µg protein/lane) onto 10% tris-glycine gels (10-well or 15-well gels). Run the gels at 140 V for 1.5 h.
2. Transfer onto nitrocellulose membranes at 125 V for 2 h, keeping the transfer buffer cool. Alternatively, carry out the transfer overnight at 25 V.
3. Rinse membranes in water, and then block with blocking solution for a minimum of 1 h (blocking can occur overnight at 4°C).
4. Rinse membranes 3× for 5 min in TBST.
5. Incubate in primary antibody solution for a minimum of 3 h (this step can go overnight). Wash membranes for 5 min in TBST.
6. Incubate in secondary antibody solution for 1 h. Rinse 3× for 15 min in TBST.

7. Detect signal with enhanced chemiluminescence reagents (Amersham). Let membranes sit in ECL reagent for 1 min. Dab dry and then place into sheet protectors. Expose and develop onto Kodak BioMax Light film.

8. Quantitate by densitometry.

3.2. Immunohistochemistry Analysis of PMA-Stimulated Whole Blood (modified from Chow et al. [5])

3.2.1. Peripheral Blood Collection and Handling Procedures

1. Withdraw a 2-mL sample of whole blood into a purple-top evacuated tube containing ethylenediamine tetraacetic acid (EDTA) anticoagulant.

2. Gently invert the tube eight times to assure complete mixing with the EDTA solution. DO NOT SHAKE. Samples must remain at room temperature from the time of blood collection through preparation.

3. Dispense 1 mL undiluted blood to the bottoms of two 50 mL polypropylene tubes. Avoid contaminating the sides of the tubes with blood.

4. Add a final concentration of 400 n*M* PMA (diluting a 1000X stock solution) to one tube, DMSO for negative controls). Keep at 37°C for 5 min.

5. Add 20 mL of distilled water to each tube. After 30 s (timing is critical) add 2.2 mL of 10X strength PBS to each tube and vortex immediately.

6. Immediately centrifuge at 800*g* for 4 min at room temperature. Aspirate the hemoglobin-containing supernatant as thoroughly as possible.

7. Wash cells in 1 mL of 1X strength PBS.

8. Centrifuge again at 800*g* for 4 min at room temperature.

9. Aspirate the supernatant and resuspend the cells in 100 µL of 2% formaldehyde. Mix and hold at 37°C for 10 min.

10. Place on ice for 3 min and then add 1.8 mL of ice-cold 100% methanol, followed by vortex mixing. Hold on ice for 30 min.

11. Centrifuge at 800*g* for 4 min at room temperature.

12. Aspirate the supernatant.

13. Add 300 µL of 1X strength PBS and mix.

14. Load 150 µL of cells onto cytofunnel preassembled in cytoclip with silane slide using a wide bore tip and spin at 40*g* for 4 min, medium acceleration at room temperature.

15. Air dry for 10 min or let sit overnight at 4°C.

16. Block in mouse IgG 1 µg/mL (Sigma) (2 mg/mL stock), prepared in 1% ovalbumin, 1% BSA in PBS. Incubate for 1 h at room temperature.

17. Wash 3× in 1X PBS.

18. Incubate in primary antibody solution (Promega; polyclonal diluted 1 : 500 in 1% ovalbumin, 1% BSA in PBS) for 1 h at room temperature.

19. Wash 3× in 1X PBS.

20. Incubate in secondary antibody (Molecular Probes; Alexa fluor 488 goat anti-rabbit IgG Fab fragment conjugate; 2 mg/mL stock); 0.5 µg/mL in 1% ovalbumin, 1% BSA in PBS.
21. Wash 3× in 1X PBS.
22. Cover slip with 1 drop of Aqua-poly mounting media (Polysciences).

Representative data are shown in **Figures 2** and **3**.

3.3. Flow Cytometry Analysis of PMA-Stimulated T-Cells

A protocol for whole blood assay has been described *(5)*. Here we detail a procedure for Jurkat T-cells.

1. Serum-starved Jurkat cells (10^6/mL) are incubated in the presence or absence of MEK inhibitor as described in **Subheading 3.1.1.**
2. Stimulate with 100 n*M* PMA for 10 min at 37°C.
3. Spin down cells in an Eppendorf centrifuge.
4. Follow **steps 9–12** from **Subheading 3.2.1.**
5. Resuspend to give 10^6 cells/100 µL PBS and 4% FBS. For positive control, incubate in Promega pMAPK polyclonal antibody diluted 1:100 for 1 h. Wash in 2 mL PBS and 4% FBS. Incubate in Molecular Probes Alexa Fluor 488 goat anti-rabbit IgG Fab fragment (0.5 µg/mL) for 1 h. Wash in 2 mL of PBS and 4% FBS. For negative control, incubate in rabbit IgG solution (1 µg/mL) for 1 h. Wash in 2 mL of PBS and 4% FBS. Incubate in Molecular Probes Alexa Fluor 488 goat anti-rabbit IgG Fab Fragment (0.5 µg/mL) for 1 h. Wash in 2 mL PBS and 4% FBS.
6. Run samples on flow cytometer.

4. Notes

1. Western analysis of pMAPK levels (**Fig. 1**) is a straightforward, relatively rapid method of quantitation that is most appropriate for homogeneous tissues. These assays are particularly amenable to the preclinical evaluation of murine tumors and human xenografts. However, Western immunoblotting may not be the method of choice for analysis of clinical samples, owing to dilution of total cellular protein with stromal tissue. Immunohistochemistry analysis (**Fig. 3**) offers the advantage of distinguishing tumor cells from stromal cells.
2. Flow cytometric assays (**Fig. 4**) represent an alternative methodology for determination of pMAPK levels and are particularly suitable to analysis of blood cells *(5)*. However, high protein concentrations in whole blood may pose complications, contributing to the relatively poor stimulation of MAPK that has been observed upon addition of PMA *(6)*.

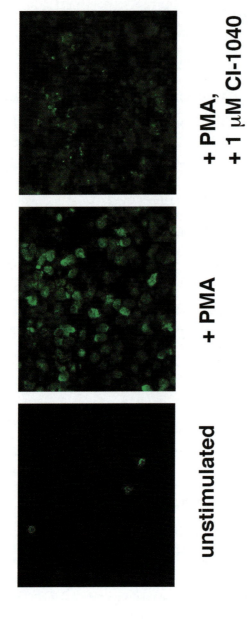

unstimulated

+ PMA

+ PMA,
+ 1 µM CI-1040

Fig. 2. Immunohistochemical analysis of PMA-stimulated whole blood.

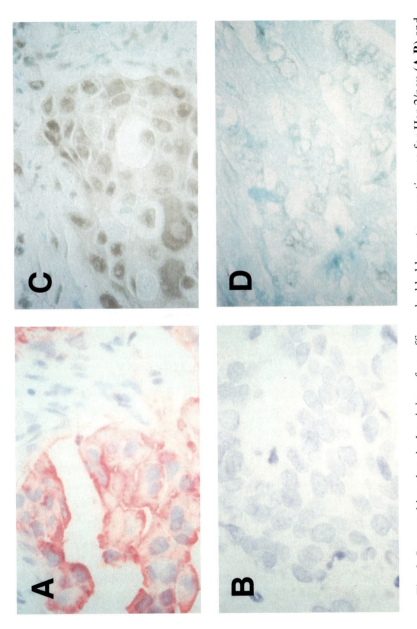

Fig. 3. Immunohistochemical staining of paraffin embedded breast cancer tissues for Her-2/neu (**A,B**) and pMAPK (**C,D**). Images shown in **A** and **B** correspond to the tissues depicted in **C** and **D**, respectively. Data were provided courtesy of Sarah Bacus, Ventana Medical Systems, Inc., QDL, Westmont, IL.

37

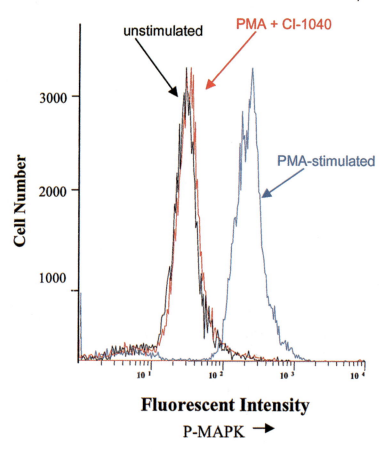

Fluorescent Intensity

P-MAPK ➡

Fig. 4. Assessment of pMAPK levels in PMA-stimulated Jurkat cells by flow cyto-metric assay. The MEK inhibitor CI-1040 was added at a final concentration of 0.3 μ*M*.

References

1. Cobb, M. H. (1999). MAP kinase pathways. *Prog. Biophys. Mol. Biol.* **71,** 479–500.
2. Lewis, T. S., Shapiro P. S., and Ahn, N.G. (1998). Signal transduction through MAP kinase cascades. *Adv. Cancer Res.* **74,** 49–139.
3. Kolch, W. (2000) Meaningful Relationships: the regulation of the Ras/Raf/MEK/ERK pathway by protein interactions. *Biochem. J.* **351,** 289–305.
4. Sebolt-Leopold J. S., Dudley D. T., Herrera R., et al. (1999) Blockade of the MAP kinase pathway suppresses growth of colon tumors in vivo. *Nat. Med.* **5,** 810–816.
5. Chow, S., Patel, H., and Hedley, D. W. (2001) Measurement of MAK kinase activation by flow cytometry using phospho-specific antibodies to MEK and ERK: potential for pharmacodynamic monitoring of signal transduction inhibitors. *Cytometry (Communications in Clinical Cytometry)* **46,** 72–78.
6. Herrera, R., unpublished observations.

3

Assays for Cyclin-Dependent Kinase Inhibitors

Adrian M. Senderowicz and Tyler Lahusen

1. Introduction

Cyclin-dependent kinases (CDK) are serine/threonine kinases that regulate cell cycle control and progression (*1,2*). A CDK holoenzyme complex is active if associated with its cyclin partner and if the complex is phosphorylated at specific activating residues (threonine 160/161) (*1,2*). The progression through the cell cycle is mediated by the sequential activation of CDKs during different phases of the cycle. The G1/S phase transition of the cell cycle is mediated by phosphorylation of the Retinoblastoma gene product (Rb) by CDK4 and/or CDK6 (G1/S checkpoint), leading to the release of bound E2F from Rb and allowing the transcription of genes by "free E2F" necessary for S phase progression. During late G1 phase, CDK2/cyclin E complex phosphorylates several substrates including Rb. On the other hand, CDK2/cyclin A complex is active throughout S phase. For cells to progress to mitosis, CDK1 (CDC2) must be "activated," and activated cdc2 phosphorylates substrates required for mitosis (*3*).

Modulation of cdk function can be achieved by direct effects on the cdk catalytic subunit, "direct cdk inhibitors," or by modulation of pathways necessary for the activation of cdks, "indirect cdk inhibitors" (*4,5*). Examples of the first group include flavopiridol, UCN-01, paullones, hymenialdisine, roscovitine, and indirubins (*4–8*). These compounds, when included in cdk in vitro kinase reactions (*see* **Subheading 3.1.**), decrease the capacity of cdks to phosphorylate its substrates.

In contrast, the indirect cdk inhibitors (such as rapamycin, lovastatin, antisense against cdks or cyclins and the like) do not have the capacity, when included in cdk in vitro kinase reactions (*see* **Subheading 3.1.**), to decrease the

From: *Methods in Molecular Medicine, vol. 85: Novel Anticancer Drug Protocols*
Edited by: J. K. Buolamwini and A. A. Adjei © Humana Press Inc., Totowa, NJ

phosphorylation of cdk substrates *(4,5,9)*. However, these compounds could lead to loss in cdk activity in intact cells owing to modulation of upstream pathways required for cdk activation (*see* **Subheading 3.1.**). Moreover, based on the known role of cdks in the phosphorylation of specific endogenous substrates, we can assess the cellular effects of these compounds by Western blot using phospho-specific antibodies that recognize cdk phosphorylated substrates (*see* **Subheading 3.2.**). Finally, the cellular consequence of cdk inhibition is manifested by the block in cell cycle progression; this effect can be determined by the assessment of the DNA content as measured by FACS analysis (*see* **Subheading 3.3.**).

2. Materials

All chemicals used should be of the highest quality and water should be de-ionized. Most reagents were obtained from Sigma. Mammalian cells are grown in a 5% CO_2 humidified incubator at 37°C, and should be handled in sterile conditions at all times in a laminar flow-hood.

1. 1.5-mL microfuge tubes.
2. 15-mL centrifuge tubes.
3. 50-mL centrifuge tubes.
4. Cell scraper.
5. 100-mm cell culture plates.
6. 5-mL polystyrene round-bottom tube.
7. Deionized water.
8. Absolute ethanol.
9. Phosphate-Buffered Saline (PBS), pH 7.4.
10. β-Mercaptoethanol.
11. Dimethyl Sulfoxide (DMSO).
12. Ponceau S: (0.1% Ponceau Solution in 5% acetic acid).
13. Tween 20 (Sigma).
14. Tris-HCl, pH 7.4.
15. Ethylene diamine tetraacetic acid (EDTA), 0.5 *M*.
16. Bromodeoxy uridine (BrdU) 50 m*M* stock in water, heat at approx 37°C to get into solution.
17. RNase A (DNase free).
18. Propidium Iodide (50 µg/mL in PBS).
19. Gammabind G Sepharose (Amersham).
20. Anti-Rabbit and Mouse IgG (Amersham).
21. Phospho-specific Rb antibodies (Cell Signalling Technology).
22. Enhanced chemiluminescent reagent (Amersham).
23. Bovine Serum Albumin (BSA).
24. Purified Full-length Rb protein (QED Biosciences) or GST-Rb (Santa Cruz).

25. Histone H1 (Sigma).
26. Kinase lysis buffer (final concentration): 1 M HEPES, 0.5 M EDTA, 0.5% NP-40, 1 mM NaF, 10 mM β-glycerophosphate; protease inhibitor cocktail: 200 mM sodium orthovanadate, 100 mM dithiothreitol (DTT), 100 mM aminoethyl benzene sulfonyl fluoride (AEBSF), 20 μg/mL Aprotinin, 20 μg/mL Leupeptin.
27. Kinase reaction buffer (final concentration): 50 mM HEPES, 10 mM MgCl$_2$, 5 mM MnCl$_2$, 2.5 mM ethylene glycol tetraacetic acid (EGTA), 0.4 mM Na vanadate, 1 mM β-glycerophosphate, NaF, 1 mM DTT, ATP (CDK1/2 50 μM, CDK4/6 5 μM).
28. Immunoblot washing buffer (TNE): (20X) 1 M Tris-HCl, pH 7.5, 50 mM EDTA, NaCl 1 M; (1X) add 0.1% Tween.
29. Electrophoresis buffer: 25 mM Tris, 192 mM glycine, and 0.1% sodium dodecyl sulfate (SDS), pH 8.3.
30. Transfer buffer: 25 mM Tris-HCl, 192 mM glycine, and 20% methanol.
31. Kodak Bio-Max MR autoradiography film.
32. Autoradiography cassette.
33. PhosphorImager screen (Amersham).
34. Saran Wrap.
35. Whatman filter paper.
36. PVDF immublotting transfer membrane (Millipore).
37. Paraformaldehyde: Heat 1 g in H$_2$O at 65°C for 15 min and then add a few drops of 10 N NaOH; finally add 5 mL 10X PBS (Make fresh for each use).
38. LDS/SDS Sample Buffer: 4X Invitrogen; 2X SDS Quality Biological.
39. Mouse anti-BrdU (clone B44, Becton Dickinson).
40. Donkey anti-mouse IgG Cy3-conjugated antisera (Jackson Immunochemicals).
41. Vectashield mounting medium with DAPI (Vector Laboratories, cat. No. H-1200).
42. Precast tris-glycine polyacrylamide mini-gels (Invitrogen).
43. Antibodies against cdk1 (Life Technologies), cdk2, cdk4, and cdk6 (Santa Cruz).
44. Purified active CDK 1/cyclin B1 (Life Technologies), active CDK2/cyclinA (Upstate Biotechnology).
45. Gel electrophoresis unit (Invitrogen).
46. Immunoblot transfer unit (Hoefer TE 22 Mini Tank Transphor Unit; Amersham).
47. Poly-D-Lysine (Roche).

3. Methods

3.1. Measuring Cyclin-Dependent Kinase (CDK) Activity In Vitro

Kinase assays are carried out with endogenous kinase immunoprecipitated from cells (*see* **Subheading 3.1.2.**) or directly with purified recombinant kinase (*see* **Note 3**).

3.1.1. Lysis of Mammalian Cells

1. Plate cells in 100 mm dishes so that at the time of treatment, the cells will be 50–60% confluent.
2. Wash cells 2× with cold PBS and remove all residual PBS.
3. Add 100–250 µL of lysis buffer and scrape cells to one side.
4. Collect lysate in microcentrifuge tubes and continue lysis for 15 min.
5. Clarify lysate by centrifugation at 13,000g for 20 min to remove insoluble debris. Remove lysate to another microfuge tube without disturbing pellet.
6. Make protein standard with 1 µg/µL BSA. Aliquot and store at –20°C.
7. Prepare protein standard reagent (Bio-Rad Protein Assay Reagent 1:5 vol/vol with water).
8. Add 2, 4, 5, 7.5, 10, and 15 µg protein to 3 µL lysis buffer for standard curve. Sample protein lysate should be in the range from 2–4 µg/µL. Analyze with 3 µL lysate in duplicates.
9. Read at 595 nm on a spectrophotometer.

3.1.2. Immunoprecipitation

1. Lyse cells and determine the protein concentration as in **Subheading 3.1.1.**
2. Use 200–500 µg protein for the immunoprecipitation and 1–3 µg of antibody for 1 h at 4°C on a rotator.
3. Capture antibody by adding 25 µL Gammabind G Sepharose for 30 min while rotating; wash 2× with lysis buffer containing 100 mM NaCl for CDK1/2 and 500 mM for CDK4/6. Centrifuge at 5000g for 3 min after each wash to pellet beads. Remove and discard supernatant with a pipet tip connected to a vacuum without disturbing beads.
4. Wash 1× with kinase buffer for the final wash.

3.1.3. In Vitro CDK Assay

Because this assay requires the use of radioactive material, care must be taken to limit exposure and to prevent contamination of the laboratory. Keep proteins always at 4°C. Avoid freeze and thaw of proteins because of the loss of kinase activity!

1. To the pelleted beads (or to purified recombinant cdk/cyclins), add 25 µL of kinase reaction buffer (*see* **Subheading 2., item 28**).
2. If a chemical compound being tested is dissolved in DMSO, the concentration should not exceed 0.01% of the reaction mixture.
3. Add 50 µM ATP for CDK1/2 or 5 µM ATP for CDK 4/6; 10 µCi of [γ-^{32}P]ATP (300 Ci/mmol) and 2 µg histone H1 for CDK 1/2 or 1 µg of full-length Rb for CDK4/6 (*see* **Notes 1** and **2**).
4. Incubate for 30 min at 30°C with shaking. Terminate by adding 4% SDS-sample buffer. Heat sample at 95°C for 5 min.

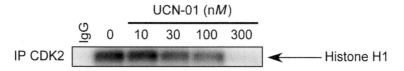

Fig. 1. In vitro cdk kinase assays. HN12 squamous head and neck carcinoma cells were treated with the CDK inhibitor UCN-01 for 24 h, harvested and kinase assay performed as described in **Subheading 3.1.** As a control for specificity (negative control), unrelated IgG was used in place of the CDK2 antibody for the immunoprecipitation. The substrate used in the kinase reaction is histone H1. Clear dose-dependent loss in H1 phosphorylation is shown.

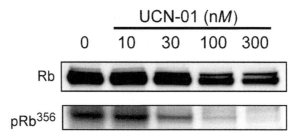

Fig. 2. Determination of cdk activity by western blots against phospho-Rb antibodies. Parallel lysates from **Figure 1** were run in SDS gel and immunoblotted as described in **Subheading 3.2.** In the upper band, an antibody recognizes total Rb levels and in the lower band, an antibody that recognizes only the phosphorylation of Rb at a CDK2 phosphorylation site, threonine[356] *(10)*. Clear dose-dependent loss in Rb phosphorylation is shown.

5. Resolve samples by polyacrylamide gel electrophoresis, 8% for Rb and 12% for histone H1.
6. Set power supply to 100 V and stop before dye front runs off gel. Remove gel from electrophoresis unit and place on filter paper. Cover with Saran Wrap.
7. Dry gel with a gel dryer for 45 min to 1 h at 80°C.
8. Expose film to autoradiography film and/or PhosphorImager screen.
9. Develop film in film developer and/or phosphorimager (*see* **Fig. 1**).

3.2. Measuring CDK Activity in Intact Cells by Using Phospho-Specific Antibodies Against Endogenous CDK Substrates

If a chemical compound inhibits cdks in vitro, then it will be necessary to determine the phosphorylation status of the CDK substrate. Thus, either direct or indirect small molecule cdk inhibitors should lead to loss in the phosphorylation of endogenous substrates such as Rb, vimentin, NPAT, or p70S6 kinase *(10–14)* (*see* **Fig. 2**).

3.2.1. Polyacrylamide-Gel Electrophoresis

1. Prepare protein lysate to a concentration of 1 μg/μL.
2. Add protein to SDS-sample buffer (2X + 5% β-Mercaptoethanol or 4X + 10%) and add lysis buffer up to 25 μL.
3. Heat sample at 95°C for 5 min. Cells should be lysed and the protein concentration determined as in **Subheading 3.1.1.**
4. Load samples on to a 4–20% gradient or 8% tris-glycine polyacrylamide mini-gel.
5. Initially, set power supply to 100 V, and then after 15 min increase the voltage to 150 V.
6. Saturate polyvinylidine fluoride (PVDF) membrane in methanol for 1 min and then in tris-glycine buffer for 5 min.
7. Remove gel and place into tris-glycine buffer.
8. Set up sandwich from transfer unit. First, place cassette in transfer buffer; second, place filter paper on sponge; third, place gel on to filter paper; fourth, place PVDF membrane on to gel; fifth, remove any bubbles from underneath membrane; sixth, place wet filter paper on to membrane; seventh, place sponge on to filter, last, close sandwich cassette and place in transfer unit.
9. Transfer should be done at 4°C, at 80 V for 2 h or at 15 V for approximately 15 h.
10. Remove membrane from transfer unit.
11. Wash membrane in PBS.
12. Check transfer efficiency and protein loading by Ponceau S staining for 1 min.
13. Rinse with PBS to observe protein staining.
14. Wash out the Ponceau S stain with TNE wash buffer for a few min.

3.2.2. Immunoblotting

1. Block PVDF membrane with 4% milk in TNE overnight at 4°C or for 30 min at room temperature while rocking.
2. Rinse 1× with TNE buffer.
3. Incubate with primary antibody at room temperature for 1 h or at 4°C overnight while rocking.
4. Rinse 1× with TNE.
5. Wash membrane 2× for 5 min each time with TNE.
6. Incubate with horseradish peroxide (HRP)-conjugated secondary antibody for 30 min at room temperature while rocking.
7. Rinse 1× with TNE.
8. Wash membrane 2× for 5 min each time with TNE.
9. Incubate with enhanced chemiluminescence (ECL) reagent for 1 min.
10. Expose film. Determine optimal exposure of film.

3.3. Effects of CDK Modulation on Cell Cycle Progression

Small molecules that cause a loss in cdk activity should arrest cells at different phases of the cell cycle. One traditional method used to determine

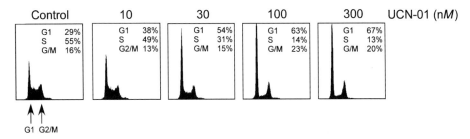

Fig. 3. Cell cycle analysis of UCN-01 treated cells by propidium iodide staining. Region between G1 and G2/M represents the S phase region.

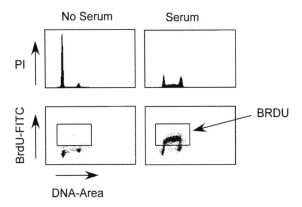

Fig. 4. BrdU and PI determination by FACS analysis. MCF10A breast immortalized cell lines were serum starved for 24 h (left panel) and then serum stimulated for 18 h (right panel). Upper panels represent PI labeling and lower panels represent BrdU incorporation. As shown in the upper panels, serum starved cells have 1% of S phase in comparison to serum (58%). Similarly, in the lower panels, serum starved cells have 1% of BRDU positive cells compared with 57% of cells stimulated with serum.

the percentage of cells in each phase is measuring DNA content by FACS analysis (*see* **Fig. 3**). Also, the determination of S phase can be obtained by BrdU incorporation (DNA synthesis) (*see* **Fig. 4**).

3.3.1. Assessment of DNA Content by FACS Analysis with Propidium Iodide

1. Plate attached cells in 100 mm dishes so that they are 40–50% confluent (approx 5.0×10^5 cells) upon treatment. For suspension cells, plate approx 4×10^5 cells/mL. At least 1.0×10^6 cells are needed for the assay.
2. Harvest attached cells by trypsinization for 3–5 min. Collect trypsinized cells with 4°C PBS. Centrifuge at 800*g* in a 15-mL tube. Suspension cells are collected directly into a 15-mL tube.

3. Wash 1× with PBS and centrifuge.
4. Resuspend pellet in 1 mL PBS and add 4 mL of –20°C absolute EtOH (Add ethanol in pulses of 1 mL each with repeater pipet while vortexing tube).
5. Place samples at –20°C for minimum of 24 h and maximum up to 1 mo.
6. When sample is to be analyzed, centrifuge cells and remove ethanol. Wash 1× with PBS.
7. Resuspend the cell pellet in 500 µL of 50 µg/mL propidium iodide solution in PBS plus 100 µg/mL RNase. Transfer to a 5-mL round-bottom tube.
8. Incubate for 1 h at 37°C. Analyze with a flow cytometer in the FL2 channel (*see* **Note 4** and **Fig. 3**).

3.3.2. Using FACS Analysis to Measure DNA Synthesis (S-Phase) by BrdU Incorporation

1. Plate cells as described in **Subheading 3.3.1.**
2. Pulse cells with 50 µ*M* of BrdU 1 h before harvesting.
3. Follow **Steps 1–6** from **Subheading 3.3.1.** on cell cycle analysis.
4. Slowly, add 500 µL of 2 *M* HCl/0.5% triton X-100 a few drops at a time while maintaining a vortex. Incubate for 30 min at room temperature.
5. Centrifuge the cells at 800*g* for 5 min. Aspirate the supernatant and resuspend in 1 mL of 0.1 *M* $Na_2B_4O_7$. Centrifuge at 800*g* for 5 min.
6. Resuspend approx 10^6 cells in 1 mL of 0.5% Tween 20/1% BSA/PBS. Centrifuge at 800*g* for 5 min.
7. Add 300 µL Tween/BSA/PBS and 20 µL of Anti-BrdU FITC. Incubate for 30 min at 37°C.
8. Centrifuge cells at 800*g* for 5 min. Resuspend in 1 mL of PBS containing 5 µg/mL propidium iodide.
9. Analyze on a flow cytometer. On a Becton Dickinson flow cytometer the FL1 channel will measure BrdU FITC and the FL2 channel will measure propidium iodide. Create a dot-plot and set the X-axis as FL2 and the Y-axis as FL1 (*see* **Fig. 4**).

3.3.3. Using Immunofluorescence to Measure DNA Synthesis (S-phase) by BrdU Incorporation

1. Autoclave glass cover slips and place into wells of 6-well plate. Add 1 mL of poly-ᴅ-lysine to each well. Leave for 5 min and then wash 1× with PBS.
2. Plate approx 2×10^5 cells in each well.
3. Pulse cells with 50 µ*M* of BrdU 1 h before harvesting cells.
4. At harvest time, remove medium and wash 1× with PBS.
5. Fix cells in 2% paraformaldehyde for 20 min. Wash 1× with PBS. At this point, the cells may be stored at 4°C for up to 1 wk. Add 1 mL of Triton/BSA/PBS solution for 10 min.
6. Wash 1× with PBS containing calcium and magnesium. Add 100 units of DNase I in 1 mL calcium and magnesium containing PBS for 1 h at 37°C.

7. Wash cover slips 2× with PBS. Add 80 µL 1:100 anti-BrdU in Triton/BSA/PBS solution to cover slip and incubate for 30 min at 37°C in a humidified chamber.
8. Wash 2× with PBS. Add 80 µL of 1:500 anti-mouse conjugated Cy3 to cover slip for 30 min at 37°C in a humidified chamber.
9. Wash 2× with PBS. Put one drop of mounting medium containing 4,6-diamino-2-phynylindole (DAPI) to a glass slide. After aspirating PBS from cover slip, carefully pick up cover slip with forceps and place down with the cells contacting the medium. The slides should be kept at 4°C in the dark until analysis for up to a week.
10. Stained cells can be visualized with a fluorescent microscope.

4. Notes

1. It is important to mention that when comparing the inhibitory potencies (IC_{50}) of different small molecule cdk inhibitors, the concentration of ATP in each reaction is of paramount importance as these small molecule cdk inhibitors compete with substrate (ATP). Thus, if the in vitro kinase reaction is performed with very high ATP concentrations, the potency is much lower than when the same compound is tested at lower ATP concentrations. Therefore, the only accurate way to compare these compounds is through the determination of a K_i with respect to ATP. This value is a constant and does not vary with ATP concentration. For example, we can calculate the $K_{i\ app}$ using this formula: $K_i = IC_{50}/(1 + S/K_m)$, where S is the ATP concentration and K_m is the concentration of substrate (ATP) that leads to half-maximal velocity. If the ATP concentration used is lower than the K_m, then the IC_{50} is similar to the $K_{i\ app}$ (*9*).
2. To determine if a small molecule inhibits cdk activity by competition with ATP, kinase reactions should be done in the presence of increasing amounts of ATP while maintaining constant the amounts of kinase, substrate, and inhibitor. Moreover, in order to determine if the inhibitor competes with substrate, increasing amounts of substrate should be tested in the presence of fixed amounts of kinase, ATP, and inhibitor.
3. Cdk1 (cdc2) kinase activity from endogenous sources: The number of cells with G2/M DNA content is low (<15% total) in most exponentially growing cells, thus, the activity of cdc2 is quite low. To enrich cells with G2/M content (and active cdc2), aphidocolin-synchronized cells (arrested in S phase) can be released into media; and cells should be harvested approx 12 h later (depending on the cell line), when cdc2 becomes active.
4. Set up a plot with the parameters: Forward Scatter (FSC) on the X-axis and Side Scatter on the Y-axis. The second plot will be a histogram with FL-2 as DNA-Area. Fl-2 should be adjusted so that the G1 peak falls on channel 200 and then the G2/M peak will be at channel 400.

References

1. Morgan, D. O. (1995) Principles of CDK regulation. *Nature* **374,** 131–134.
2. Morgan, D. O. (1997) Cyclin-dependent kinases: engines, clocks, and microprocessors. *Annu. Rev. Cell Dev. Biol.* **13,** 261–291.

3. Sherr, C. J. (1996) Cancer cell cycles. *Science* **274,** 1672–1677.
4. Senderowicz, A. M. and Sausville, E. A. (2000) Preclinical and clinical development of cyclin-dependent kinase modulators. *J. Natl. Cancer Inst.* **92,** 376–387.
5. Senderowicz, A. (2000) Small molecule modulators of cyclin-dependent kinases for cancer therapy. *Oncogene* **19,** 6600–6606.
6. Hoessel, R., Leclerc, S., Endicott, J. A., et al. (1999) Indirubin, the active constituent of a Chinese antileukaemia medicine, inhibits cyclin-dependent kinases. *Nat. Cell Biol.* **1,** 60–67.
7. Meijer, L. and Kim, S. H. (1997) Chemical inhibitors of cyclin-dependent kinases. *Methods Enzymol.* **283,** 113–128.
8. Meijer, L., Thunnissen, A. M., White, A. W., et al. (2000) Inhibition of cyclin-dependent kinases, GSK-3beta and CDK1 by hymenialdisine, a marine sponge constituent. *Chem. Biol.* **7,** 51–63.
9. Senderowicz, A. M. (2001) Cyclin-Dependent kinase modulators: a novel class of cell cycle regulators for cancer therapy, in *Cancer Chemotherapy & Biological Response Modifiers* (Giaccone, G. G., Schilsky, R. L., and Sondel, P. M. eds.), Elsevier Science, Oxford, UK, Annual Vol. 19 (in press).
10. Kitagawa, M., Higashi, H., Jung, H. K., et al. (1996) The consensus motif for phosphorylation by cyclin D1-Cdk4 is different from that for phosphorylation by cyclin A/E-Cdk2. *EMBO J.* **15,** 7060–7069.
11. Weinberg, R. A. (1995) The retinoblastoma protein and cell cycle control. *Cell* **81,** 323–330.
12. Zhao, J., Dynlacht, B., Imai, T., Hori, T., and Harlow, E. (1998) Expression of NPAT, a novel substrate of cyclin E-CDK2, promotes S-phase entry. *Genes Dev.* **12,** 456–461.
13. Papst, P. J., Sugiyama, H., Nagasawa, M., Lucas, J. J., Maller, J. L., and Terada, N. (1998) Cdc2-cyclin B phosphorylates p70 S6 kinase on Ser411 at mitosis. *J. Biol. Chem.* **273,** 15,077–15,084.
14. Meijer, L., Borgne, A., Mulner, O., et al. (1997) Biochemical and cellular effects of roscovitine, a potent and selective inhibitor of the cyclin-dependent kinases cdc2, cdk2 and cdk5. *Eur. J. Biochem.* 243, 527–536.

4

Identifying Inhibitors of ATM
and ATR Kinase Activities

Jann N. Sarkaria

1. Introduction

The Ataxia Telangiectasia *mutated* (ATM) and the ATM and Rad3-related (ATR) proteins function in partially overlapping DNA damage checkpoint pathways that orchestrate the cellular response to DNA damage. Both proteins belong to a growing family of serine/threonine-directed kinases that contain C-terminal kinase domains bearing significant sequence homology to those of mammalian and yeast phosphoinositide 3-kinases *(1)*. In response to genotoxic insults, these kinases phosphorylate a number of key proteins that control cell cycle progression and DNA repair *(2)*. ATM and ATR-mediated phosphorylation of the tumor suppressor protein p53 and the associated Mdm2 protein result in accumulation and transcriptional activation of p53. The subsequent p53-mediated up-regulation of p21[cip1/waf1] protein levels results in inhibition of G_1 cyclin-dependent kinases and prevents cells from entering S-phase with unrepaired DNA damage. In a similar pathway, damage-dependent phosphorylation of the checkpoint proteins Chk1 and Chk2 ultimately results in the radiation-inducible arrest of cells in G_2 through their downstream effects on Cdc25C. Likewise, ATM and ATR regulate the repair of DNA damage through phosphorylation of putative DNA repair proteins like BRCA1, NBS1, and BLM *(3–5)*.

The importance of the ATM protein kinase in the cellular response to genotoxic stress is highlighted by the severe pathologies associated with germ-line homozygous mutations of the *atm* gene in the Ataxia Telangiectasia (A-T) syndrome *(1,6)*. One of the hallmark features of this syndrome is the profound sensitivity to ionizing radiation displayed by patients affected by

From: *Methods in Molecular Medicine, vol. 85: Novel Anticancer Drug Protocols*
Edited by: J. K. Buolamwini and A. A. Adjei © Humana Press Inc., Totowa, NJ

A-T. Likewise, cells lacking normal ATM or ATR function exhibit multiple cell cycle arrest defects and hypersensitivity to ionizing radiation. Based on these observations, it has been speculated that small molecule inhibitors of ATM and/or ATR should sensitize tumor cells to the lethal effects of ionizing radiation or commonly used chemotherapeutic agents. In fact, we and others have shown that caffeine inhibits ATM and ATR kinase activities at concentrations associated with the sensitizing effects of this drug *(7–9)*. Although radiosensitizing concentrations of caffeine are lethal in humans, these studies suggest that selective small molecule inhibitors of ATM or ATR will be useful adjuvant therapeutic agents *(10)*.

The identification of novel ATM and ATR inhibitors has been hampered because catalytically active versions of these kinases cannot be efficiently overexpressed in bacterial or insect cell systems. Because purified recombinant kinases are not readily available, direct high-throughput kinase inhibitor screens for ATM or ATR have yet to be described. Instead, cell-based screens have been used to identify compounds that abrogate ATM- or ATR-dependent signaling pathways *(11,12)*. Promising compounds from these screens can then be tested in in vitro assays for inhibition of relevant kinases. In this review, we describe a specific protocol for ATM and ATR immune-complex kinase assays and their application to the identification of potential small-molecule inhibitors.

2. Materials

All chemicals are reagent grade materials and all solutions are made in de-ionized H_2O unless otherwise specified. The lysis and kinase base buffers are stored at 4°C (*see* **Note 1**).

1. Microcentrifuge tubes, cell scraper, 27-gauge needle, 18-gauge needle.
2. 100-mm Tissue culture dishes.
3. Phosphate-buffered saline (PBS).
4. Base lysis buffer: 20 mM HEPES, pH 7.4, 0.1 M NaCl, 10 mM NaF, 1.5 mM MgCl$_2$, 1 mM ethylene glycol tetraacetic acid (EGTA), and either 0. 2% Tween 20 for ATM or 1% TritonX-100 for ATR.
5. Stock solution of 1 M β-glycerol phosphate, pH ~7.4, dissolved in water and stored at 4°C.
6. Freshly prepared solution of 1 M dithiothreitol (DTT) in H_2O.
7. Protease and phosphatase inhibitors made at a 1000X concentration and stored at –20°C. (a) 10 mg/mL aprotinin dissolved in H_2O; (b) 5 mg/mL leupeptin dissolved in H_2O; (c) 5 mg/mL pepstatin dissolved in methanol; (d) 20 μM microcystinLR dissolved in methanol.
8. Bradford protein concentration assay reagent.
9. Protein A-Sepharose beads rehydrated in PBS.

10. Buffered salt solution: 0.6 M NaCl, 0.1 M Tris-HCl, pH 7.4.
11. Kinase base buffer: 10 mM HEPES, pH 7.4, 50 mM NaCl, 10 mM MgCl$_2$.
12. Freshly-made 1 mM ATP dissolved in H$_2$O.
13. Fresh, frozen [γ-^{32}P] ATP (specific activity: 4500 Ci/mmol).
14. Stock solution of 1 M MnCl$_2$ stored at –20°C for not more that 2 mo.
15. ATM peptide substrate. PHAS-1 (Stratagene) or N-terminal p53-GST fusion protein stored at –80°C.
16. 4X sodium dodecylsulfate (SDS) sample buffer.
17. Refrigerated microcentrifuge.
18. Sodium dodecylsulfate-polyacrylamide gel electrophoresis (SDS-PAGE) apparatus and reagents, polyvinylidene fluoride (PVDF) membrane and electro-transfer apparatus.

3. Methods

The catalytic activity of the ATM and ATR protein kinases can be measured in immune-complex kinase assays following immunoprecipitation of ATM or ATR from a variety of sources, including cultured cells, solid tumors, and organ tissues. Likewise, these assays can be performed on endogenous protein or epitope-tagged recombinant proteins that are transiently or stably expressed in mammalian or insect cell lines. The basic protocol involves cell lysis in a non-ionic detergent-containing buffer followed by immunoprecipitation. Immunoprecipitates are serially washed in lysis buffer, high-salt buffer, and kinase buffer to remove contaminating proteins and then incubated in a kinase reaction buffer that contains an appropriate peptide substrate and [γ-^{32}P] ATP. The ATM and ATR kinases catalyze the transfer of the gamma-phosphate from ATP onto select serine or threonine residues of the substrate. The efficiency of this phosphotransferase reaction is evaluated by measuring the incorporation of ^{32}P into the peptide substrate using either phosphorimaging or scintillation counting. The kinase assays for ATM and ATR are essentially identical with the exception of the detergent used in the lysis buffer. Therefore, the protocol detailed below is relevant for both of these kinase assays with the minor modifications noted in the text.

3.1. Immunoprecipitation

The success of any immune complex kinase assay depends on the efficient immunoprecipitation of catalytically active kinase (*see* **Note 2**). For the ATM kinase assay, the catalytic activity of the protein is especially sensitive to the detergents used during cell lysis. We have had good success in recovering active ATM using 0.2% Tween-20 in our lysis buffer. In contrast, the addition of 0.5% TritonX-100 or NP-40 to the lysis or wash buffers results in complete loss of ATM kinase activity. Because of the relatively mild conditions used, one of three methods of gentle mechanical disruption are used to facilitate complete cell lysis: (1) repetitive freeze-thaw cycles, (2) sonication, or (3) scraping. In contrast to ATM, the catalytic activity of ATR is unaffected by either TritonX-100 or NP-40, and we routinely use 0.5–1% TritonX-100 in the lysis buffer for our ATR kinase assays.

1. Prepare the complete lysis buffer by adding the following to the base lysis buffer (*see* **Subheading 2., Step 4**): (a) protease inhibitors—1:1000 dilution of stock aprotinin, leupeptin, pepstatin; (b) phosphatase inhibitors—1:1000 dilution of microcystinLR and 1:100 dilution of β-glycerol phosphate (10 mM final concentration); (c) reducing agent—1:1000 dilution of DTT (1 mM final concentration)

   Store on ice until ready for use. Also place an appropriate amount of lysis base buffer, buffered salt solution and kinase base buffer on ice in anticipation of the wash steps at the end of the immunoprecipitation (*see* **Step 8**).

2. The cells must be washed free of media prior to lysis. Use $4.0–10.0 \times 10^6$ cells per sample. Rinse adherent cells grown on tissue culture dishes twice with a generous amount of PBS. Tilt the dishes on their side and suction off the remaining PBS before placing the plates on a bed of ice. For cells grown in suspension, centrifuge the cells for each sample, resuspend the cell pellet in 1 mL of PBS, and transfer to 1.5-mL microcentrifuge tubes. Centrifuge and wash once more in 1 mL of PBS. Remove the PBS and place the nearly dry pellet on ice.

3. For adherent cells, add 300 µL of complete lysis buffer to each sample and vigorously scrape the cells off the plate into the lysis buffer. Transfer the lysate into microcentrifuge tubes and vortex for 10 sec. For suspension cells, add 1 mL complete lysis buffer to the individual tubes, resuspend thoroughly by pipetting, and then sonicate on ice with 3 bursts of 5 sec each at full power. Incubate on ice a total of 15 min. Because the ATR lysis buffer uses TritonX-100 instead of Tween 20, mechanical disruption of the cells is not necessary in the ATR assay.

4. To separate soluble proteins from insoluble cellular material, centrifuge the cell lysates in a refrigerated microcentrifuge at 18,000g at 4°C for 5 min. Transfer the lysate to new pre-chilled centrifuge tubes on ice and bring the volume of each sample up to 1 mL using complete lysis buffer.

5. Add an appropriate amount of ATM/ATR antibody or a non-specific control antibody to the relevant samples. Incubate the samples on ice for 2 h, inverting the tubes every 30 min to mix the samples.

6. Aliquot 15 µL of packed Protein A-Sepharose beads into a new set of tubes, add 1 mL of lysis base buffer and centrifuge at 7000g for 30 sec. Remove the supernatant and place the tubes on ice.

7. Transfer the lysate into the new tubes containing Protein A-Sepharose beads and rotate them at 4°C for 30 min.

8. Centrifuge samples at 7000g for 30 sec, aspirate the lysate and wash the beads twice with 1 mL of ice-cold lysis base buffer. Then wash the beads once with

1 mL of ice-cold buffered salt solution and twice with 1 mL of kinase base buffer.

3.2. Kinase Assay Reaction

The kinase activities of both ATM and ATR are dependent on the presence of $MnCl_2$ in the reaction buffer. In addition to both $MnCl_2$ and $MgCl_2$, the reaction buffer contains a reducing agent (DTT), non-radioactive ATP, [γ-^{32}P]ATP, and a polypeptide substrate. Several substrates have been identified for ATM and these include the N-terminus of p53 and the eIF-4E-binding protein (PHAS-1) *(3)*. Potential kinase inhibitors can be evaluated by pre-incubating ATM/ATR immune-complexes with appropriate concentrations of inhibitors and then adding the kinase reaction mixture to the beads. Following incubation of the kinase reaction, the reaction products are spotted onto phosphocellulose paper or resolved by SDS-PAGE. Inhibition of ATM/ATR kinase activity then is assessed by measuring changes in the incorporation of ^{32}P into the substrate by scintillation counting or phosphorimaging.

1. Prior to washing the immunoprecipitates (*see* **Subheading 3.1.**, **Step 8**), add the following components to the kinase base buffer (final concentration in parentheses)—non-radioactive ATP (20 μM), DTT (2 mM), $MnCl_2$ (20 mM), and substrate (1 μg per reaction). Do not add the radioactive ATP at this step. It will be added immediately before assembling the kinase reaction in **Step 4**. At this time, any potential kinase inhibitors to be tested in these assays should be diluted to appropriate concentrations in kinase base buffer in separate tubes.
2. Remove the majority of the buffer from the beads washed in **Subheading 3.1.**, **Step 8** with an 18-gauge needle. Then, using a 27-gauge needle attached to suction, briefly dry the beads by placing the needle directly into the beads. Close the cap and place each sample on ice.
3. After drying all samples, immediately add 20 μL of kinase base buffer or appropriate drug dilutions in base buffer to the beads and incubate on ice for 15 min.
4. During the drug incubation in the previous step, thaw the [γ-^{32}P]ATP on ice and add 20 μCi/reaction to the 2X kinase reaction mix. At the completion of the drug incubation, aliquot 20 μL of this 2X kinase reaction mix into each sample, pipet several times to mix, and return to ice. After all the kinase reactions have been assembled, transfer them to a 30°C water bath and incubate for 10–40 min (*see* **Notes 3** and **4**).
5. At the end of the incubation, transfer the tubes to ice. If the reaction products will be separated on SDS-PAGE, then add 15 μL of 4X SDS sample buffer to stop the kinase reaction and boil the samples for 5 min. Depending on the substrate used, it may be possible to assess substrate phosphorylation by spotting samples onto Whatman P-81 phosphocellulose paper. This would allow the rapid assessment of the kinase assay results by scintillation counting (*see* **Note 5**). In this case,

stop the reaction by adding an equal volume of 30% acetic acid. Spot duplicate aliquots onto Whatman P-81 phosphocellulose paper and immediately place in a 100 mL of 15% acetic acid/10 mM sodium pyrophosphate. Wash the samples 4X in this solution (5 min/wash), rinse the papers briefly in acetone followed by petroleum ether, and allow them to air dry.

6. Following resolution of reaction products by SDS-PAGE, transfer the proteins onto nylon membranes and assess substrate phosphorylation by phosphorimaging or autoradiography. For reaction products spotted onto P-81 paper, the radioactivity of these samples can be assessed by phosphorimaging or liquid scintillation counting.

4. Notes

1. The kinase activities of ATM and ATR are relatively finicky and attention to detail is critical for a successful kinase assay. Samples should be maintained at 0°C whenever possible. All buffers used in the protocol should be ice-cold prior to use and all tubes should be cooled on ice before cell lysate is transferred into them. The storage and handling of the [γ-^{32}P]ATP label is also critical for an adequate kinase signal. We routinely use [γ-^{32}P]ATP preparations that are stored at −20°C and are less than 1 wk beyond the reference date provided by the manufacturer. Allowing the [γ-^{32}P]ATP to warm above 0°C prior to the kinase assay typically results in a very poor outcome. Therefore, the radioactive ATP should be thawed on ice and aliquoted into single-use amounts after receipt from the manufacturer. Although more convenient, we have not tested the [γ-^{32}P]ATP formulations that can be stored at 4°C.

2. The selection of appropriate cell lines and antibodies for the immunoprecipitation of ATM or ATR are clearly important. For ATM assays, we use 2 μg of the Protein G purified Ab-3 (cat. no. PC116) from Oncogene Research-Calbiochem to immunoprecipitate ATM from the A549 lung carcinoma cell line. ATR is abundantly expressed in the K562 erythroblastoid leukemia cell line and is efficiently immunoprecipitated with a rabbit antibody raised against ATR *(13)* that is now marketed by Oncogene Research-Calbiochem as the Ab-1 ATR/FRP antibody (cat. no. PC128). Alternatively, epitope-tagged versions of ATM or ATR can be expressed in mammalian or insect cells and immunoprecipitated with an appropriate epitope-specific antibody.

3. The optimal length of incubation for a kinase reaction will vary between laboratories depending on the conditions established for the assay and the goals of the experiment. When comparing relative kinase activities between samples, then a preliminary time course experiment should be performed to identify the linear range for the assay. Alternatively, if linearity is not important, then the reaction can be carried out for 30–40 min to maximize phosphorylation of the substrate.

4. Minimizing the variability of ATM or ATR kinase levels between samples is important for obtaining reproducible results. When evaluating potential kinase

inhibitors, we routinely pool the cell lysates from all samples in a pre-chilled tube and then aliquot equal amounts of lysate into the sample tubes. Alternatively, differences in kinase levels between samples can be minimized by equalizing the amount of soluble protein used for each immunoprecipitation.

5. Using phosphocellulose paper is a convenient method for measuring ^{32}P incorporation into the kinase substrate and we have used this method successfully with the PHAS-1 polypeptide substrate *(14)*. Because background from the [^{32}P]ATP label can be problematic, it is best to resolve the reaction products by SDS-PAGE when first establishing the conditions for a kinase assay and then switch to phosphocellulose paper for subsequent experiments. Background can be reduced by using sodium pyrophosphate in the wash buffer and by placing the samples in the wash buffer immediately after spotting the reaction products.

Acknowledgments

This work was supported by the Mayo Foundation, Mayo Cancer Center, and by a grant from the National Institutes of Health (CA80829). Many thanks to Dr. Jeffrey Eshleman for his careful review of this manuscript.

References

1. Lavin, M. F. (1999) ATM: the product of the gene mutated in ataxia-telangiectasia. *Int. J. Biochem. Cell Biol.* **31,** 735–740.
2. Zhou, B. B. S. and Elledge, S. J. (2000) The DNA damage response: putting checkpoints in perspective. *Nature* **408,** 433–439.
3. Kastan, M. B. and Lim, D. S. (2000) The many substrates and functions of ATM. *Nat. Rev. Mol. Cell Biol.* **1,** 179–186.
4. Ababou, M., Dutertre, S., Lecluse, Y., Onclercq, R., Chatton, B., and Amor-Gueret, M. (2000) ATM-dependent phosphorylation and accumulation of endogenous BLM protein in response to ionizing radiation. *Oncogene* **19,** 5955–5963.
5. Tibbetts, R. S., Cortez, D., Brumbaugh, K. M., et al. (2000) Functional interactions between BRCA1 and the checkpoint kinase ATR during genotoxic stress. *Genes Dev.* **14,** 2989–3002.
6. Canman, C. E. and Lim, D. S. (1998) The role of ATM in DNA damage responses and cancer. *Oncogene* **17,** 3301–3308.
7. Blasina, A., Price, B. D., Turenne, G. A., and McGowan, C. H. (1999) Caffeine inhibits the checkpoint kinase ATM. *Curr. Biol.* **9,** 1135–1138.
8. Sarkaria, J. N., Busby, E. C., Tibbetts, R. S., et al. (1999) Inhibition of ATM and ATR kinase activities by the radiosensitizing agent, caffeine. *Cancer Res.* **59,** 4375–4382.
9. Zhou, B. B. S., Chaturvedi, P., Spring, K., et al. (2000) Caffeine abolishes the mammalian G(2)/M DNA damage checkpoint by inhibiting ataxia-telangiectasia-mutated kinase activity. *J. Biol. Chem.* **275,** 10,342–10,348.
10. Eshleman, J. S. and Sarkaria, J. N. (2001) ATM as a target for novel radiosensitizers. *Sem. Rad. Oncol.* **11,** 316–327.

11. Roberge, M., Berlinck, R. G. S., Xu, L., et al. (1998) High-throughput assay for G(2) checkpoint inhibitors and identification of the structurally novel compound isogranulatimide. *Cancer Res.* **58,** 5701–5706.
12. Jiang, X., Lim, L. Y., Daly, J. W., Li, A. H., Jacobson, K. A., and Roberge, M. (2000) Structure-activity relationships for G2 checkpoint inhibition by caffeine analogs. *Int. J. Oncol.* **16,** 971–978.
13. Tibbetts, R. S., Brumbaugh, K. M., Williams, J. M., et al. (1999) A role for ATR in the DNA damage-induced phosphorylation of p53. *Genes Dev.* **13,** 152–157.
14. Sarkaria, J. N., Tibbetts, R. S., Busby, E. C., Kennedy, A. P., Hill, D. E., and Abraham, R. T. (1998) Inhibition of phosphoinositide 3-kinase related kinases by the radiosensitizing agent wortmannin. *Cancer Res.* 58, 4375–4382.

III

ANGIOGENESIS AND METASTASIS PROTOCOLS

5

The Rat Aortic Ring Assay for In Vitro Study of Angiogenesis

Ronald S. Go and Whyte G. Owen

1. Introduction

Angiogenesis is necessary for growth and metastasis of cancer. It is comprised of several distinct steps, including degradation of extracellular matrix, cell migration, proliferation, and structural reorganization *(1)*. Inhibition of angiogenesis has been shown in pre-clinical studies to suppress tumor growth *(2–4)*. Currently, the use of anti-angiogenic therapy in cancer is under intensive investigation *(5)*. Several in vitro and in vivo assays are available to study angiogenesis, each with its own advantages and limitations *(6)*. In vivo assays simulate the natural process but are often complicated by inflammatory host responses that may interfere with angiogenesis. Variables are more likely to be controlled using in vitro assays. However, these assays are performed using undefined media supplemented with serum, which in itself is very much angiogenic *(7)*. In addition, most in vitro assays are designed only to look at selective phases (endothelial cell migration and proliferation) of angiogenesis.

The rat aortic ring assay, developed by Nicosia et al., is unique in that it integrates the advantages of both in vivo and in vitro systems *(8)*. It is a useful assay to test angiogenic factors or inhibitors in a controlled environment. More importantly, it recapitulates all of the necessary steps involved in angiogenesis. In this quantitative method of studying angiogenesis, ring segments of rat aorta are embedded in a three-dimensional matrix composed of fibrin or collagen, and cultured in a defined medium devoid of serum and growth factors. Microvessels sprout spontaneously from the cut surfaces of the aortic rings. This angiogenic process is triggered by the dissection procedure and mediated by endogenous growth factors produced from the aorta *(9,10)*. Microvessels

From: *Methods in Molecular Medicine, vol. 85: Novel Anticancer Drug Protocols*
Edited by: J. K. Buolamwini and A. A. Adjei © Humana Press Inc., Totowa, NJ

are counted manually or quantified using computer-assisted image analysis. Test agents can be added to the culture medium to assay for angiogenic or anti-angiogenic activity.

2. Materials

1. Rats, 1–2 mo old.
2. Dissecting instruments.
3. MCDB 131 culture medium (Clonetics, San Diego, California).
4. Culture dishes, 100 × 15 mm.
5. 1.5% agarose (type VI-A) solution.
6. Puncher. This has two concentric rings with diameters of 10 mm and 17 mm. It can be made with either nylon or metal.
7. Fibrinogen solution, 3 mg/mL. Prepare fresh.
8. Thrombin solution, 5 NIH U/mL.
9. Epsilon-aminocaproic acid (EACA).
10. L-glutamine.
11. Triple antibiotics (penicillin, streptomycin, amphotericin B).
12. Inverted microscope.
13. Digital camera.

3. Methods

3.1. The Rat Aortic Ring Assay

This rat aortic ring assay involves three steps: preparation of the aorta, making agarose culture wells, and culture of the aortic rings. The agarose culture wells serve as molds for the fibrin or collagen matrix. The entire assay should be prepared using aseptic technique and takes about 3 h to finish.

3.1.1. Preparation of the Aorta

1. Isolate the thoracic and abdominal aorta from the sacrificed rat. Handle the aorta only at its ends and avoid trauma to the body of the aorta.
2. Transfer aorta to a culture dish containing MCDB 131 culture medium.
3. Remove the surrounding fibro-adipose tissues.
4. Cut away the proximal and distal 2-mm segments of the aorta.
5. Cut the aorta into 1-mm ring sections and rinse in 5–8 washes of MCDB 131 culture medium. Make sure all blood residues are removed.

3.1.2. Making the Agarose Culture Wells

1. Pour 30 mL of agarose solution into each culture dish.
2. Once the agarose solution solidifies, use the puncher to make concentric rings. Each dish provides six to seven agarose culture wells.
3. Transfer four culture wells into each culture dish.

3.1.3. Culturing of the Aortic Rings

1. Coat the bottom of each agarose well with 150 μL of clotting fibrinogen solution. The latter is made by adding 20 μL of thrombin solution into 1 mL of fibrinogen solution at room temperature. The solution needs to be dispensed within 1 min of mixing.
2. Embed aortic rings into the fibrin-coated agarose wells, one ring per well (*see* **Note 1**).
3. Fill up all the agarose wells completely with another freshly prepared clotting fibrinogen solution.
4. Cut away agarose wells after fibrin solidifies.
5. Add 10 mL of supplemented MCDB 131 culture medium into each petri dish. The MCDB 131 culture medium is supplemented with L-glutamine (1.5 mg/mL), penicillin (100 U/mL), streptomycin (100 μg/mL), amphotericin B (0.25 μg/mL), and EACA (300 μg/mL).
6. Keep the cultures at 37°C with 5% CO_2.
7. Change the culture medium every 3 d.

3.2. Quantification of Microvessel Growth

Quantification can be performed either by visually counting the number of microvessels present at the end of the experiment, or by using computer-assisted image analysis (*see* **Note 2**). The latter will be described in this section. Because the periaortic adipose tissues cannot always be removed completely and can interfere with image analysis, it is necessary to take an image on d 0 as a baseline.

1. Adjust appropriate microscope lighting and settings. Use the same settings throughout the experiment (*see* **Note 3**).
2. Mount digital camera on microscope and take pictures of the aortic rings on d 0 and d 12. A picture of rat aortic ring culture taken on d 12 is shown in **Fig. 1A**.
3. Download pictures into computer.
4. Convert images into grayscale. Commercially available picture software such as Adobe Photoshop (San Jose, California) or NIH image software (available for free from the National Institute of Health web site) can be used.
5. Manually delete everything in the picture other than the microvessels (**Fig. 1B**) and invert the remaining image (**Fig. 1C**). Microvessels should now appear as black.
6. Use NIH image to calculate the integrated density of the resulting images. Vessel pixel integrated density (VPID) is calculated by multiplying the number of pixels in the subtracted images by the difference of the mean and background gray scale.
7. Subtract VPID of d 0 from d 12. The difference is an indirect measure of the amount (total surface area and density) of microvascular growth (*see* **Note 4**).
8. Analyze results.

A

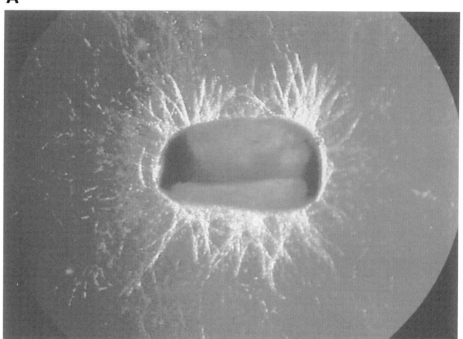

B

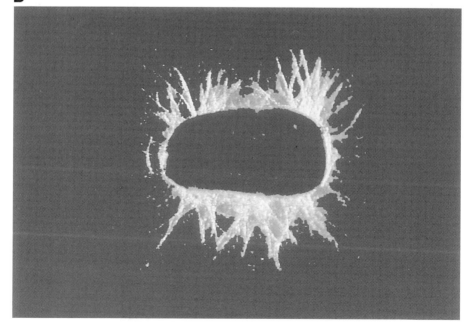

C

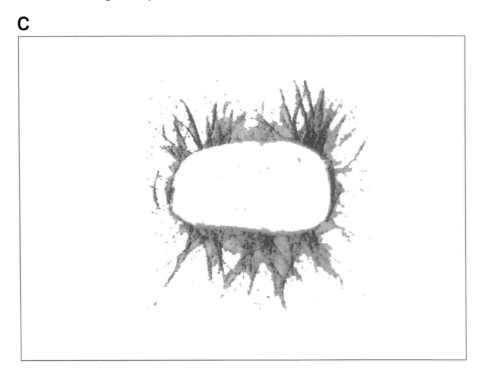

Fig. 1. Quantification of microvessels using computer-assisted image analysis. An image of rat aortic ring culture taken on day 12 is shown (**A**). Image management software is used to delete the body of the rat aorta to leave behind an image of microvessels (**B**). The remaining image is inverted to render the microvessels black (**C**). The vessel pixel integrated density is then calculated.

4. Notes

1. It is preferable to embed the aortic rings on their sides (they appear as rectangles) in the three-dimensional matrix rather than on their ends (open rings). This provides optimal visualization of microvascular growth, as the microvessels mostly arise from the cut surfaces and grow along the axis of the lumen. When the rings are placed on their ends, the microvessels would appear to be growing towards the observer.

2. By the end of the week, an average of 25–50 microvessels can be seen to sprout from each aortic ring in control cultures. However, when the cultures are supplemented with growth factors, the microvessels can increase several folds in number and are superimposed upon each other. This makes quantification using direct microscopic visualization difficult, if not impossible. In addition, manual counting does not take into account the length or width of the microvessels. Thus computer-assisted image analysis may be preferable.

3. Because of the nature of computer-image analysis, the importance of maintaining the same microscopic settings throughout the entire experiment cannot be overemphasized. In particular, the amount of illumination should be standardized for the entire experiment. The microvessels are thin and transparent and thus appear bright in the photomicrograph.

4. Spontaneous angiogenesis in the rat aortic rings is usually minimal and self-limited. We have found the rat aortic ring assay to be a more sensitive assay to test for angiogenic compared to anti-angiogenic agents. The sensitivity can be improved by supplementing small amounts of growth factor (e.g., 50 ng/mL of basic fibroblast growth factor or 0.5% serum) to the control and experimental cultures when anti-angiogenic agents are being tested.

References

1. Kumar, R., Yoneda, J., Bucana, C. D., and Fidler, I. J. (1998) Regulation of distinct steps of angiogenesis by different angiogenic molecules. *Int. J. Oncol.* **12,** 749–757.
2. O'Reilly, M. S., Holmgren, L., Shing, Y., et al. (1994) Angiostatin: a novel angiogenesis inhibitor that mediates the suppression of metastases by a Lewis lung carcinoma. *Cell* **79,** 315–328.
3. Fotsis, T., Zhang, Y., Pepper, M. S., et al. (1994) The endogenous oestrogen metabolite 2-methoxyoestradiol inhibits angiogenesis and suppresses tumor growth. *Nature* **368,** 237–239.
4. O'Reilly, M. S., Pirie-Shepherd, S., Lane, W. S., and Folkman, J. (1999) Anti-angiogenic activity of the cleaved conformation of the serpin antithrombin. *Science* **285,** 1926–1928.
5. Ferrara, N. and Alitalo, K. (1999) Clinical applications of angiogenic growth factors and their inhibitors. *Nat. Med.* **5,** 1359–1364.
6. Cockerill, G. W., Gamble, J. R., and Vadas, M. A. (1995) Angiogenesis: models and modulators. *Int. Rev. Cytol.* **159,** 113–160.
7. Go, R. S. and Owen, W. G. (2000) Very low concentrations of rat plasma and rat serum stimulate angiogenesis in the rat aortic ring assay. *Fibrinolysis Proteol.* **19** (Suppl 1), 45.
8. Nicosia, R. F. and Ottinetti, A. (1990) Growth of microvessels in serum-free matrix culture of rat aorta: a quantitative assay of angiogenesis in vitro. *Lab. Invest.* **63,** 115–122.
9. Villaschi, S. and Nicosia, R. F. (1993) Angiogenic role of endogenous basic fibroblast growth factor released by rat aorta after injury. *Am. J. Pathol.* **143,** 181–190.
10. Nicosia, R. F., Lin, Y. J., Hazelton, D., and Qian, X. H. (1997) Endogenous regulation of angiogenesis in the rat aorta model: role of vascular endothelial growth factor. *Am. J. Pathol.* 151, 1379–1386.

6

Real Time In Vivo Quantitation of Tumor Angiogenesis

Gregory I. Frost and Per Borgström

1. Introduction

Animal models are crucial to further our understanding of tumor biology. For many years, observation chambers, implanted in various animal species, have been used for intravital microscopy of tumor microcirculation. As far back as 1943, Algire described the adaptation of the transparent chamber technique to the mouse *(1)*. From the introduction of a subsequent paper by Algire et al. *(2)*, the following paragraph is quoted:

> "Recently, in vivo techniques have been developed which make it possible to make microscopic observations of the development of the blood supply of tumor transplants in the mouse. It has also been possible to obtain a quantitative expression of the morphological changes as they occur over a prolonged period. . . . The results presented indicate (i) that the rapid growth of tumor transplants is dependent upon the development of a rich vascular supply, and (ii) that an outstanding characteristics of the tumor cell is its capacity to elicit continuously the growth of new capillaries."

Algire thus concluded in 1945 that tumors were angiogenesis-dependent. Subsequent reports, using intravital microscopic techniques are very sporadic. In 1965, Goodall et al. described a transparent chamber model inserted in the cheek pouch of the hamster *(3)* Yamura et al., developed a transparent chamber in the rat skin *(4)*. In a study by Wolf and Hubler in 1975 *(5)*, a transparent acrylic hamster cheek-pouch chamber was used to investigate the elaboration of a tumor angiogenic factor (TAF) by human cutaneous neoplasms, from which they concluded:

From: *Methods in Molecular Medicine, vol. 85: Novel Anticancer Drug Protocols*
Edited by: J. K. Buolamwini and A. A. Adjei © Humana Press Inc., Totowa, NJ

"Tumor angiogenic factor appears to induce direct stimulation of endothelial cell mitosis and may be essential for survival of nutritionally ravenous neoplastic tissues. The interference with TAF has therapeutic implications."

Transparent chambers have been instrumental in the understanding of tumor biology. With the development of molecular biology techniques such as spontaneously fluorescent proteins (GFP, RFP), and elaborate image analysis software, it is now much easier to generate quantitative data. Such systems can clarify tumor microcirculatory phenomena, and mechanisms underlying anti-angiogenic and anti-tumor activities that are poorly understood using traditional histopathology.

Multi-cellular tumor spheroids are being used with increasing frequency in various aspects of tumor biology. There are many similarities in the growth and cellular characteristics for different types of tumor cells grown as multi-cellular spheroids. Once implanted into the chamber system, spheroid peripheral layers proliferate, with central cells non-cycling or forming necrotic cores. They are formed from monolayer tumor cells by various in vitro methods (e.g., liquid-overlay, spinner flask, and gyratory rotation systems). Because of the cellular organization in spheroids, they often recreate in vivo tumors much more closely than two-dimensional in vitro models *(6–9)*.

We have developed an intravital microscopic model, which is based on the dorsal skin fold chamber technique in mice. We use multi-cellular spheroids as the source for transplants *(10)*. The use of tumor spheroids as the source of transplants allows precise determination of tumor size to be implanted. Usually, spheroids are prepared from 25,000–50,000 tumor cells using liquid overlay techniques, which minimize variations within animals in the same groups. The system allows continuous measurements of both growth and angiogenesis of the small tumor spheroids. We used this system to evaluate various therapeutic interventions on several mouse and human cancer cell lines *(11)*. In those studies, we used a rhodamine based in vivo dye (CMTMR) to determine tumor growth. However, we found that the CMTMR labeling lasted at most for two weeks. Moreover, macrophages, which had engulfed tumor cells, became fluorescent as well, making it very difficult to assess the true tumor area.

Green fluorescent protein, GFP, is a spontaneously fluorescent protein isolated from coelenterates such as the Pacific jellyfish, *Aequoria victori (12)*. When expressed ectopically in mammalian cells, fluorescence from wild type GFP is typically distributed throughout the cytoplasm, but excluded from the nucleolus and vesicular organelles *(13)*. However, highly specific intracellular localization including the nucleus *(14)*, mitochondria *(15)*, secretory pathway *(16)*, plasma membrane *(17)*, and cytoskeleton *(18)* can be achieved via fusions both to whole proteins and to individual targeting sequences. The enormous

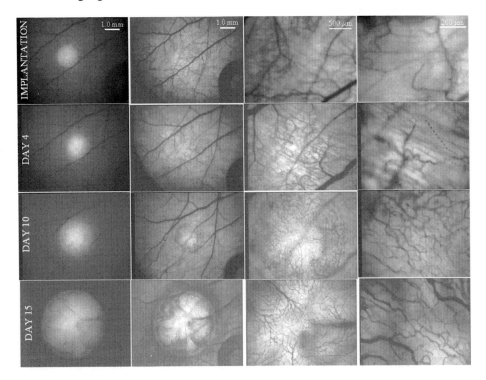

Fig. 1. Microphotographs obtained from dorsal skinfold chamber in 6 wk nu/nu mouse implanted with HT1080 fibrosarcoma tumor spheroids transduced with the Histone H2B-GFP fusion protein. The left column using fluorescence microscopy illustrates the utility of GFP in determining tumor area. Panels to the right are photomicrographs with increasing magnification obtained using transillumination of blue filtered light (BG12), for enhancement of red blood cells, demonstrating the intense angiogenic activity of these micro-tumors.

flexibility of GFP as a noninvasive marker in living cells allows for numerous other applications such as a cell lineage tracing, reporter of gene expression, and as a potential measure of protein–protein interactions (*19*). Kanda et al. (*20*) developed a highly sensitive method for observing chromosome dynamics in living cells. They fused the human Histone H2B gene to the gene encoding the GFP, which was transfected into human HeLa cells to generate a stable line constitutively expressing H2B-GFP. The H2B-GFP fusion protein was incorporated into chromatin without affecting cell cycle progression. We have generated cDNA encoding a Histone H2B-GFP fusion protein under the 5'LTR in the LXRN retroviral cassette, and have introduced it into a number of human as well as murine cancer cell lines by retroviral transduction. **Figure 1**

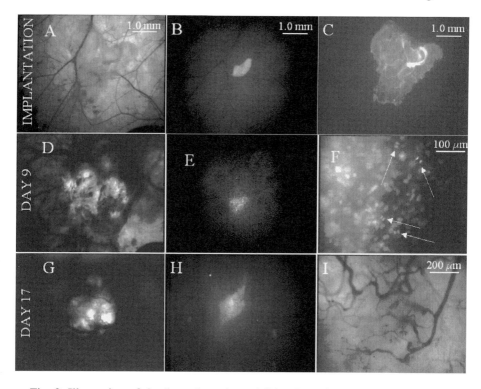

Fig. 2. Illustration of the "pseudo-orthotopic" implantation of murine TRAMP-C2 prostate carcinoma cells in dorsal skinfold chambers in C57/BL6 mice. A small piece of anterior prostate with an area of approx 3 mm^2 was pre-labeled in vitro with a rhodamine based dye (CMTMR) (**C**). A tumor spheroid (H2B-GFP transduced TRAMP-C2 cells), were applied on top of the prostate tissue (**B**). Panels **E** and **H** illustrate the growth of TRAMP-C2 cells within the prostate tissue graft. Panel **F** shows numerous mitotic figures in anaphase, and in panel **I**, the intense angiogenic activity obtained with the "pseudo-orthotopic" system can be readily visualized. The left column was obtained using filtered blue light enhancing red blood cells.

illustrates the growth characteristics of multi-cellular tumor spheroids obtained from the human fibrosarcoma cell line, HT1080 implanted in dorsal skinfold chambers in nude mice.

The use of well defined tumor spheroids also permits the introduction of stroma together with the spheroids. We have used this technique to create a pseudo-orthotopic milieu for murine prostate tumor cells in dorsal skinfold chambers. We implant small pieces (<5 mm^2) of murine prostate labeled with CMTMR from a donor mouse, and carefully apply tumor spheroids obtained from TRAMP-C2 cells, transduced with Histone H2B-GFP, on top of the prostate tissue (*see* **Fig. 2**).

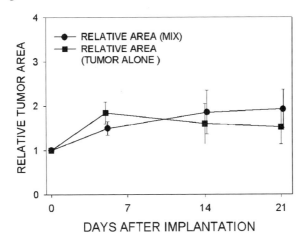

Fig. 3. Comparison of growth characteristics of TRAMP-C2 tumor spheroids (Tumor alone), and TRAMP-C2 spheroids implanted with prostate tissue (Mix). When TRAMP-C2 spheroids are implanted without prostate tissue, cells become very invasive without significant increases in cell number. During the first five days, the tumor area A_T increases by 64%, however the total photo intensity I_T simultaneously decreases with 70%, implying that the increase in area is due mainly to migration of tumor cells, i.e., such that density is significantly lower at d 5 compared to at implantation (*see* **Fig. 6**).

Mixing prostate tissue with the murine TRAMP-C2 cell line (Transgenic Adenocarcinoma Mouse Prostate), we have obtained more physiological growth characteristics as compared to implantation of TRAMP-C2 spheroids alone (*see* **Fig. 3**). The TRAMP-C2 cell line is derived from a transgenic mouse model in which mice develop spontaneous prostate tumors. TRAMP mice develop a distinct pathology in the dorso-lateral epithelium of the prostate by 10 wk of age. By 12 wk, they have widespread infiltration of the prostate and by wk 24 exhibit well-differentiated prostate tumors *(21)*.

The greatest advantage of the chamber technique is that it allows the study of cancer in the context of the host. For instance, tumors are frequently infiltrated by numerous tumor associated macrophages (TAMs) that can be found within the tumor mass or surrounding the tumor. TAMs influence diverse processes such as angiogenesis, tumor cell proliferation, and metastasis during tumor progression. In a variety of tumor types, the number of TAMs associate with poor prognosis *(22)*. However, TAMs can also participate in the immunologic anti-tumor defense mechanism through cytotoxic activities, such as direct cellular cytotoxicity and the release of cytokines and reactive oxygen species. The local injection of 10 µL of 1% RITC-dextran into the chamber permits

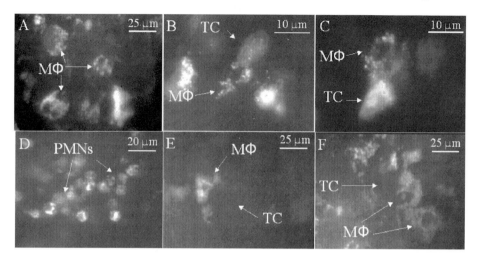

Fig. 4. As an additional feature, the innate immune system such as tumor associated macrophages (TAMs), can be visualized through the injection of RITC-labeled dextran into the chamber. Scavenger receptors on TAMs result in high levels of RITC-dextran endocytosis, which can be visualized in vesicles within 24 h. (TC; tumor cell, MΦ; macrophage, PMN; granulocyte).

visualization of tumor-TAM interactions. Scavenger receptor expression on TAMs result in the uptake of large amounts of Rhodamine labeled material. **Figure 4** illustrates the anti-tumor response encountered after implantation of tumor spheroids of the human prostate carcinoma cell line PC3. In a recent study, we found that the inability to effectively exclude the innate immune system by encapsulation was the main impediment to the survival of small human prostate micro-tumor xenografts. This suggest that the complex interactions between tumor cells and TAMs, pivotal in tumor biology, are extensively perturbed by "foreign" human tumor cells implanted in immunodeficient mice *(23)*. The ability of our model to continuously assess mitotic and apoptotic indices was an important feature in discovering that the tumors were dying "from the outside in," i.e., mitotic cells were confined to the center of the tumor, and numerous apoptotic cells to the periphery. This finding rules out death of tumor cells because of lack of angiogenesis within the central tumor mass.

2. Materials

All surgical procedures are performed in a sterile laminar flow hood. Dorsal skinfold chambers and surgical instruments are autoclaved before use. Saline used to keep tissue moist during surgical preparation is mixed with gentamicin

(50 µL/mL). Small circular Band Aids are applied on the backside of the chamber after surgery to prevent scratching. Other materials used are:

1. 7.3 mg ketamine hydrochloride and 2.3 mg xylazine/100 g body weight.
2. DMEM 4.5 g/L glucose, supplemented with pyruvate, glutamine nonessential amino acids, and gentamicin (50 µg/mL).
3. Genprobe PCR mycoplasma detection kit.
4. 1% Rhodamine-B isothiocyanate-dextran 70S.
5. CellTracker™ Orange CMTMR (5-(and-6)-(((4-chloromethyl) benzoyl)amino) tetramethylrhodamine).
6. 96-well round bottom sterile tissue culture plates.
7. 1% Agarose in Dulbecco's modified Eagle medium (DMEM).
8. Angiogenic tumor cell line transduced with H2BeGFP.

3. Methods
3.1. Animal Model and Surgical Techniques

The dorsal skinfold chamber in the mouse (*see* **Fig. 5**) is prepared as described previously *(24)*. Male mice (25–35 g body weight) are anesthetized (7.3 mg ketamine hydrochloride and 2.3 mg xylazine /100 g body weight, ip) and placed on a heating pad. Two symmetrical titanium frames are implanted into a dorsal skinfold, so as to sandwich the extended double layer of skin. A 15 mm full thickness layer is excised. The underlying muscle (M. cutaneous max.) and subcutaneous tissues are covered with a glass cover slip incorporated in one of the frames. After a recovery period of 2–7 d, tumor spheroids are carefully placed in the chamber.

3.2. Generation of H2B-eGFPN1 Cell Lines

Human Histone H2B-eGFP, a kind gift from Dr. Kanda (Salk Institute, La Jolla, CA) was excised from the Sal-I Not-I sites in the BOS H2BGFP-N1 vector. The H2B-eGFP retroviral vector was generated by cutting first with Not-I followed by Mung-Bean Nuclease digestion to remove the overhanging end. The fragment was gel purified followed by Sal-I digestion. The resultant Sal-I/blunt fragment was cloned into the Sal-I Hpa-I sites in the LXRN retroviral vector (Clontech, Palo Alto, CA). VSVG pseudotyped retrovirus is generated by transfecting GP293 GagPol expressing 293 cells (available from Clontech) in T75 flasks at 75% confluence with 5 µg of this resultant L-H2BGFP-RN-L vector with 5 µg VSV-G vector (Clontech) and harvesting viral supernatants 48 h posttransfection. Retroviral supernatants can be used immediately or concentrated by centrifugation at 50,000g and stored at –80°C until use. Tumor cells are transduced with VSVG-pseudotyped H2B-GFP LXRN viral supernatant for 48 h in 8 µg/mL polybrene followed by election in

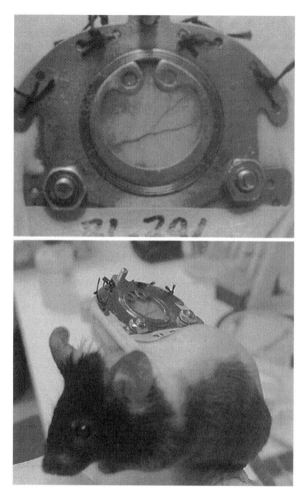

Fig. 5. Photos illustrating the dorsal skinfold chamber system in mice.

300 µg/mL G418 for 2 wk. Pooled H2B-GFP expressing tumor cells are usually heterogeneous by fluorescent microscopy, but can be FACS sorted if necessary. Most cells used for chamber studies are passaged in DMEM with 4.5 g/L glucose, supplemented with pyruvate, glutamine, and non-essential amino acids containing gentamicin (50 µg/mL) and maintained in a humidified 5% CO_2 atmosphere at 37°C. Cells are routinely tested for mycoplasma contamination with the Genprobe mycoplasma detection kit.

3.3. Preparation of Tumor Spheroids

Liquid overlay plates are generated using 1% Molecular Biology grade agarose melted in DMEM in a microwave. The melted agarose solution is plated into round bottom 96-well plates at 50 µL/well and allowed to cool at room temperature. Tumor cells grown as pre-confluent monolayers are trypsinized and diluted to a final volume of 250,000 tumor cells/mL. Viability is determined using Trypan blue dye. The tumor suspensions are dispersed 100 µL/well into the 96-well agarose coated round bottom plates. Spheroids are allowed to compact for 48 h and picked from the plates with a pipet followed by transfer into serum free media immediately before implantation into chambers.

3.4. Intravital Microscopy

Fluorescence microscopy is performed using a Mikron Instrument Microscope (Mikron Instrument, San Diego, CA) equipped with epi-illuminator and video-triggered stroboscopic illumination from a xenon arc (MV-7600, EG&G, Salem, MA). A silicon intensified target camera (SIT68, Dage-MTI, Michigan City, IN) is attached to the microscope. A Hamamatsu image processor (Argus 20) with firmware version 2.50 (Hamamatsu Photonic System, USA) is used for image enhancement and to capture images to a computer. A Leitz PL1/0.04 objective is used to obtain an overview of the chamber and for determination of tumor size. A Zeiss long distance objective ×10/0.22 is used to capture images for calculation of vascular parameters. A Zeiss Achroplan ×20/0.5 W objective is used for capturing images for calculation of mitotic and apoptotic indices.

Our system permits evaluation of the following parameters:

3.4.1. Parameters Related to Tumor Growth/Regression and Tumor Cell Motility

By default, Image-Pro expresses spatial measurements in terms of pixels. A Spatial command is used to change the terms in which Image-Pro reports such measurements. This command is used to measure objects in terms of mm or µm. Spacial calibrations are made for all different objectives being used.

After choosing the proper special calibration, tumor area (AT) is defined as number of pixels with photo density above 75 (256 gray levels), i.e.,

$$A_T = \sum_{k=75}^{255} A_k$$

Since TRAMP-C2 tumors are very heterogenous (*see* **Fig. 6**), changes in A_T do not directly reflect tumor growth. To take into account variations of tumor cell intensity with in the tumor area, we define total intensity I_T as,

$$I_T = \sum_{k=75}^{255} A_k * k$$

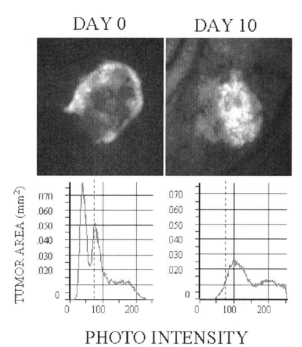

PHOTO INTENSITY

Fig. 6. Tumor area A_T is defined as the sum of all pixels with photo intensity above 75 (256 gray levels), and total Intensity I_T as the sum of he product of photo intensity and number of pixels with that intensity for pixels with intensity above 75. An increase in A_T without corresponding increase in I_T reflects migration rather than growth.

and relative intensity for Day X relative to Day 0 is defined as,

$$(\mathbf{I_{rel}})\textbf{DAYX} = (I_T)_{DAYX}/(I_T)_{DAY0}$$

Relative tumor cell density $(\mathbf{D_T})$ is defined as,

$$\mathbf{D_T} = I_T/A_T.$$

Calculation of these parameters permits evaluation of tumor growth/ shrinkage (I_{REL}) as well as tumor cell motility ($\mathbf{D_T}$). Thus, treatments resulting in an increase in A_T without corresponding increase in $\mathbf{I_T}$ reflect increased tumor cell motility rather than tumor growth.

3.4.2. Mitotic and Apoptotic Indices

At each time point, two peripheral and two central X20 fields of the tumor are captured with a FITC filter using Image-Pro Plus software and an integrated frame grabber. Only mitotic figures in telophase (MI) are included in the

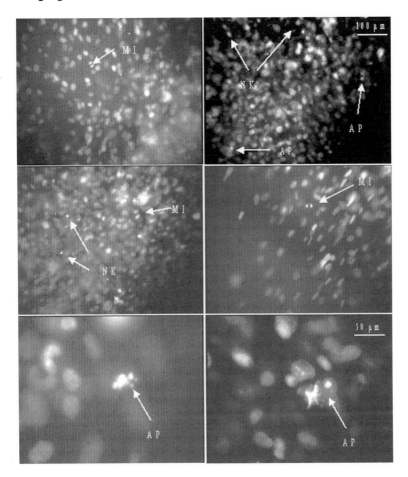

Fig. 7. Photomicrographs illustrating the usefulness of H2B-GFP transduced cells. The ability of our system to continuously assess apoptotic and mitotic indices is of great importance to clarify the mechanisms underlying the anticancer effect of various treatment regimens. Temporal and spatial relation of vessel density to cell death allows a detailed quantitative evaluation of regimen effectiveness as well as inferences to direct and indirect mechanisms of action. Only mitotic figures in telophase (MI) are included in the mitotic index. Apoptotic/Pyknotic nuclei (AP) are defined as H2B-GFP labeled nuclei with a cross sectional area <30 μm^2. Nuclear karyorrhexis (NK) is included within this apoptotic index.

mitotic index to exclude potential artifact of nuclear membrane distortion. Apoptotic/Pyknotic nuclei are defined as H2B-GFP labeled nuclei with a cross sectional area <30 μm^2. Nuclear karyorrhexis (NK), easily distinguishable by the vesicular nuclear condensation and brightness of H2B-GFP, is included within this apoptotic index (*see* **Fig. 7**).

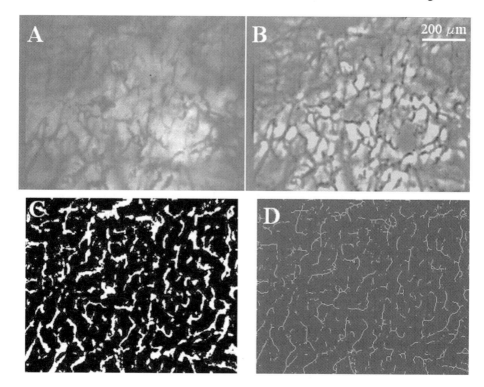

Fig. 8. To calculate vascular parameters, we use Image-Pro Plus (Media Cybernetics, MD). This software allows "flattening" of the photos to eliminate uneven illumination (**B**). The threshold feature is used to segment the picture into objects and background (**C**), from which vascular area is calculated. Finally, the picture is skeletonized (**D**), in order to calculate vascular length and vascular density.

3.4.3. Vascular Parameters

Image analysis: For each spheroid, video recordings are used to calculate length, area, and vascular density of the neovasculature being induced by the implanted tumor spheroids. Vascular parameters are analyzed off-line from the video recording using a photodensitometric computer software (Image-Pro Plus, Media Cybernetics, MD). Photomicrographs obtained with the X10 objective (*see* **Fig. 8A**), are "flattened" to reduce the intensity variations in the background pixels (**8B**). The flattened photomicrograph is cropped to eliminate distorted areas, and the thresholding feature is used to segment the picture into objects and background (**8C**). This panel is used to calculate vascular area (A_V). Finally, the picture is skeletonized (**8D**), in order to calculate vascular length (L_V). From these parameters average tumor vessel diameter D_V is calculated as A_V/L_V, and vascular density (Δ_V) is calculated as L_V per tumor area.

Acknowledgment

We thank Dale Winger for expert assistance with all surgical procedures. This work was supported by Grants from NCI (no. 1RO 1CA79004–03), and from the Department of Defense Prostate Cancer Research Program (no. DAMD17–99–1–9010).

References

1. Algire, G. H. (1943) An adaptation of the transparent chamber technique to the mouse. *J. Nat. Cancer Inst.* **4,** 1–11.
2. Algire, G. H. and Chakley, H. W. (1945) Vascular reactions of normal and malignant tissues in vivo. I. Vascular reactions of mice to wounds and to normal and neoplastic transplants. *J. Natl. Cancer Inst.* **6,** 73–85.
3. Goodall, C. M., Sanders, A. G. and Shubik, P. (1965) Studies of vascular patterns in living tumors with a transparent chamber inserted in hamster cheek pouch. *J. Natl. Cancer Inst.* **35,** 497–521.
4. Yamura, H., Suzuki, M., and Sato, H. (1968) Transparent chamber in the rat skin for studies on microcirculation in cancer tissue. *J. Natl. Cancer Inst.* **41,** 111–124.
5. Wolf, J. E. and Hubler, W. R. (1975) Tumor angiogenic factor and human skin tumors. *Arch. Dermatol.* **111,** 321–327.
6. Mueller-Klieser, W. (2000) Tumor biology and experimental therapeutics. *Crit. Rev. Oncol. Hematol.* **36,** 123–139.
7. de Ridder, L., Cornelissen, M., and de Ridder, D. (2000) Autologous spheroid culture: a screening tool for human brain tumour invasion. *Crit. Rev. Oncol. Hematol.* **36,** 107–122.
8. Desoize, B., Gimonet, D., and Jardiller, J. C. (1998) Cell culture as spheroids: an approach to multi-cellular resistance. *Anticancer Res.* **18,** 4147–4158.
9. Santini, M. T., Rainaldi, G., and Indovina, P. L. (1999) Multi-cellular tumour spheroids in radiation biology. *Int. J. Radiat. Biol.* **75,** 787–799.
10. Torres-Filho, I. P., Hartley-Asp, B., and Borgstrom, P. (1995) Quantitative angiogenesis in a syngeneic tumor spheroid model. *Microvasc. Res.* **49,** 212–226.
11. Borgstrom, P., Gold, D. P., Hillan, K. J., and Ferrara, N. (1999) Importance of VEGF for breast cancer angiogenesis in vivo: implications from intravital microscopy of combination treatments with an anti-VEGF neutralizing monoclonal antibody and doxorubicin. *Anticancer Res.* **19,** 4203–4214.
12. Morin, J. and Hastings, J. (1971) Energy transfer in a bioluminescent system. *J. Cell Physiol.* **77,** 313–318.
13. Cubitt, A., Heim, R., Adams, S., Boyd, A., Gross, L., and Tsien, R. (1995) Understanding, improving and using green fluorescent proteins. *TIBS* **20,** 448–455.
14. Kanda, T., Sullivan, K. F., and Wahl, G. M. (1998) Histone-GFP fusion protein enables sensitive analysis of chromosome dynamics in living mammalian cells. *Curr. Biol.* **8,** 377–385.

15. Rizzuto, R., Brini, M., De Giorgi, F., Rossi, R., Heim, R., Tsien, R., and Pozzan, T. (1996) Double labeling of subcellular structures with organelle-targeted GFP mutants in vivo. *Curr. Biol.* **6,** 183–188.

16. Kaether, C. and Gerdes, H. (1995) Visualization of protein transport along the secretory pathway using green fluorescent protein. *FEBS Lett.* **369,** 267–271.

17. Marshall, J., Molloy, R., Moss, G., Howe, J., and Hughes, T. (1995) The jellyfish green fluorescent protein: a new tool for studying ion channel expression and function. *Neuron* **14,** 211–215.

18. Kahana, J., Schapp, B., and Silver, P. (1995) Kinetics of spindle pole body separation in budding yeast. *Proc. Natl. Acad. Sci. USA* **92,** 9707–9711.

19. Mitra, R., Silva, C., and Youvan, D. (1996) Fluorescence resonance energy transfer between blue-emitting and red-shifted excitation derivatives of the green fluorescent protein. *Gene* **173,** 13–17.

20. Kanda, T., Sullivan, K. F., and Wahl G. M. (1998) Histone-GFP fusion protein enables sensitive analysis of chromosome dynamics in living mammalian cells. *Curr. Biol.* **8,** 377–385.

21. Greenberg, N. M., DeMayo, F., Finegold, M. J., et al. (1995) Prostate cancer in a transgenic mouse. *Proc. Natl. Acad. Sci. USA* **92,** 3439–3443.

22. Lissbrant, I. F., Stattin, P., Wikstrom, P., Damber, J. E., Egevad, L., and Bergh, A. (2000) Tumor associated macrophages in human prostate cancer: relation to clinicopathological variables and survival. *Int. J. Oncol.* **17,** 445–451.

23. Frost, G. I., Dudouet, B., Lustgarten, J., and Borgström, P. The roles of epithelial mesynchymal interactions and the innate immune response on the tumorigenicity of human prostate carcinoma cell lines grown in immuno-compromised *Mice.* Submitted.

24. Lehr, H., Leunig, M., Menger, M. D., and Messmer, K. (1993) Dorsal skinfold chamber technique for intravital microscopy on striated muscle in nude mice. *Am. J. Pathol.* 143, 1055–1062.

7

Use of Tumor-Activated Hepatic Stellate Cell as a Target for the Preclinical Testing of Anti-Angiogenic Drugs Against Hepatic Tumor Development

Elvira Olaso and Fernando Vidal-Vanaclocha

1. Introduction

The prognosis of patients with advanced liver tumors is very poor, regardless of current treatment schedules based on surgery and/or chemotherapy. Anti-angiogenic therapy represents one of the most promising target-oriented therapeutic approaches. However, because of organ-specific differentiation of liver microvasculature *(1)*, the use of non organ-specific models of angiogenesis may not be adequate for screening candidate anti-angiogenic compounds, and only a few preclinical models that are able to provide clinically relevant therapeutic options are available.

Hepatic tumor angiogenesis depends on a complex interaction among microvascular endothelial cells (the sinusoidal endothelial [HSE] cells) and pericyte-like cells (the hepatic stellate cells [HSCs]). First, tumor-derived factors promote the recruitment of HSCs to nonclinically detectable avascular tumor foci (<400 µm in diameter). Thereafter, HSC-mediated deposition and remodeling of tumor-associated extracellular matrix *(2,3)*, and the release of soluble factors contribute to the chemotactic migration and growth of hepatocellular carcinoma *(4,5)* and metastatic cancer cells *(6,7)*.

We have reported *(8)* that infiltration of tumor-activated HSC precedes HSE cell recruitment in prevascular micrometastases. Thereafter, HSCs and HSE cells co-localize within neoangiogenic capillaries and their numerical densities correlate with hepatic metastasis (*see* **Fig. 1**). Mechanistically, hypoxia and tumor-derived soluble factor(s) promote the production of vascular endothelial

From: *Methods in Molecular Medicine, vol. 85: Novel Anticancer Drug Protocols*
Edited by: J. K. Buolamwini and A. A. Adjei © Humana Press Inc., Totowa, NJ

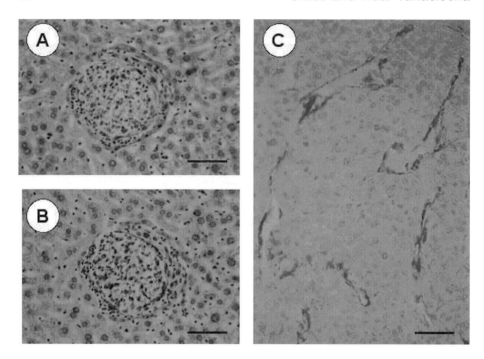

Fig. 1. **(A)** A single CD31 expressing cell in an avascular micrometastasis obtained after intrasplenic injection of C26-CC cells. **(B)** Same micrometastasis stained for alpha-smooth muscle actin expression. **(C)** Alpha-smooth muscle actin expression in a vascularized micrometastasis obtained after intrasplenic injection of B16M cells. Scale bar: 100 μm **(A,B)** and 25 μm **(C)**.

growth factor (VEGF) by recruited HSCs, which in turn increases HSE cell migration, proliferation, and survival. Thus, tumor-activated HSCs may create a pro-angiogenic microenvironment, which plays a key regulatory role in the HSE cell recruitment during the transition of liver metastasis from an avascular to a vascular stage. Interestingly, TNP-470, a semisynthetic analog of fumagillin that inhibits HSC proliferation and activation *(9)*, also inhibits primary and secondary hepatic tumors *(10,11)*. Moreover, administration of an inhibitor of angiogenic tyrosine kinase receptors improved the survival of mice bearing colon cancer liver metastases by decreasing HSC-coverage of angiogenic tracts *(12)*.

HSC may constitute a key cellular target for the preclinical testing of anti-angiogenic drugs against hepatic tumor development. Thus, we propose a two-step assay for the screening of anti-angiogenic drugs during experimental hepatic tumor development: (i) *In situ* analyses on HSC recruitment and co-localization with neo-angiogenic tracts (vascular coverage) during liver tumor development, and (ii) in vitro analyses of pro-angiogenic activation of tumor-activated HSCs and functional assessment of their effects on primary cultured HSE cells.

2. Materials

1. Male mice, 4–8 wk old.
2. Surgical instruments.
3. Hank's Balanced Salt Solution (HBSS).
4. Tumor cell lines: B16 melanoma (B16M), syngenic with C57Bl/6J mouse; C26 murine colon carcinoma (C26-CC) and BNL murine hepatocellular carcinoma (BNL-HCC), both syngeneic with Balb/c mouse.
5. Equipment for immunohystochemical analyses: Integrated image analysis system (Olympus Microimage 4.0 capture kit) connected to an Olympus BX51TF microscope. Monoclonal antibody against human ASMA (Sigma Chemicals) and polyclonal antibody against rat PECAM-1 (CD31, BD Pharmingen). Vectastain ABC-AP kit and avidin/biotin blocking solution kit (both from Vector Laboratories). Fab-goat anti-mouse IgG (Jackson Laboratories).
6. Equipment for mouse liver sinusoidal cells isolation (HSE cells and HSCs): Perfusion pumps and tubing; refrigerated centrifuge; pronase, collagenase, and DNase enzymes for *in situ* tissue digestion (Roche Pharmaceuticals), and metrizamide for cell separation through isopycnic gradient (Boehringer-Ingelheim).
7. Standard reagents and equipment for tissue culture: Dulbecco's modified eagle medium (DMEM), fetal calf serum (FCS), and antibiotics (100 units/mL penicillin and 100 mg/mL streptomycin, Gibco), culture-grade collagen type I (Becton-Dickinson).
8. Enzyme-linked immunosorbent assay (ELISA) kit for VEGF detection in supernatants of cultured cells (R&D).
9. Modified Boyden chambers suitable for cell migration assay (Becton-Dickinson).
10. Zinc fixative solution: 0.1 M Tris-HCl, pH 7.4, 0.5 g calcium acetate, 5 g zinc acetate, 5 g zinc chloride, adjusted to pH 6.75.
11. TUNEL-based apoptosis detection system (ApoAlert DNA Fragmentation Assay, Clontech).

3. Methods

3.1. Assessment of Tumor-Angiogenesis During Murine Hepatic Tumor Development

3.1.1. Experimental Hepatic Tumor Models

1. Hepatic metastases are produced by intrasplenic injection of viable cancer cells (i.e., B16M; C26-CC).
2. Position an anesthetized mouse on its right side and make a small subcostal incision.

3. Inject a standard inoculum of 3×10^5 viable tumor cells suspended in 0.1 mL of Ca^{2+}- and Mg^{2+}-free Hank's balanced salt solution (HBSS) into the upper pole of the exposed spleen with a 27-gauge needle. Then close both the abdominal wall musculature and the skin in one layer. Assess cell viability before injection using the Trypan blue exclusion test. Multifocal hepatocellular carcinoma foci are produced after intrahepatic injection of BNL-HCC cells (2×10^6 cells in 0.1 mL of HBSS) into anesthetized mouse. Ten mice are used per experimental group.

4. Sacrifice mice by cervical dislocation on the 12th (for B16M), 20th (for C26-CC), or 30th (for BNL-HCC) day after the injection of cancer cells (*see* **Note 1**).

3.1.2. Anti-Angiogenic Treatment Schedules

1. Pre-angiogenic tumor treatment schedule: Inject mice daily with the anti-angiogenic compound from d 1 to 7 for B16M, d 1 to 10 for C26-CC, or d 1 to 15 for BNL-HCC, after the injection of cancer cells. Sacrifice the mice on the last day.

2. Post-angiogenic tumor treatment: Inject mice daily with anti-angiogenic compound from d 7 to 12 for B16M, d 10 to 20 for C26-CC, or d 16 to 30 for BNL-HCC, after cancer cell injection. Sacrifice the mice on the last day.

3. Inject control animals daily with the same volume of the vehicle in which the drug is dissolved.

3.1.3. Immunohistochemical Evaluation of Endothelial Cell and Pericyte Recruitment in Tumor Tissue

1. Dissect livers at each time point, cut tissue slices not more than 3 mm in thickness, and incubate in zinc fixative solution for 8 h, at room temperature.

2. Using the Ventana NexES system (Ventana Medical Systems), perform a haematoxylin/eosin stain, PECAM-1 (CD31, as marker of endothelial cells) and alpha-smooth muscle actin (ASMA, as marker of activated HSCs *[13]*) expression analysis on 4 µm-thick paraffin sections from the zinc-fixed tumor tissue samples (five groups, separated 500 µm), as follows: (i) Preincubate slides at room temperature with Fab-goat anti-mouse IgG for 1 h, followed by a 1:20 dilution of FCS in PBS for 30 min, and avidin and biotin blocking solutions for 15 min each; (ii) Incubate slides with 1:25 dilutions of either anti-ASMA (1 h) or anti-CD31 antibodies (overnight at 4°C). Secondary goat anti-rat IgG (1:66 dilution, against anti-CD31 antibody) and goat anti-mouse IgG (1:200 dilution, against anti-ASMA antibody) antibodies are used. Irrelevant mouse IgG is used as negative control. (iii) Finish the staining with VECSTAIN ABC-AP Reagent plus the Vector Red Alkaline Phosphatase Substrate detection kit following the manufacturer's instructions.

3.1.3.1. ANALYSIS

The number and average diameter of tumor foci and the density of intra- and peri-tumoral CD31-expressing microvessels and ASMA-expressing pericytes are quantified with the aid of an integrated image analysis system (Olympus Microimage 4.0 capture kit) connected to an Olympus BX51TF microscope. Metastatic foci are arbitrarily divided into groups according to their average diameter (50, 100, 200, 400, 800, 1600, 3200 µm). Next, metastasis density (foci number per 100 mm^3) and the percentage of liver volume occupied by metastases are determined *(14)*. An angiogenic index is calculated as the microvessel density per unit of tumor tissue surface. Light intensity-based densitometry and color discrimination between reddish staining of CD31-expressing cells, brown staining of ASMA-expressing pericytes, and blue tissue background produced by mild hematoxylin counterstaining allows accurate determination of average tissue densities of recruited microvessels in analyzed tumor specimens. The correlation between ASMA-expressing cell density and intrametastatic capillary density for each metastatic size subgroup is analyzed by means of a regression analysis.

3.2. In Vitro Determination of Pro-Angiogenic Activities of Hepatic Stellate Cells

After primary cultures of HSCs are exposed to the anti-angiogenic compound and to tumor-derived soluble factors. The ability of tumor-activated HSCs to sustain angiogenesis is tested in 3 ways: (i) by HSC migration assay performed using tumor-derived soluble factors as chemoattractants; (ii) by ELISA on the level of VEGF in HSC-conditioned media (CM); and (iii) by HSE cell survival and migration assays in response to HSC-CM.

1. *Generation of Tumor- and HSC-Conditioned Media:* Subconfluent cultures of cancer cells are maintained for 24 hr in serum-free media. Primary HSC cultures (*see* **Notes 1** and **2**) are serum-starved for 12 h and then incubated for up to 24 h in the presence or absence of tumor-CM. Anti-angiogenic compounds are added to HSCs prior to the addition of tumor-CM. Conditioned Media are briefly centrifuged to eliminate cell debris and stored at –80°C.

2. *Cell Migration Assays:* 2.5×10^5 HSE or 1×10^5 HSC cells are allowed to migrate across collagen type I-coated inserts *(15)* (*see* **Note 2**). Tumor-CM is added to the lower compartment (for HSC chemotaxis assay). For HSE cell migration assay, HSC-CM is added to the upper and lower compartments. All cells are allowed to migrate for up to 48 h. Migrated cells are fixed in 100% methanol, stained with 0.2% crystal violet, and counted in 10 random high-power fields per membrane. Data is expressed relative to the migration of cells in wells containing DMEM plus 0.5% FCS in both the upper and lower chambers.

3. *VEGF Measurement:* The levels of VEGF in the conditioned media are analyzed using a commercial ELISA kit (R&D).

4. *Detection of Apoptotic HSE Cells:* Serum-starved HSE cells are maintained in the presence or absence of conditioned media from untreated and tumor-CM-treated HSCs. Cell survival is analyzed at various time points using a TUNEL-

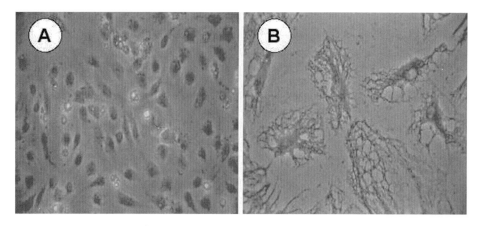

Fig. 2. (**A**) Primary culture of hepatic sinusoidal endothelial (HSE) cells. (**B**) Desmin expression in a primary culture of hepatic stellate cells (HSCs).

based assay (Clontech) following the manufacturer's instructions. Results are expressed as the ratio of TUNEL-positive cells versus propidium iodide-positive nuclei per high field power.

4. Notes

1. These time points were chosen because they allowed us to observe a significant amount of tumor foci of a variety of sizes (i.e., micrometastases ranging from 50–3000 mm in diameter) in each analyzed liver section.

2. Isolation and primary culture of hepatic sinusoidal endothelial and stellate cells: HSE cells and HSCs are isolated from adult mouse liver by in situ digestion followed by density gradient centrifugation as follows *(16,6)*: the liver from an anesthesized mouse is perfused through the portal vein (1 mL/min) with 5 mL of HBSS, followed by 10 mL 0.1% pronase in HBSS and 15 mL of HBSS containing 0.08% collagenase and 0.03% pronase. The liver is minced and stirred in 13 mL of HBSS containing 0.03% pronase, 0.04% collagenase and 0.0003% type I deoxyribonuclease at 37°C for 10 min, at pH 7.4. Cells are suspended in DMEM and poured gently on top of a double layer of 10% and 17.5% (w/v) metrizamide in HBSS. After a 15 min centrifugation at 800g, HSCs are collected from the 10% layer and HSE cells from the 17.5% layer. Cells are cultured in collagen-coated (0.5×10^6 HSE cells/cm^2) or uncoated wells (0.5×10^5 HSC cells/cm^2) in basal DMEM culture medium supplemented with 10% FCS and antibiotics, and allowed to recover for 24 h (HSE cells) or 48 h (HSCs) prior to analysis (*see* **Fig. 2**). For cell migration assays, both HSE and HSC cells are directly delivered into 0.3 cm^2 inserts coated with collagen type I (10–100 mg/cm^2 for 30 min at 37°C).

3. Quiescent versus activated HSCs: Under normal physiological conditions of the liver, HSC cells show a quiescent phenotype. Progressive HSC activation, as

defined by *de novo* expression of ASMA filaments, loss of vitamin A, proliferation and increased extracellular matrix production *(16)*, occurs spontaneously during in vitro culture on plastic. Thus, freshly isolated primary cultures are recommended for the study of HSC activation by tumor-derived factors.

4. In vitro treatment schedule: The length of the incubation time with the anti-angiogenic compound must be determined empirically. Incubation periods shorter than 24 h are advised, as primary cultures usually suffer when cultured under serum-free conditions for more than one day.

References

1. Vidal-Vanaclocha, F. (1997) The Hepatic Sinusoidal Endothelium: functional aspects and phenotypic heterogeneity, in *Functional Heterogeneity of Liver Tissue: From Cell Lineage Diversity To Sublobular Compartment-Specific Pathogenesis* (Vidal-Vanaclocha, F., ed.), R G Landes, Austin, TX, pp. 69–108.
2. Terada, T., Makimoto, K., Terayama, N., Suzuki, Y., and Nakanuma, Y. (1996). Alpha-smooth muscle actin-positive stromal cells in cholangiocarcinomas, hepatocellular carcinoma and metastatic liver carcinoma. *J. Hepatol.* **24,** 706–712.
3. Theret, N., Musso, O., Turlin, B., et al. (2001) Increased extracellular matrix remodeling is associated with tumor progresssion in human hepatocellular carcinoma. *Hepatology* **34,** 82–88.
4. Mouvoisin, A., Bisson, C., Si-Tayeb, K., Balabaud, C., Desmouliere, A., and Rosenbaum, J. (2002) Involvement of matrix metalloproteinase type-3 in hepatocyte growth factor-induced invasion of human hepatocellular carcinoma cells. *Int. J. Cancer* **97,** 157–162.
5. Faouzi, S., Lepreux, S., Bedin, C., et al. (1999) Activation of cultured rat hepatic stellate cells by tumoral hepatocytes. *Lab. Invest.* **79,** 485–493.
6. Olaso, E., Santisteban, A., Bidaurrazaga, J., Gressner, A. M., Rosenbaum, J., and Vidal-Vanaclocha, F. (1997) Tumor-dependent activation of rodent hepatic stellate cells during experimental melanoma metastasis. *Hepatology* **26,** 634–642.
7. Shimizu, S., Yamada, N., Sawada, T., et al. (2000) In vivo and in vitro interactions between human colon carcinoma cells and hepatic stellate cells. *Jpn. J. Cancer Res.* **91,** 1285–1292.
8. Santisteban, A., Olaso, E., Bidaurrazaga, J., Rosenbaum, J., and Vidal-Vanaclocha, F. (1999) Tumor-activated hepatic stellate cells upregulate in vitro proliferation and tubulization of sinusoidal endothelial cells and constitutes a stromal support for neoangiogenesis in murine melanoma hepatic metastasis, in *Cells of the Hepatic Sinusoid* (Wisse, E., Knook, D. L., De Zanger, R. and Fraser, R., eds), Vol 7, Kupffer Cell Foundation, Leiden, pp. 41–42.
9. Wang, Y. Q., Ikeda, K., Ikebe, T., et al. (2000) Inhibition of hepatic stellate cell proliferation and activation by the semisynthetic analogue of fumagillin TNP-470 in rats. *Hepatology* **32,** 980–989.
10. Tanaka, T., Konno, H., Matsuda, I., Nakamura, S., and Baba, S. (1995) Prevention of hepatic metastasis of human colon cancer by angiogenesis inhibitor TNP-470. *Cancer Res.* **55,** 836–839.

11. Yoshida, T., Kaneko, Y., Tsukamoto, A., Han, K., Ichinose, M., and Kimura, S. (1998) Suppression of hepatoma growth and angiogenesis by a fumagillin derivative TNP470: possible involvement of nitric oxide synthase. *Cancer Res.* **58,** 3751–3756.

12. Shaheen, R. M., Tseng, W., Davis, D. W., et al. (2001) Tyrosine kinase inhibition of multiple angiogenic growth factor receptors improves survival in mice bearing colon cancer liver metastases by inhibition of endothelial cell survival mechanism. *Cancer Res.* **61,** 1464–1468.

13. Bachem, M. G., Meyer, D., Schaefer, W., et al. (1993) The response of rat liver perisinusoidal lipocytes to polypeptide growth regulators changes with their transdifferentiation into myofibroblast-like cells in culture. *Hepatology* **18,** 40–52.

14. Vidal-Vanaclocha, F., Fantuzzi, G., Mendoza, L., et al. (2000) IL-18 regulates IL-1beta-dependent hepatic melanoma metastasis via vascular cell adhesion molecule-1. *Proc. Natl. Acad. Sci. USA* **97,** 734–739.

15. Olaso, E. and Friedman, S. L. (1998) Molecular regulation of hepatic fibrogenesis. *J. Hepatology* **29,** 836–847.

16. Olaso, E., Ikeda, K., Eng, F. J., et al. (2001) DDR2 receptor promotes MMP-2-mediated proliferation and invasion by hepatic stellate cells. *J. Clin. Invest.* 108, 1369–1379.

8

Cell Motility, Adhesion, Homing, and Migration Assays in the Studies of Tyrosine Kinases

Martin Sattler, Elizabeth Quackenbush, and Ravi Salgia

1. Introduction

The malignant potential of many cancers is characterized by the rate of metastsis. Metastasis is a multistep process that in general requires detachment from the original tissue, migration through the vascular endothelium, circulation in the blood, attachment to the inner blood vessel wall and penetration into surrounding tissue *(1)*. For example, lung cancer cells have a very high rate of metastasis with cells invading virtually every organ in the body with a predilection to brain, bone, bone marrow, liver and adrenal glands. There are intrinsic abnormalities of cell motility of these lung cancer cells with increased propensity to invade and metastasize to the other organs *(2)*. Most of the cell motility processes are tightly regulated by tyrosine kinases *(3)* and protein tyrosine phosphatases *(4)*. In malignant cells, these crucial pathways can be brought out of balance through constitutive activation of growth factor receptors and their associated kinases or through formation of tyrosine kinase oncogenes. Overexpression and activation of receptor tyrosine kinases (RTKs) has been found in non small cell lung cancer (NSCLC) cells, including epidermal growth factor receptor (EGFR), HER2/neu, c-Met, and in small cell lung cancer (SCLC) cells, including c-Kit and c-Met receptors *(5)*. The downstream targets of these kinases can involve cytoskeletal proteins which are important in cell motility, cell migration and invasion. It is also known that the tyrosine kinase oncogene BCR/ABL, the transforming protein in chronic myeloid leukemia (CML), is a potent kinase for inducing increased cell motility (membrane ruffling, filipodia formation, lamellopodia formation, and formation of uropod)

From: *Methods in Molecular Medicine, vol. 85: Novel Anticancer Drug Protocols*
Edited by: J. K. Buolamwini and A. A. Adjei © Humana Press Inc., Totowa, NJ

and migration over extracellular matrix components such as fibronectin *(6)*. Tyrosine kinases are novel therapeutic targets against many cancers. As an example, the tyrosine kinase inhibitor STI-571 (Gleevec, Novartis) is being effectively used in CML, targeting the BCR/ABL tyrosine kinase *(7)*. Also, ZD-1839 (Iressa, Astra Zeneca) is being used in clinical trials in NSCLC, targeting the epidermal growth factor (EGF)-receptor tyrosine kinase *(8)*. It is important to realize that tyrosine kinases and their downstream targets play a crucial role in the migration of cells, and this chapter will describe common methodologies for studying the role of tyrosine kinases using SCLC, NSCLC, and CML cells as typical examples. The motility of cancer cells can be studied by time-lapse video microscopy (TLVM), adhesion to various extracellular matrix components via adhesion assays, migration via chemotactic assays, and mechanisms of metastasis to the bone marrow via intra-vital microscopy.

1.1. Time-Lapse Video Microscopy

Time-lapse video microscopy has enhanced our understanding of cell behavior in terms of cell motility. Cell motility plays a key role in both normal physiology and various disease processes. Many animal cells can move through or over a substrate along a chemotactic gradient, and in the absence of such a gradient, cells tend to move randomly over the substratum *(9)*. The actin cytoskeleton is widely accepted as the basic engine for crawling/gliding. The initial protrusive structure (filopodia and lamellipodia, for example) contains dense arrays of actin filaments with their barbed ends (fast growing, or plus ends) oriented in the direction of protusion *(10)*. The simplest protrusive structures are filopodia, composed of thin cylinders. Lamellipodia contain webs of actin filaments. Most motile cells and cultured fibroblasts have been shown to move using lamellipodia *(11)*, while hematopoietic cells typically move through small pseudopods *(12,13)*.

Protrusive structures move out away from the main body of the cell by one of two processes. One such process is elongation, where new actin polymers can be generated only by polymerization onto existing barbed ends; and the other is nucleation followed by elongation, where newly nucleated filaments are attached to the barbed ends of existing polymers *(11)*. In motile cells, however, new actin polymerization at the leading edge occurs continually at a steady state and must be balanced by depolymerization elsewhere. After the protrusive structure adheres to a substrate, usually in crawling cells, traction helps to move the rest of the cell body in the direction of the protrusion *(11)*. Cells that do not adhere to a substratum permanently, such as leukocytes, can move 10–60 times faster than adherent cells such as fibroblasts *(14)*. The suspension cells exert less drag forces, and protrusion itself may be sufficient enough to move the cell forward *(11)*.

De-adhesion and tail retraction occurs as the last process in cell motility. In this process the actin cytoskeleton in the back of the cell is broken down and the actin monomers recycled for potential use in the front of the cell for protrusion and traction of the cell. One of the key events regulating cell motility is polymerization of actin, formation of actin stress fibers, and focal adhesion. It has been shown that inactivating tyrosine kinases decreases cell motility *(15–17)*.

1.2. Adhesion Assay

Alterations in integrin-mediated signaling, as well as factors affecting the condition of the matrix, can lead to cellular transformation. Normal cells can potentially be distinguished from transformed cells by the extent to which they will adhere to its underlying substratum *(18–20)*. The adhesion assay is a simple in vitro method used to determine the rate or strength of adhesion of different cell types to extracellular matrix proteins. Cells are labeled with the fluorescent dye Calcein-acetoxymethyl ester and the number of bound cells correlated with the fluorescence recorded. The total amount of incorporated Calcein may vary between different cell lines or cell types, but this does not affect the assay. Unlike normal cells, cancer cells tend to secrete less fibronectin, have poorly developed stress fibers, and bind weakly to the extracellular matrix, giving them a rounded appearance. The apparent effects of differential integrin expression on cell anchorage, adhesion, and fibronectin deposition influence cell motility and invasion *(18–20)*. Consistent with this, the tyrosine kinase Src-containing recombinant retrovirus (ZSV)-transformed F2408 rat cells exhibit downregulation of cellular fibronectin and an integrin receptor, implicating integrin and/or the extracellular matrix in suppression of v-Src transformation of these cells *(21)*. In a similar fashion, other tyrosine kinases have been shown to have similar effects on adhesion as v-Src.

1.3. Transwell Migration

Cell migration can be assessed using in vitro chemotaxis systems, such as the Boyden chamber, Neuro Probe plate, or Transwell insert system *(22–24)* (*see* **Fig. 1**). These devices typically consist of an upper and lower chamber that are separated by a microporous, polycarbonate membrane. Cells are placed in the upper chamber and their response to a chemotactic gradient, created by placing a chemoattractant in the lower chamber, is measured by quantitating the number of cells that appear in the lower chamber or that adhere to the underside of the membrane. The membrane can be coated with extracellular matrix proteins, such as collagen or fibronectin, or with endothelial cells (EC) that have been allowed to grow to confluence on the membrane. EC-coated

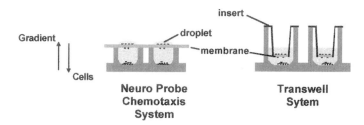

Fig. 1. Comparison of the Neuro Probe Chemotaxis and the Transwell System. The Neuro Probe system for chemotaxis consists of a polycarbonate membrane that snaps over a customized 96-well microtiter plate. The Transwell system consists of a polycarbonate membrane insert that separates a lower compartment from an upper Transwell chamber. The lower wells contain enough chemoattractant solution to make contact with the underside of the membrane, creating a gradient (direction indicated by arrow) between the well and the cell-containing droplet on the surface of the membrane or the Transwell insert. The droplet in the Neuro Probe system is maintained by a coating of hydrophobic ink that surrounds the circular area of membrane directly above each well. Cells migrate from the droplet or the transwell insert through the membrane (as indicated by the arrow), and may drop into the lower well or adhere to the underside of the membrane.

membranes are considered to be a more physiologic surface for leukocyte adhesion and migration, and human umbilical vein endothelial cell monolayers (HUVEC) are most frequently used *(25)*. Immortalized cell lines or freshly isolated cells can be used to mimic as closely as possible the in vivo mechanism being investigated, such as tumor metastasis, constitutive lymphocyte homing, or neutrophil migration to inflamed tissues *(24,25)*. Despite being widely used to model cell adhesion and migration, in vitro chemotaxis systems have many limitations. For example, many of the molecules needed for proper adhesion and diapedesis may not be present on either the EC or the cells of interest, the EC monolayer may not form a physiologic barrier to diffusion of the chemokine, and/or cell adhesion may not be properly generated without the hemodynamic forces that result from blood flow in vivo *(26,27)*.

1.4. In Vivo Homing Assay

Cells have various receptors that are important in homing to specific organs. As an example, the HIV T-tropic chemokine receptor CXCR4 with its ligand SDF-1α is required for hematopoietic progenitor cells to home to the bone marrow and lymph nodes. To study homing mechanisms, SDF1-α has been injected into the spleen of mice, and the homing of hematopoietic progenitor cells such as FDCP-1 have been well documented *(28)*. In BCR/ABL transformed cell lines, SDF1-α-induced homing to the spleen is altered compared

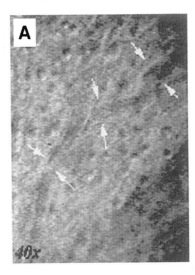 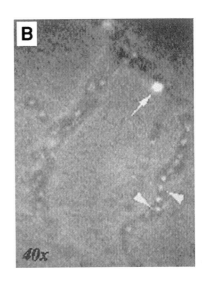

Fig. 2. Acridine Orange-labeled Fetal Cells in the Microvasculature of the Murine Yolk Sac at day 14 of Gestation. Acridine Orange was injected into the internal jugular vein of a pregnant mouse (day 14 of gestation), post exteriorization of the fetus for IVM (unpublished IVM experimental model). The unlabeled microvascular bed of the yolk sac is shown in panel **A**. The acridine dyes are small (MW 670), weakly acidophilic compounds that readily diffuse through cell membranes and strongly accumulate in acidic cell compartments, such as lysosomes, and weakly in the nucleus by intercalating with DNA and RNA. Acridine Orange crosses the placenta within seconds of injection into the anesthetized mother and sufficiently labels fetal cells, as shown in panel **B**. The majority of cells within the vessel are nucleated red blood cells (arrowheads), along with rare white blood cells (arrows).

to untransformed cells *(29)*. These types of assays can also be utilized to study how solid tumor cells, such as lung cancer cells, can metastasize to the lymph nodes and bone marrow using various chemokines. Here we describe a homing assay that examines the ability of ex vivo-labeled cells to home to an ectopically placed chemoattractant, in this case SDF-1α in the spleen.

1.5. Intravital Microscopy

In the past several years, intravital microscopy (IVM) has been used with increasing sophistication to visualize complex biological interactions in microvascular beds of many different animal species (*see* **Fig. 2**). Several IVM models of normal and pathological cell behavior have been developed, and it has become a powerful tool for determining the in vivo relevance of in vitro observations *(30)*. For example, fibrosis, angiogenesis, ischemia-reperfusion, inflammation, and cell trafficking/metastasis have been studied by IVM

(31–34). To date, the microcirculation of almost all organs (and recently the murine fetus) have now been analyzed by the invaluable technique of IVM.

With few exceptions, surgical preparations for IVM result in the upregulation of inflammatory molecules that may affect the parameter being quantitated, and the majority of standard models are not amenable to serial measurements over long periods of time. Technical advances, such as the use of implanted chambers that allow for repeated measurements over days in awake animals, have improved our ability to monitor the effects of compounds on cell behavior *(35)*. Furthermore, the use of video-triggered, strobe-generated epi-illumination (for fluorescent analysis) has allowed leukocyte-endothelial cell interactions to be clearly visualized, quantitated and manipulated with less phototoxicity. Much of what we have learned about cell trafficking has been acquired through IVM *(36)*.

An IVM setup is often customized to accommodate the specific needs of the individual laboratory, thus, a detailed understanding of the multiple uses and technical aspects of IVM can be found in additional references *(31–38)*. Nonetheless, there are many general features shared by different setups. A typical IVM set up consists of a microscope equipped with infinity-corrected water-immersion optics, light source (brightfield and/or fluorescent), a camera and image processor, and a recording system *(37)*. Analysis of videotaped events can be performed on- or off-line, depending on the parameter being measured and the system used. Hemodynamic parameters, vascular morphology, and leukocyte-endothelial cell interactions (i.e., percent of rolling and adherent cells) can be accurately quantitated by IVM *(38)*.

2. Materials

2.1. Time-Lapse Video Microscopy

2.1.1. Reagents

1. Tissue Culture plates (60 × 15 mm, Becton Dickinson Labware, Franklin Lakes, NJ).
2. Phosphate buffered saline (Mediatech, Herndon, VA).
3. Human plasma fibronectin (Gibco BRL, Life Technologies, Rockville, MD).
4. 0.1% (w/v) Poly-L-Lysine solution (Sigma, St. Louis, MO).

2.1.2. Time-Lapse Video Microscopy Equipment Found in a Standard Set-Up

1. An Olympus IX70 inverted microscope (Olympus, Lake Success, NY) with Hoffman optics (×10/20/40); the microscope is mounted on a vibration-free base (*see* **Fig. 3**).
2. Incubator (Omega temperature control device, Washington, PA), with 5% (v/v) CO_2 supply and humidity control.

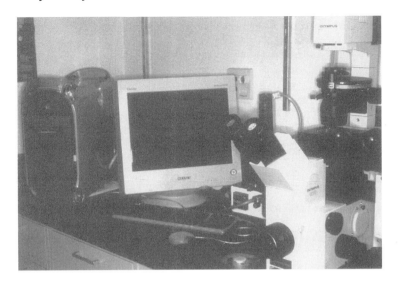

Fig. 3. Standard Set-up of the Time-lapse Video Microsopy (TLVM) Equipment. An Olympus IX70 inverted microscope (right) with Hoffman optics and incubator (Omega temperature control device) is mounted on a vibration-free base. The microscope is protected from outside light sources and operated in a darkened room. Images are captured with a digital video camera (not shown) and transfered directly to a Macintosh G4 computer (left). The monitor (middle) enables real-time imaging of the digitalized microscopy data.

3. Images are captured with an Optronics DEI-750 3CCD digital color video camera (Optronics Engineering, Galeta, CA); the microscope is operated in a darkened room, protected from outside light sources.
4. The images are recorded with a Sony SVT-S3100 time-lapse S-VHS video recorder or transfered directly to a connected Macintosh G4 computer.
5. For image presentation, captured images can be printed with the Sony Color Video Printer UP-5600MD, presented on a video monitor, or transformed into a quicktime movie.
6. Because of their small size, very little intracellular detail can be appreciated with standard phase microscopy, although it is entirely satisfactorily used to perform the assays described in the methods section. In general, the intracellular detail with time-lapse video microscopy using Hoffman optics is much better than with phase, and the generation of pseudopods, the membrane ruffling, and the de-adhesion of trailing edges of cells can be studied in more detail.

2.2. Adhesion Assay

2.2.1. Reagents

1. Phosphate buffered saline (PBS, Mediatech, Herndon, VA).
2. Human plasma fibronectin (Gibco BRL, Life Technologies, Rockville, MD).

3. Costar 96-well polystyrene tissue culture treated black clear-bottom plate (Corning Inc., Corning, NY).
4. RPMI1640 (Mediatech, Herndon, VA).
5. Bovine serum albumin (BSA) (Sigma, St. Louis, MO).
6. Calcein-AM (Molecular Probes, Eugene, OR).

2.2.2. Equipment Required for Adhesion Assay

The number of labeled cells bound to the bottom of the microtiter plates can be analyzed with a standard 96-well fluorescence plate reader such as the SPECTRAmax-GEMINI XS (Molecular Devices, Sunnyvale, CA), connected to a Pentium II PC and controlled by the SOFTmax Pro Vers. 3.1 software (Molecular Devices, Sunnyvale, CA).

2.3. Transwell Migration

2.3.1. Chemotaxis Systems

1. Neuro Probe Chemotaxis systems (Neuro Probe, Cabin John, MD) (*see* **Note 1**).
2. Costar Transwell system (Costar, Cambridge, MA) (*see* **Note 2**).
3. Boyden Microchamber (Neuro Probe, Cabin John, MD (*see* **Note 3**).

2.3.2. Reagents

Cell preparations are resuspended in Hank's Balanced Buffered Saline (HBSS) solution with 1% BSA, or in the culture medium in which the cells are grown. If using tissue culture medium, the percentage of fetal calf serum (FCS) should not exceed 2% during the incubation. Chemoattractants are diluted in the same medium as the cells, and the ideal concentration needs to be determined by titration for each chemoattractant tested. Wells can be coated with different extracellular matrix proteins, such as collagen, fibronectin or vitronectin, depending on the cell type to be tested.

1. Fibronectin 50 µg/mL (GIBCO BRL, Life Technologies, Rockville, MD).
2. HBSS or tissue culture medium of choice (Mediatech, Herndon, VA).
3. BSA, 10% stock. Keep sterile and at 4°C.
4. Sterile FCS, heat inactivated at 55°C for 45 min.
5. 199 medium (GIBCO BRL, Life Technologies, Rockville, MD).

2.4. In Vivo Homing Assay

2.4.1. Reagents

1. Dulbecco's Modified Eagle's Medium.
2. HEPES.
3. FCS.
4. TRITC (Molecular Probes, Eugene, OR).
5. Calcein-AM (Molecular Probes).

6. C57BL/6 mice of both sexes.
7. Physiological saline.
8. Ketamine-HCl.
9. Xylazine.
10. Histopaque-1077 (Sigma).

2.4.2. FACS Equipment Required in a Standard Set-Up

FACScan flow cytometer (Becton Dickinson, San Jose, CA).

2.5. Intravital Microscopy

Reagents that alter cell or vessel behavior in vivo can be injected or applied topically (known as superfusion), depending upon the microvascular bed analyzed. Topical reagents do not penetrate encapsulated tissues such as peripheral lymph nodes, in high concentrations. However, the cremaster muscle and mesenteric vasculatures can be successfully superfused with reagents dissolved in isotonic solutions. Any reagent used in IVM should be isotonic, endotoxin-free, and administered in a volume that does not cause cardiac dysfunction, which will alter hemodynamic profiles.

2.5.1. Reagents

1. Bicarbonate-buffered saline: 132 mM NaCl, 4.7 mM KCl, 2 mM CaCl$_2$, 1.2 mM MgCl$_2$, 18 mM NaHCO$_3$, equilibrated with 5% CO$_2$ in N$_2$ to adjust pH to 7.35.
2. For visualization of plasma distribution: FITC-dextran (of varying molecular weights) at 20 mg/kg body weight in physiologic saline. A molecular mass of 150 kDa is most commonly used, as it is well-retained within the vasculature.
3. Endogenous cells can be labeled with rhodamine 6G (single bolus intravenously of 0.15 mg/kg in physiologic saline).

2.5.2. IVM Equipment Found in a Standard Set-Up

1. A microscope with infinity-corrected water-immersion optics (×2.5/10/20/40/63/100; ocular of 10); microscope is mounted on a vibration-free base.
2. Light sources: (i) for transillumination: a variable volt, 150-watt halogen lamp is brought under the stage through a fiber-optic cable. Hemoglobin absorbs light in the blue spectrum, thus, a blue-green filter is commonly used; (ii) For epi-illumination: the light source will vary depending upon the fluorescent marker. Intense markers, such as FITC-dextran can be visualized with a variable 12-volt, 100-watt halogen light source, whereas weaker signals (e.g., rhodamine 6G) must be visualized with a 100-watt mercury vapor lamp. Phototoxicity is lessened by using a video-triggered stroboscopic epi-illumination light source that delivers two, intense, closely-spaced flashes of light.
3. Filter sets are available for use with epi-illumination. A standard filter block contains separate positions for FITC-dextran, rhodamine 6G and for transillumination.

4. Microscopic images are captured with a black and white or color camera and stored on videotape. Images are analyzed off-line by means of computer-assisted microcirculation analyzing systems. Vessel lengths and diameters, capillary/venular red blood cell velocities, functional capillary density, rolling fractions and sticking cell fractions can all be determined off-line, which eliminates increased exposure to the light source and phototoxicity.

3. Methods

3.1. Video Microscopy

3.1.1. Preparation of Cells and Microscopy

1. Incubate cell culture plates with poly-L-lysine, human plasma fibronectin in PBS, or other extracellular matrix proteins for 18 h at 4°C.
2. Wash the plates twice with PBS immediately before use.
3. Resuspend the cells at 0.1×10^6 cells/mL in culture medium and transfer 1–2 mL of cell suspension to the cell culture plate.
4. Turn on the temperature control unit 30 min before the experiment, allowing time for the incubation chamber to warm up.
5. Adjust the magnification on the microscope so that a few single cells or clusters of cells are clearly visible. Coordinate the Hoffman Modulation Contrast unit with the magnification (HMC40 with ×40 magnification works usually the best). In the first hour of taping, check and re-adjust the focus if necessary.
6. Once focused, adjust the sharpness, brightness and contrast with the CCD camera control unit. Finally, pick the time mode to record in, e.g., tape adherent cells such as the NSCLC cell line CALU-1 at ×240 or non-adherent cells such as the SCLC cell line NCI-H69 at ×480. Four hours recording at ×480 will tape about 1 min of video, viewed at ×2.

3.1.2. Data Analysis

Cell motility for hematopoietic cells (such as Ba/F3, pre-B cells dependent on IL-3 for survival) is quite different from that for SCLC cells such as H69 cells. Ba/F3 cells are individual and their cell movement over a course of time (distance and speed) and the rate of formation and retraction of filopodia/lamellipodia/uropod can be calculated by taking the video images, converting them to "quicktime" movies, then downloading into the NIH Image Analysis type of program. The images are analyzed for the various quantitations required by computer off-line with the Scion Image 1.62c software (for MacOS 7.5 to 9.0), basically identical to the program designed by Wayne Rasband at the National Institute of Health (NIH) and can be downloaded free of charge from the Scion Image Corporation website (http://scioncorp.com/frames/fr_scion_products.htm). 300–500 cells tend to reflect the average behavior of the particular cell line. The study of SCLC cell motility offers interesting challenges, since these cells move in clusters, as our data show. However, the study of the cluster may provide unique insights into the in vivo behavior of SCLC cells, as well as other solid tumors, especially in the context of solid tumor metastasis. In the NIH Image Analysis program (using Macros), several different methods can be utilized to quantify the cell motility of SCLC cellular clusters.

1. *Cluster cell movement:* clusters of cells can be grouped together by tracing the cluster, frame by frame (usually for a 240 min real-time experiment, our videotape is for 2 min, and there are 120 frames we capture in a quick-time movie) for each time point, and the movement of the cluster over a course of time is reflected in a cartoon pictorial with a graph of several cluster movements over time.
2. *Cluster centroid movement:* The cluster motion can be grouped together as a centroid (which can be calculated for any individual cell or a group of cells), and this can be plotted over time.
3. *Cluster centroid distance and speed:* The centroid distance moved over time on an average will reflect the speed of the cells.
4. *Single cell movement within the cluster:* There is movement within the cluster itself, and as seen in our video images, we can identify each of the cells in the cluster, calculate the centroid of each cell as compared to the centroid of the cluster, and determine the movement (distance) of each single cell centroid in reference to the cluster centroid, and plot that over time. This gives a quantitation of how individual cells move in a cluster.
5. *Measurement of actin projections:* The various actin projections, such as filopodia, lamellipodia, and uropod can be calculated over a course of time by taking frame-by-frame pictures and calculating the rate of formation and retraction of these structures. Then, average rates can be determined.
6. *Quantitative measurements of distance moved beyond TLVM:* Slides coated with colloidal gold have been used to measure crawling of a variety of cell types, as moving cells leave trails in the coating which can be measured with a micrometer, expressing the data as "mm/h."

3.2. Adhesion Assay

3.2.1. Preparation of Cells and Plates

1. Dissolve human plasma fibronectin (5 µg/mL) in PBS.
2. Coat 96-well tissue culture plate with 100 µL of fibronectin solution (or other extracellular matix proteins) for 18 h at 4°C.
3. Wash the plate twice with PBS.
4. Add 100 µL of adhesion medium (0.2% (w/v) BSA in RPMI 1640 culture medium) and incubate for 2 h at 37°C.
5. Incubate cells in 5 µM Calcein-AM for 30 min at 37°C.
6. Wash cells twice with adhesion medium and resuspend at 5×10^5 cells/mL.

3.2.2. Cell Adhesion Assay

1. Add 100 µL cell suspension per well (n = 4) to a 96-well plate.
2. Spin the plate for 10 sec at 200*g*.
3. Incubate for 30 min to 2 h at 37°C. (The incubation time has to be determined empirically for each cell line since cells can not only differ in the overall amount of adherent cells but also in the rate of adherence to fibronectin.)
4. Carefully remove medium and add 200 µL adhesion medium.
5. Repeat **step 4** three times.
6. Add 200 µL of PBS per well (adding medium instead of PBS tends to create more bubbles that must be removed before reading the plate).
7. Measure fluorescence with $\lambda_{excitation}$ = 494 nm and $\lambda_{emission}$ = 517 nm.

3.2.3. Data Analysis

The change in cell adhesion correlates directly with the change in fluorescence and a percent decrease in adhesion can be calculated as the percent in change in fluorescence compared to the control. For example, an appropriate control would be a cell treated with solvent compared to a cell treated with a tyrosine kinase inhibitor.

3.3. Transwell Migration Assay

3.3.1. Transendothelial Migration of Cells in Costar Transwell Inserts

1. Coat Transwell inserts (with 5 µ*M* pores) with 100 µL of sterile fibronectin (50 µg/mL in HBSS) for 2 h at 37°C. Remove excess fibronectin solution and allow inserts to dry.
2. For each insert, plate 2×10^5 non-confluent HUVEC cells (*see* **Note 4**) at 37°C in 100 µL of complete 199 medium supplemented with 20% heat inactivated FCS. After 24 h, remove excess medium and cover monolayers with sterile, serum-free medium alone; keep plates at 37°C in preparation for chemotaxis.
3. *Prepare cells for chemotaxis:* Cells should be washed three times in sterile medium containing 2% FCS or in HBSS containing 1% BSA; resuspend at a concentration of 5×10^6/mL (2.5×10^6/mL for freshly isolated neutrophils) and keep at 37°C while preparing the plates.
4. Dilute chemoattractants appropriately (*see* **Note 5**) and load 600 µL into each well. Set up wells in triplicate, and include wells that have medium alone as a negative control.
5. Gently remove the medium from the HUVEC-coated inserts and place each insert into a well, taking care not to trap air bubbles underneath the insert. Add 100 µL of the cell suspension to each insert and incubate at 37°C for the desired length of time of chemotaxis: 4 h for lymphocytes, 3 h for cultured cells, 2 h for monocytes and 1 h for neutrophils.
6. Harvest the cells from the lower chamber and count on a hemocytometer or cell sorter.

3.3.2. Data Analysis

Migrating cells can be quantitated in a number of ways, e.g., the underside of the membrane in the Boyden microchamber can be stained with vital dyes and adherent cells can be scored as number of cells/field of view with a microscope (×400). Alternatively, cells that drop off the membrane into the lower chamber can be scored in a hemocytometer chamber or they can be assessed by flow cytometry. Flow cytometry is particularly useful if more than one cell subset is present in the migrating population, as different populations can be identified by their forward and side scatter characteristics. The input population can also be labeled with fluorescent dyes for analysis of migrating cells by ELISA or flow cytometry. The chemotactic index (CI), a measure of the specificity of migration, is determined by dividing the number of cells that migrate to the chemoattractant by the number of cells that migrate to control.

3.4. In Vivo Homing Assay

3.4.1. Labeling of Cells

1. Wash cells three times in Dulbecco's Modified Eagle's Medium (DMEM, BIOWHITTAKER) containing 20 mM HEPES and 1% FCS, pH 7.4.
2. Resuspend cells at 20× 10^6/mL and then incubate for 20 min with TRITC (30 µg/mL) or Calcein-AM (200 nM).
3. Label cells for 20 min at 37°C and mix frequently during the incubation.
4. Wash cells with an equal volume of fresh FCS (or 20% BSA) and pellet cells at 1000g for 10 min. Check viability of cells and re-warm them at 37°C for 15 min before injection. The labeling time may be shortened if viability is impaired.

3.4.2. Injection of Cells into Mice

1. For homing experiments, anesthetize C57BL/6 mice of both sexes by intraperitoneal injection of physiological saline containing ketamine-HCL (100 mg/mL) and xylazine (10 mg/mL).
2. Cannulate the left carotid artery with PE-10 polyethylene tubing to allow injection of cells into the descending aorta. Save an aliquot of injected cells for analysis of intensity of labeling.
3. Just prior to cell injection, make a left flank incision.
4. Inject the exposed spleen with 50 µL of PBS alone or PBS containing 1 µg of SDF-1α using an insulin syringe. Close the flank incision with surgical glue or by sutering.
5. Pool labeled cells for injection (total volume of 0.5 mL, containing 10^7 cells). Inject the cells slowly, over a 15–20 min period and allow the animals to awake.
6. After three hours, sacrifice the animals and harvest spleen, lungs, bone marrow, and peripheral blood (via cardiac puncture).

3.4.3. FACS Analysis

1. Prepare single cell suspensions from minced tissues by gently passing them through a 70 μm nylon mesh.
2. Separate single cell suspensions on a Histopaque-1077 gradient. Wash the cell populations recovered at the gradient interface in DMEM. Pellet and fix in 4% paraformaldehyde for analysis on a FACScan flow cytometer.
3. Count the residual fluorescent cells present in the catheter after injection to determine the frequency of each cell line in the input population.
4. Analyze $5–10 \times 10^6$ cells for each tissue and quantitate fluorescent cells within a gated region whose borders are determined from the injected pool.

3.4.4. Data Analysis

The percentages of gated cells recovered in each organ will be corrected for differences in the percentages of each labeled in the input cell type population.

3.5. Methods for Intravital Microscopy

3.5.1. Anesthetizing and Cannulating Mice

1. Adult mice (pregnant or nonpregnant) are anesthetized with a mixture of ketamine (100 mg/kg) and xylazine (10 mg/kg) in normal saline, injected intraperitoneally. Animals are monitored during filming by tail pinches and whisker flicking.
2. The anesthetized mouse is placed on a 37°C heating blanket and the temperature is monitored by a rectal thermometer. Hair is removed from the anterior neck and flank or abdomen, depending on the tissue to be visualized. A commercial hair remover can be used, but it should be tested first for any adverse skin effects.
3. To cannulate the internal jugular vein, a midline incision is made in the anterior neck and the edges of the skin are spread slightly with forceps. Without disrupting the vasculature, the internal jugular vein is visualized through separation of surrounding fat and tissue.
4. Two separate pieces of suture material are passed under the jugular vein, and the suture more proximal to the cranium is used to tie off the jugular vein.
5. The jugular vein is grasped with a fine forceps and a small incision is made in it with a fine spring microscissors. The PE-10 tubing (gently pulled out to a thinner diameter) is inserted into the jugular vein (circa 5 mm in length), and the second suture is tied around the now-catheterized vein, to hold the catheter in place.
6. The suture is clipped close to the knot and surgical glue is used to close the incision around the catheter. The artery (femoral or carotid) is cannulated in an identical manner, except blood flow is temporarily impeded with a surgical clip distal to the vessel incision site, prior to making the incision, to allow for catheter placement in a blood-free field.

3.5.2. Surgical Preparation of the Tissue of Interest

The tissue of interest is surgically accessed/exteriorized and the preparation is kept moist by immersion in bicarbonate-buffered saline solution, at 37°C. Depending upon the tissue to be exposed, cannulation and surgery require approximately one hour. Each IVM model has distinct surgical steps required for exposure of the tissue. Here, we describe the preparation of the mesenteric vasculature and lymph node *(38)*.

1. The animal is laid on its side and the peritoneal cavity is opened by a midline incision with a thermocauter to prevent local bleeding. A few loops of the ileum (proximal to the appendix) and its attached mesentery are exteriorized gently with saline-moistened cotton-tipped applicators.
2. The mesenteric tissue and intestinal loop are laid flat on a clean glass slide placed on a customized Plexiglas stage. A large ring of vacuum grease on the slide is drawn around the tissue to form a well, and the tissue is superfused with pre-warmed (37°C) bicarbonate-buffered saline. Mesenteric lymph nodes are contained within the fatty tissue of the mesentery and require dissection of any overlying fat in order to visualize the internal vascular tree.
3. The tissue is kept moist by constant superfusion with pre-warmed, buffered saline. The water-immersion objective is slowly brought down over the preparation to bring venules and arterioles into view. Arterioles are defined as vessels with divergent bifurcations.
4. Test compounds, fluorescent markers and/or donor cells are injected in appropriate vehicle through the internal jugular catheter or femoral or carotid artery in small boluses (50 µL per bolus, with total the volume injected not to exceed 10% of the animal's blood volume). Allow for hemodynamic equilibration between boluses (minimum of 15 min). After filming, the anesthetized animal is euthanized without being allowed to awaken.

3.5.3. Data Analysis

Digital or analog images are analyzed off-line using computer-assisted microcirculation analyzing systems *(37,39,40)*. Microscopic images can be captured by a black and white analog video camera coupled to an image intensifier. They can also be captured with real-time digital recording equipment and Premiere 5.1 software (Adobe Systems, San Jose, CA, USA) *(41)*. Hemodynamic parameters (e.g., rolling fraction, sticking fraction, mean blood flow velocity, centerline cell velocity, bulk blood flow, and cell wall shear rate) are determined by examining multiple representative vessels (25 or more) and scoring ≥10 consecutive cells/vessel, depending on the parameter being measured *(34)*. Luminal cross diameters are determined for the same vessels in which leukocyte-endothelial interactions are scored *(34)*.

4. Notes

1. The Neuro Probe system consists of a polycarbonate filter of varying pore size that snaps onto a matching 96-well microtiter plate. Cells are loaded on top of the microporous filter, directly over the wells, in droplets whose shape is maintained by a hydrophobic ink coating that surrounds bare circles on the filter. The size of the droplet (30 μL maximum, containing 1.25×10^5 cells), surface area of the filter's circles, and volume of the lower wells (25–30 μL) makes this system ideal for small numbers of cells and limited quantities of chemoattractants. However, there are fewer migrating cells for analysis. Both the underside of the membrane and the lower well contents can be scored, and the filter and plate can be read by an ELISA plate reader as a unit or independently if fluorescently-labeled cells are used.

2. The Costar Transwell system consists of cup-shaped inserts with polycarbonate filter bottoms of varying pore size (3, 5, and 8 μM) that fit into 6-, 12- or 24-well plates. Cells are placed in the insert and 600 μL of chemoattractant is placed in the lower well. Avoid trapping air bubbles under the bottom of the insert by slowly lowering it into the well at an angle. At the end of the experiment, migrating cells in the lower well are harvested for analysis. It is more difficult to score cells that adhere to the underside of the membrane with this system, although the filter can be cut away from the insert and viewed under a microscope, if necessary.

3. The traditional Boyden microchamber system consists of two plates that are held together tightly to create 48 upper and lower chambers when a polycarbonate membrane is inserted between the plates. The upper chamber can hold up to 50 μL of cells (at 4×10^6/mL) and the lower chamber holds 30 μL of chemoattractant. The advantage of the Boyden chamber is that the removable filter's upper surface can be scraped to remove residual input cells that did not migrate to the underside.

4. HUVEC are isolated from fresh umbilical veins by digestion in collagenase, as previously described *(25)*.

5. The optimal concentration of a chemoattractant can vary from 1 ng/mL to >1μg/mL, and a titration curve should be established for each reagent tested.

References

1. Fidler, I. (1995) Modulation of the organ microenvironment for treatment of cancer metastasis. *J. Natl. Cancer Inst.* **87,** 1588–1592.
2. Wang, W.-L., Healy, M. E., Sattler, M., et al. (2000) Growth inhibition and modulation of kinase pathway of small cell lung cancer cell lines by the novel tyrosine kinase inhibitor STI571. *Oncogene* **19,** 3521–3528.
3. Porter, A. C. and Vaillancourt, R. R. (1999) Tyrosine kinase receptor-activated signal transduction pathways which lead to oncogenesis. *Oncogene* **17,** 1343–1352.
4. Angers-Loustan, A., Cote, J. F., and Tremblay, M. L. (1999) Roles of protein tyrosine phosphatases in cell migration and adhesion. *Biochem. Cell. Biol.* **77,** 493–505.

5. Salgia, R. and Skarin, A. T. (1999) Molecular and cellular biological abnormalities in lung cancer and the potential for novel therapeutics, in *Multimodality Treatment of Lung Cancer* (Skarin, A. T., ed.), Marcel Dekker, New York, NY, pp. 3–25.

6. Salgia, R., Li, J. L., Ewaniuk, D. S., et al. (1997) BCR/ABL induces multiple abnormalities of cytoskeletal function. *J. Clin. Invest.* **100,** 46–57.

7. Mauro, M. J. and Druker, B. J. (2001) Chronic myelogenous leukemia. *Curr. Opin. Oncol.* **13,** 3–7.

8. Baselga, J. and Averbuch, S. D. (2000) ZD1839 ('Iressa') as an anticancer agent. *Drugs* 60, 33–40.

9. Ehrengruber, M. U., Deranleau, D. A. and Coates, T. D. (1996) Shape oscillations of human neutrophil leukocytes: characterization and relationship to cell motility. *J. Exp. Biol.* **199,** 741–747.

10. Small, J. V. (1988) The actin cytoskeleton. *Electron Microsc. Rev.* **1,** 155–174.

11. Mitchison, T. J. and Cramer, L. P. (1996) Actin-based cell motility and cell locomotion. *Cell* **84,** 371–379.

12. Stossel, T. P. (1994) The machinery of blood cell movements. *Blood* **84,** 367–379.

13. Stossel, T. P. (1993) On the crawling of animal cells. *Science* **260,** 1086–1094.

14. Oliver, T., Lee, J. and Jacobson, K. (1994) Forces exerted by locomoting cells. *Semin. Cell Biol.* **5,** 139–147.

15. Naccache, P. H., Gilbert, C., Caon, A. C., et al. (1990) Selective inhibition of human neutrophil functional responsiveness by erbstatin, an inhibitor of tyrosine protein kinase. *Blood* **76,** 2098–2104.

16. Bennett, P. A., Dixon, R. J. and Kellie, S. (1993) The phosphotyrosine phosphatase inhibitor vanadyl hydroperoxide induces morphological alterations, cytoskeletal rearrangements and increased adhesiveness in rat neutrophil leucocytes. *J. Cell Sci.* **106,** 891–901.

17. Azuma, E. K., Kitagawa, S., Yuo, A., et al. (1993) Activation of the respiratory burst and tyrosine phosphorylation of proteins in human neutrophils: no direct relationship and involvement of protein kinase C-dependent and -independent signaling pathways. *Biochim. Biophys. Acta* **7,** 213–223.

18. Chiquet-Ehrismann, R. (1993) Tenascin and other adhesion-modulating proteins in cancer. *Semin. Cancer Biol.* **4,** 301–310.

19. McCarthy, J. B., Skubitz, A. P., Iida, J., Mooradian, D. L., Wilke, M. S. and Furcht, L.T. (1991) Tumor cell adhesive mechanisms and their relationship to metastasis. *Semin. Cancer Biol.* **2,** 155–167.

20. Stetler-Stevenson, W. G., Aznavoorian, S. and Liotta, L. A. (1993) Tumor cell interactions with the extracellular matrix during invasion and metastasis. *Annu. Rev. Cell Biol.* **9,** 541–573.

21. Inoue, H., Tavoloni, N. and Hanafusa, H. (1995) Suppression of v-Src transformation in primary rat embryo fibroblasts. *Oncogene* **20,** 231–238.

22. Tanabe, S., Luo, Y., Quackenbush, E. J., Berman, M. A., Jacobs, K. and Dorf, M. (1997) Identification of a new mouse β-chemokine, TCA4, expressed in thymic medulla with activity on mesangial cells. *J. Immunol.* **159,** 5671–5679.

23. Salgia, R., Quackenbush E. J., Ewaniuk, D., et al. (1999) BCR/ABL-transformed hematopoietic cells have reduced chemotaxis to the chemokine SDF-1α. *Blood* **94,** 4233–4246.

24. Roth, S. J., Woldemar Carr, M. and Springer, T. A. (1995) C-C chemokines, but not the C-X-C chemokines interleukin-8 and interferon-γ inducible protein-10, stimulate transendothelial chemotaxis of T lymphocytes. *Eur. J. Immunol.* **25,** 3482–3488.

25. Lidington, E., Nöhammer, C., Dominguez, M., Ferry, B. and Rose, M. L. (1996) Inhibition of the transendothelial migration of human lymphocytes but not monocytes by phosphodiesterase inhibitors. *Clin. Exp. Immunol.* **104,** 66–71.

26. von Andrian, U. H. and Mackay, C. R. (2000) Advances in immunology: T-cell function and migration—two sides of the same coin. *N. Engl. J. Med.* **343,** 1020–1034.

27. Ley, K. and Gaehtgens, P. (1991) Endothelial, not hemodynamic differences are responsible for preferential leukocyte rolling in rat mesenteric venules. *Circ. Res.* **69,** 1034–1041.

28. Aiuti, A., Webb, I.J., Bleul, C., Springer, T. and Gutierrez-Ramos, J. C. (1997) The chemokine SDF-1 is a chemoattractant for human CD34+ hematopoietic progenitor cells and provides a new mechanism to explain the mobilization of CD34+ progenitors to peripheral blood. *J. Exp. Med.* **185,** 111–120.

29. Salgia, R., Quackenbush, E., Lin, J., et al. (1999) The BCR/ABL oncogene alters the chemotactic response to stromal-derived factor-1alpha. *Blood* **94,** 4233–4246.

30. Menger, M. D., Richter, S., Yamauchi, J. I. and Vollmar, B. (1999) Intravital microscopy for the study of the microcirculation in various disease states. *Ann. Acad. Med. Singapore* **28,** 542–546.

31. Vollmer, B., Siegmund, S. and Menger, M. D. (1998) An intravital fluorescence microscopic study of hepatic microvascular and cellular derangements in developing cirrhosis in rats. *Hepatology* **27,** 1544–1553.

32. Borgstrom, P., Hillan, K. J., Sriramarao, P. and Ferrara, N. (1996) Complete inhibition of angiogenesis and growth of microtumors by anti-vascular endothelial growth factor neutralizing antibody: novel concepts of angiostatic therapy from intravital videomicroscopy. *Cancer Res.* **56,** 4032–4039.

33. Horie, Y., Wolf, R., Miyasaka, M., Anderson, D. C. and Granger, D. N. (1996) Leukocyte adhesion and hepatic microvascular responses to intestinal ischemia/reperfusion in rats. *Gastroenterology* **111,** 666–673.

34. von Andrian, U. H. (1996) Intravital microscopy of the peripheral lymph node microcirculation in mice. *Microcirculation* **3,** 287–300.

35. Lehr, H. A., Leunig, M., Menger, M. D., Nolte, D. and Messmer, K. (1993) Dorsal skinfold chamber technique for intravital microscopy in nude mice. *Am. J. Pathol.* **143,** 1055–1062.

36. von Andrian, U. H. and Mackay, C. R. (2000) Advances in immunology: T-cell function and migration—two sides of the same coin. *N. Engl. J. Med.* **343,** 1020–1034.

37. Harris, A. G., Hecht, R., Peer, F., Nolte, D. and Messmer, K. (1997) An improved intravital microscopy system. *Microcirculation* **17,** 322–327.
38. Ley, K. and Gaehtgens, P. (1991) Endothelial, not hemodynamic differences are responsible for preferential leukocyte rolling in rat mesenteric venules. *Circ. Res.* **69,** 1034–1041.
39. Pries, A. (1988) A versatile video image analysis system for microcirculatory research. *Int. J. Microcir. Clin. Exp.* **7,** 327–345.
40. Steinbauer, M., Harris, A. G. Abels, C. and Messmer, K. (2000) Characterization and prevention of phototoxic effects in intravital fluorescence microscopy in the hamster dorsal skinfold model. *Langenbeck's Arch. Surg.* **385,** 290–298.
41. Becker, M. D., Nobiling, R., Planck, S. R. and Rosenbaum, J. T. (2000) Digital video-imaging of leukocyte migration in the iris: intravital microscopy in a physiological model during the onset of endotoxin-induced uveitis. *J. Immunol. Methods* 240, 23–37.

9

Inflammatory Response of Tumor-Activated Hepatic Sinusoidal Endothelium as a Target for the Screening of Metastasis Chemopreventive Drugs

Lorea Mendoza and Fernando Vidal-Vanaclocha

1. Introduction

The pathogenesis of cancer dissemination and metastasis involves a cascade of interdependent events *(1)*. These are regulated by complex host-tumor cell interaction mechanisms, such as cancer cell adhesion to endothelium and extracellular matrix, cancer cell migration and invasion through stromal barriers, and cancer-induced immune cell disfunction and neo-angiogenesis. Proinflammatory cytokine blockade inhibits cancer metastasis development under experimental conditions *(2,3)*, suggesting that proinflammatory mediators regulate host-tumor cell interactions contributing to arrest and implantation of disseminated cancer cells in target organs.

Cancer cell adhesion to the endothelium is a key regulatory step of prometastatic effects of inflammation *(4)*. Not surprisingly, cancer cells frequently use the same molecular tools (adhesion molecules, cytokines, chemokines, chemokine receptors) and pathways as leucocytes do to colonize at distant anatomical sites during inflammation *(5)*. Exogenous proinflammatory cytokines and bacterial endotoxins can promote cancer cell adhesion to endothelium and metastasis *(6–8)*. More importantly, elevated concentrations of proinflammatory cytokines IL-1 alpha, TNF alpha, IL-6, GM-CSF, VEGF, and IL-8 have been detected in the supernatant of human cancer cell lines *(9,10)*. The host environment promotes the constitutive activation of nuclear factor-kappaB (NF-κB) and proinflammatory cytokine expression during metastatic tumor progression of some murine cancer cells *(11)*. In addition, some tumor-derived proinflammatory cytokines can also induce cell adhesion molecule expression on endothelial cells, contributing to microvascular cancer cell adhesion *(12,13)*.

From: *Methods in Molecular Medicine, vol. 85: Novel Anticancer Drug Protocols*
Edited by: J. K. Buolamwini and A. A. Adjei © Humana Press Inc., Totowa, NJ

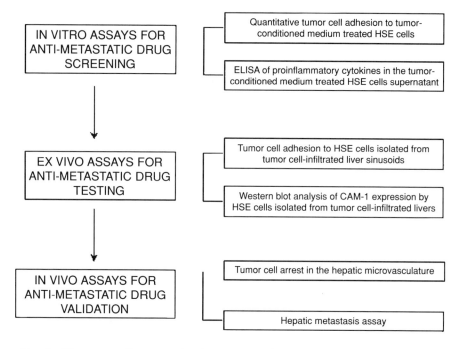

Fig. 1. Discovery of metastasis chemoprevention capacity. Biological testing of candidate antimetastatic drugs along a logical sequence of assays designed to character-ize their capacity to inhibit inflammatory responses of tumor-activated endothelial cells (hepatic sinusoidal endothelium) in vitro and ex vivo. Selected drugs are further tested for their ability to decrease circulating cancer cell arrest in the microvasculature of a target organ (liver) and to prevent metastatic implantation in vivo.

This mechanism may operate in vivo. In fact, a rapid induction of proinflam-matory cytokines and selectins in response to intrasplenic injection of different murine cancer cell type has been reported *(14)*. Thereafter, integrin receptor upregulation can be induced in tumor cell-infiltrated hepatic microvasculature *(15)*, accounting for all prometastatic activity of tumor-induced inflammatory cytokines, such as TNF-alpha, IL-1beta, and IL-18 *(8)*.

Thus, we propose the use of the inflammatory response of tumor-activated endothelial cells as a target-oriented strategy for the screening of chemical compounds with potential inhibitory effect on the mechanism of circulating cancer cell implantation in a target organ. The procedure for this biological testing of anti-metastatic activity involves the following sequence of studies. In vitro, we first determine the inhibitory effects of screened compounds on proinflammatory cytokine release, and subsequent adhesiveness of cancer cells, or endothelial cells treated with conditioned media from cancer cell cultures. Those compounds able to inhibit the above tested parameters would next be

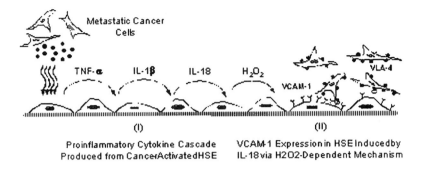

(I) Proinflammatory Cytokine Cascade Produced from CancerActivatedHSE

(II) VCAM-1 Expression in HSE Induced by IL-18 via H2O2-Dependent Mechanism

Fig. 2. Sequence of functional events occurring along the response of hepatic sinusoidal endothelium (HSE) cells to liver-infiltrating cancer cells. **(I)** Major proinflammatory cytokines are released as a hierarchical cascade from HSE cells upon activation by cancer cell-derived factors. **(II)** Interleukin-18-induced H_2O_2 accounts for VCAM-1 expression on HSE cells, and promotes adherence of VLA-4-expressing cancer cells. Cancer-endothelial cell adherence constitutes a key step for hepatic melanoma metastasis progression.

used ex vivo for determining their capacity to inhibit cell adhesion molecule expression and activity in endothelial cells isolated from tumor-infiltrated organs 18 h after cancer cell injection. Finally, to validate the antimetastatic action mechanism of most anti-adhesive compounds, we determine, in vivo, the cancer cell retention in the microvasculature of the target organ 18 h after cancer cell injection, and the metastatic foci density per unit of organ volume on d 12 after cancer cell injection (*see* **Fig. 1**).

In recent years, our research has been devoted to the study of prometastatic aspects of inflammation and, in particular, how cancer cells can usurp inflammatory response to progress along the metastatic process. In this respect, we have recently reported that the intrasinusoidal arrest of cancer cells is facilitated by tumor-derived factors increasing sinusoidal cell adhesion receptors for metastatic cells. These paracrine factors upregulate the sequential production of major proinflammatory cytokines, including IL-1beta, TNFalpha, and IL-18 in targeted endothelial cells. This upregulates VCAM-1 via H_2O_2, promoting adhesion to the endothelium of VLA-4-expressing cancer cells *(8,15)* (*see* **Fig. 2**). The relevance of the model is supported by the significant antimetastatic effects of cytokine blockade using specific soluble receptors, cell adhesion molecule interaction blockade using specific antibodies *(15)*, synthetic disintegrins *(16)*, and IL-1beta-converting enzyme (ICE) knock-out mice *(8)*.

On this basis, and because the liver is one of most frequent metastasis site organs of the human body *(17)*, the reported procedure will make use of hepatic sinusoidal endothelial (HSE) cells. These express several cell adhesion molecules in response to soluble paracrine factors released by metastatic cancer cells of different lineages *(8,14,15)*.

2. Materials

1. Male adult mice, 6–8 wk (C57Bl/6J, Balb/c).
2. Surgical instruments.
3. Nembutal.
4. Tumor cell lines: those cells able to secrete to their supernatants any endothelium-stimulating factor(s), as for example VEGF, proinflammatory cytokines, and PAF. Candidate murine cancer cell lines are: B16 melanoma cells (B16M cells), 51b-colon carcinoma cells, Pam 212 and LY2 squamous cell carcinoma cells, and the like.
5. Cell culture equipment and reagents: Hank's balance salt medium (HBSS), phosphate-buffered saline (PBS), Dulbecco's modified eagle medium (DMEM), fetal calf serum, and antibiotics (GIBCO, Grand Island, NY).
6. Hematoxylin and eosin.
7. Equipment for sinusoidal endothelial cells isolation: Perfusion equipment, enzymes (pronase E, collagenase IV, type I-DNasa), refrigerated centrifuge and metrizamide solutions for isopicnic centrifugal separation. Cells are allowed to recover for 24 h prior to analysis. Endothelial cells are cultured on collagen type I.
8. Reagents for Western Blot Analysis: RIPA buffer: 50 mmol/L Tris, pH 7.5, 150 mmol/L NaCl, 1% NP-40, 0.5% deoxycholic acid, 0.1% sodium dodecyl sulfate, 2 mmol/L ethylenediaminetetraacetic acid, 10 mmol/L NaF, 10 µg/mL leupeptin, 20 µg/mL aprotinin, 1 mmol/L phenylmethylsulfonyl fluoride. Antibodies: rat anti-mouse VCAM-1 monoclonal antibody (Serotec Ltd, Oxford), peroxidase-conjugated goat anti-rat IgG (Jackson ImmunoResearch, Baltimore, PA).
9. Equipment for retention assays: Luciferase assay kit (Promega Co, Madison, WI) and luminometer designed to read individual sample tubes (Bioorbit, LKB Wallac, Wallac Oy, Finland).
10. Equipment for adhesion assays: 2′,7′-bis-(2-carboxyethyl)-5,6-carboxyfluorescein-acetoxymethylester (BCECF-AM) solution (Molecular Probes Inc., Oregon, EEUU). Computed-assisted cell culture plate-scanning fluorimeter system.
11. Standard microdensitometer: An integrated microscopic image analysis system.
12. ELISA kits for cytokine analysis (R&D Systems, Minneapolis, MN).
13. Microplate reader.

3. Methods

3.1. In Vitro Assays for Anti-Metastatic Drug Screening

3.1.1. Quantitative Tumor Cell Adhesion to Endothelial Cells In Vitro

Time-dependent adhesion assays are carried out on a quantitative basis. For tumor cell pre-labelling, they are allowed to accumulate the non-fluorescent esterase substrate BCECF-AM (Molecular Probes, Eugene, OR) and to hydro-lyze it to its fluorescent product BCECF, which becomes trapped inside the living cells. To do this, 50 µg of BCECF-AM is dissolved in dry DMSO (5 µL) and diluted with DME medium (1.1 mL) to give 40 µg/mL. Tumor cells (5 × 10^6) are incubated in BCECF-AM solution at 37°C for 15 min. After gently washing tumor cells, they are resuspended in fresh medium (DMEM without phenol red) at a concentration of 2 × 10^6 cells/mL. Twenty-four hours post-plating primary cultured hepatic sinusoidal endothelial (HSE) cells are also used for the adhesion assay. They are incubated with tumor cell-conditioned medium (tumor-CM) in the presence or absence of inhibitors (drugs are tested at different doses and times) during 12 h. Then, the culture medium is replaced by fresh DME medium without phenol red. To determine the basal autofluorescence per well, the plates are read on a CytoFluor-2350 system (Millipore Co., Bedford, MA) using 485/22 nm excitation and the 530/25 nm emission filter at high and intermediate sensitivity settings. Then, 2 × 10^5 labeled tumor cells are added to each well of HSE cells and to collagen pre-coated control wells. However, in order to determine the exact number of cells in each well, the co-culture plates are read for a second time on the CytoFluor-system. Then, plates are incubated at 37°C and, some minutes later (it depends on the tumor cell line used in the assay), wells are washed with fresh medium (three times) and plates are read for a third time on the Cytofluor system. The number of adhered cells (registered in fluorescence arbitrary units) is expressed as percentage of the initial number of cells, and calculated for each well as follows: Fluorescence after well washing/(Fluorescence before washing—Nonspecific fluorescence before tumor cell addition). Each experiment is performed three times using three different preparations of HSE cells and three different preparations of tumor-conditioned media.

3.1.2. Measurement of Proinflammatory Cytokine Production from HSE Cells in Response to Tumor-Derived Factors In Vitro

Previously prepared untreated and tumor-CM-treated HSE cells are used. The supernatants from these cultures are collected at the end of the period of treatment with tested drugs, and prior to addition of other tumor cells to carry out the above reported adhesion assays. Then, concentrations of major pro-inflammatory cytokines (TNF-alpha, IL-1beta and IL-18) in all supernatants are measured using ELISA kits based on anti-mouse cytokine monoclonal antibodies, as suggested by the manufacturer (R&D Systems, Minneapolis, MN).

3.2. Ex Vivo Assays for Anti-Metastatic Drug Testing

3.2.1. Tumor Cell Adhesion to HSE Cells Isolated from Tumor Cell-Infiltrated Liver Sinusoids

Either three hundred thousand tumor cells in 0.1 mL HBSS or the same volume of tumor cell-free HBSS are intrasplenically injected into mice 18 h prior to HSE isolation. Before tumor cell injection, some mice of each group are treated with the test drug or its vehicle as specified by previous pharmacological and toxicological studies. The resulting HSE cells are cultured for 5 h to prevent the reversion to their original functional features. Then, adhesion assays with other BCECF-AM-labeled tumor cells are performed as described above.

3.2.2. Determination of VCAM-1 Expression in HSE Cells Isolated from Tumor Cell-Infiltrated Liver Sinusoids

VCAM-1 protein expression is determined ex vivo by Western Blot analysis. HSE cells are isolated again from mice pretreated with test drug or its vehicle and intrasplenically injected with tumor cells as described above. Then, freshly isolated HSE cells are washed with phosphate-buffered saline (PBS) and disrupted with RIPA buffer. Forty micrograms of protein is separated by 12% sodium dodecyl sulfate-polyacrylamide gel electrophoresis (SDS/PAGE) under reducing conditions and blotted onto a hybond ECL nitrocelulose membrane (Amersham Life Science, Little Chalfont, Buckinghamshire, England) using a semidry blotting apparatus (0.8 mA/cm^2, 30 min; Bio-Rad Laboratories, Richmond, CA). Blots are blocked using a 5% solution of nonfat dry milk in PBS and incubated with rat anti-mouse VCAM-1 monoclonal antibody (Serotec Ltd, Oxford) diluted 1 : 500 with PBS-5% milk during 2 h. Then, blots are washed three times (PBS/0.1% Tween 20) and the secondary antibody, peroxidase-conjugated goat anti-rat IgG (Jackson ImmunoResearch, Baltimore, PA) diluted 1 : 5000 with PBS-5% milk, is added for another 2 h. Finally, after washing the blots, VCAM-1 protein is visualized using a chemiluminescence system (Supersignal West Dura Extended Duration Substrate kit, Pierce, Rockford, USA), following the manufacturer's recommendations.

3.3. In Vivo Assays for Anti-Metastatic Drug Validation

3.3.1. Cancer Cell Arrest in the Hepatic Microvasculature In Vivo

Anti-adhesive properties during the capillary phase of metastasis are analyzed in vivo using a quantitative recording of intracapillary arrested luciferase-transfected tumor (luc-tumor) cells. First, tumor cells are permanently transfected by lipofection as previously described *(18)*, using plasmid pRc/cytomegalovirus (CMV)-luciferase, a construct containing the *Photinus pyralis* luciferase gene coding sequence under transcriptional control of the CMV promoter and the neomycin resistance gene encoding resistance to the G418 antibiotic (Life Technologies, Inc., Gaithersburg, Maryland). Mice are treated with test drug or its vehicle as specified by previous pharmacological and toxicological studies, at a dose and time necessary to inhibit the above described parameters. The mice are then intrasplenically injected with HBSS or 3×10^5 viable luc-tumor cells. Ten mice are used per experimental group. The mice are sacrificed by cervical dislocation 18 h later and livers are processed as previously described *(18)* to measure luciferase activity by chemiluminiscence using the standard luciferase assay kit (Promega Co, Madison, WI). The number of arrested cells are quantified, measuring light production using a luminometer designed to read individual sample tubes (Bioorbit, LKB Wallac, Wallac Oy, Finland) after the addition of 100 µL of luciferase assay reagent to 20 µL of each organ homogenate. Light detector measurements are expressed in relative light units (RLU), which are proportional to photon numbers. In order to evaluate linearity and sensitivity of light detection in liver homogenates, a standard plot is generated by measuring light production in a mixture which consists of a lysate from a predetermined number of tumor cells (ranging from 0 to 40×10^4 cells) and either a 20 µL aliquot from normal liver homogenate or same volume of reporter lysis buffer (RLB).

3.3.2. Hepatic Metastasis Assay

Hepatic metastases are produced by the intrasplenic injection into anesthetized mice (Nembutal, 50 mg/kg intraperitoneal) of 3×10^5 viable tumor cells suspended in 0.1 mL Hank's balanced salt solution (HBSS) *(3)*. Cell viability is assessed before injection using the Trypan blue exclusion test. One group of mice receives the test drug before tumor cell injection. Control mice receive the same volume of the vehicle in which the drug is dissolved. Mice are sacrificed by cervical dislocation on the 12th day after the injection of cancer cells. Liver tissue is processed for histology by immersion in 10% formaldehyde in phosphate buffered saline (pH 7.4) for 24 h at room temperature and are subsequently paraffin-embedded. For later morphometrical analyses, fifteen 4 µm-thick tissue sections of fixed liver (five groups, separated 500 µm) are stained with hematoxylin/eosin. An integrated image analysis system (Olympus Microimage 4.0 capture kit) connected to an Olympus BX51TF microscope is used to quantify the number, average diameter and position coordinates of metastases. Densitometric analysis of digitalized microscopic images is used to distinguish metastatic tissue from normal hepatic tissue. Previously described stereological procedures are employed *(3)* and the following parameters are calculated: the liver metastasis density, which is the number of metastases per 100 mm^3 of liver (based on the mean number of foci detected in fifteen 10×10 mm^2 sections per liver) and the liver metastasis volume (mean percentage of liver volume occupied by metastases). At least 15 mice are used per experimental group. The experiment is performed three times.

4. Notes

1. *Isolation and primary culture of HSE cells.* HSE cells are separated from mice, identified, and cultured as follows *(19)*: Hepatic tissue digestion is carried out by sequential perfusion of pronase and collagenase plus pronase solutions. The liver is then minced and stirred in another solution containing pronase, collagenase and DNase. Sinusoidal cells are separated in a 17.5% (w/v) metrizamide gradient at 800g and incubated in glutaraldehyde-treated human albumin-coated dishes for 30 min, as a selective adherence step for Kupffer cells. Non-adherent sinusoidal cells are re-plated on type I collagen-coated 24-well plates, at 1×10^6 cells/mL/well, and 2 h later are re-washed. HSE cell purity of resulting adherent sinusoidal cells is around 95% as checked by previously used identification parameters *(19)*: positive endocytosis (acetylated low density lipoprotein; ovalbumin), negative phagocytosis (1 μm latex particles), positive lectin binding site expression (wheat germ and viscum album agglutinins) and negative vitamin A storage (revealed by 328 nm UV-fluorescence). Cultures of HSE cells are established and maintained in pyrogen-free alpha-MEM supplemented with 10% FCS, 100 units/mL penicillin and 100 mg/mL streptomycin, at 37°C in a humidified atmosphere with 5% CO_2.

2. Tumor cell conditioned media (tumor-CM) are prepared as follows: 5×10^5 cells are plated in a 25 cm^2 T-flask and cultured in the above conditions for 24 h. Then, they are cultured in 5 mL serum-free medium for an additional period of 24 h (final cell density of 6×10^4 cells/cm^2) and its supernatant is collected, 25% fresh serum-free medium supplemented, and 0.22 μm-filtered. The endotoxin content of tumor-CM should be less than 20 pg/mL as measured by the *Limulus* lysate assay.

References

1. Fidler, I. J. (1989) Origin and biology of cancer metastasis. *Cytometry* **10,** 673–680.
2. Orosz, P., Echtenacher, B., Falk, W., Ruschoff, J., Weber, D., and Mannel, D. N. (1993) Enhancement of experimental metastasis by tumor necrosis factor. *J. Exp. Med.* **177,** 1391–1398.
3. Vidal-Vanaclocha, F., Amézaga, C., Asumendi, A., Kaplanski, G., and Dinarello, C. A. (1994) Interleukin-1 receptor blockade reduces the number and size of murine B16 melanoma hepatic metastases. *Cancer Res.* **54,** 2667–2672.
4. Lafrenie, R. M., Buchanan, M. R., and Orr, F. W. (1993) Adhesion molecules and their role in cancer metastasis. *Cell Biophys.* **23,** 3–89.
5. Balkwill, F and Mantovani, A. (2001) Inflammation and cancer: back to Virchow? *Lancet* **357,** 539–545.
6. Martín-Padura, I., Mortarini, R., Lauri, D., et al. (1991) Heterogeneity in human melanoma cell adhesion to cytokine activated endothelial cells correlates with VLA-4 expression. *Cancer Res.* **51,** 2239–2241.
7. Chirivi, R. G. S., Garofalo, A., Padura, I. M., Mantovani, A., and Giavazzi, R. (1993) Interleukin-1 receptor antagonist inhibits the augmentation of metastasis

induced by interleukin-1 or lipopolysaccharide in a human melanoma/nude mouse model. *Cancer Res.* **53,** 5051–5054.

8. Vidal-Vanaclocha, F., Fantuzzi, G., Mendoza, L., et al. (2000) IL-18 regulates IL-1beta-dependent hepatic melanoma metastasis via vascular cell adhesion molecule-1. *Proc. Natl. Acad. Sci. USA* **97,** 734–739.

9. Chen, Z., Colon, I., Ortiz, N., et al. (1998) Effects of IL-1alpha, IL-1Ra and neutralizing antibody on proinflammatory cytokine expression by human squamous cell carcinoma lines. *Cancer Res.* **58,** 3668–3676.

10. Köck, A., Schwarz, T., Urbanski, Z., et al. (1989) Expression and release of interleukin-1 by different human melanoma lines. *J. Natl. Cancer Inst.* **81,** 36–42.

11. Dong, G., Chen, Z., Kato, T. and Van Waes, C. (1999) The host environment promotes the constitutive activation of nuclear factor-kappaB and proinflammatory cytokine expression during metastatic tumor progression of murine aquamous cell carcinoma. *Cancer Res.* **59,** 3495–3504.

12. Burrows, F. J., Haskard, D. O., Hart, I. R., et al. (1991) Influence of tumor-derived interleukin-1 on melanoma-endothelial cell interactions in vitro. *Cancer Res.* **51,** 4768–4775.

13. Kaji, M., Ishikuro, H., Kishimoto, T., et al. (1995) E-selectin expression induced by pancreas-carcinoma-derived interleukin-1-alpha results in enhanced adhesion of pancreas-carcinoma cells to endothelial cells. *Int. J. Cancer* **60,** 715–717.

14. Khatib, A. M., Kontogiannea, M., Fallavolita, L., Jamison, B., Meterissian, S., and Brodt, P. (1999) Rapid induction of cytokine and E-selectin expression in the liver in response to metastatic tumor cells. *Cancer Res.* **59,** 1356–1361.

15. Mendoza, L., Carrascal, T., De Luca, M., et al. (2001) Hydrogen peroxide mediates vascular cell adhesion molecule-1 expression from interleukin-18-activated hepatic sinusoidal endothelium: Implications for circulating cancer cell arrest in the murine liver. *Hepatology* **34,** 298–310.

16. Danen, E. H., Marcinkiewicz, C., Cornelissen, I. M., et al. (1998) The disintegrin eristostatin interferes with integrin alpha 4 beta 1 function and with experimental metastasis of human melanoma cells. *Exp. Cell. Res.* **238,** 188–196.

17. Sugarbaker, E. V., Weingrand, D. N. and Roseman, J. M. (1982) Observations on cancer metastasis in man, in *Tumor Invasion and Metastasis* (Liotta, L. A. and Hart, I. R., eds.), Vol Nijhoff: The Jague: 427–465.

18. Rubio, N., Martinez-Villacampa, M. and Blanco, J. (1998) Traffic to lymph nodes of PC-3 prostate tumor cells in nude mice visualized using the luciferase gene as a tumor cell marker. *Lab. Invest.* **78,** 1315–1325.

19. Vidal-Vanaclocha, F., Rocha, M., Asumendi, A. and Barbera-Guillem, E. (1993) Isolation and enrichment of two sublobular compartment-specific endothelial cell subpopulations from liver sinusoids. *Hepatology* 18, 328–339.

10

Binding Assay for Selectins

Jianing Zhang and Michiko N. Fukuda

1. Introduction

Selectins form a group of C-type lectins, which bind to carbohydrates in a calcium dependent manner. Three selectins, E-, L-, and P-selectins are known. All selectins bind to sialyl Lewis X (sLe^x). E-selectin (endothelial cell adhesion molecule-1 or ELAM-1; CD62E) is expressed in the endothelial cells in response to inflammatory cytokines such as IL-1β or TNFα. E-selectin binds to the carbohydrate structure terminated by sialyl Lewis^x (sLe^x) and sialyl Lewis^a (sLe^a) *(1)*. Counter receptors recognized by E-selectin are expressed by neutrophils, monocytes, eosinophils, memory T-lymphocytes, and natural killer cells. E-selectin recruits these leukocytes to the inflammatory site. Characterization of E-selectin-deficient mice confirmed a critical role of E-selectin in acute inflammatory models *(2)*.

P-selectin (granule membrane protein GMP-140; CD62P) is found in platelets, in megakaryocytes and in the Weibel-Palade bodies of vascular endothelial cells *(3)*. P-selectin is released from these intracellular locations in less than 10 min upon stimulation with thrombin, or histamine, phorbol ester, or the calcium ionophore A23187 *(4)*. P-selectin is also transcriptionally regulated by inflammatory cytokines. P-selectin binds glycoprotein ligand, PSGL-1, containing fucosylated oligosaccharides as mucin-type core structure *(1)*.

L-selectin (MEL-14 antigen; CD62L) is present on lymphocytes and binds to sulfated sLe^x oligosaccharides of high endothelial venules in the peripheral lymph node *(1,5)*. This interaction is critical for lymphocyte recirculation from the intravascular to the lymphatic compartment.

From: *Methods in Molecular Medicine, vol. 85: Novel Anticancer Drug Protocols*
Edited by: J. K. Buolamwini and A. A. Adjei © Humana Press Inc., Totowa, NJ

Certain epithelial cancer cells express sLe^a and sLe^x as tumor-associated carbohydrate antigens *(6,17)*. In human lung and colon carcinomas, highly metastatic tumor cells express more sLe^x on the cell surface and bind more strongly to E-selectin than do their poorly metastatic counterparts *(6)*. Therefore, sLe^x may play a critical role in the metastasis of certain tumor cells. E- and P-selectins are also expressed on capillary endothelium during acute and chronic inflammation. These include immune complex-dependent acute lung injury, cardiac allografts, rheumatoid arthritis, wound sepsis, and skin inflammation. Acute inflammatory response mediated by E- or P-selectin was inhibited by sLe^x or glycopeptides containing sLe^x capping structure *(8,9)*.

The protocol described below is an in vitro assay developed by Weitz-Schmidt et al. *(10)*. We have been using this method for identifying new selectin ligands *(11)* and selectin-like carbohydrate binding protein. Standard E-, P-, and L-selectins and chemically defined and sensitive ligands are commercially available, which advances the described assay for many applications.

2. Materials
2.1. Selectins

1. Soluble and recombinant of E-, L-, and P-selectins are commercially available from Calbiochem (La Jolla, CA). One can also prepare recombinant selectins as follows *(11,12)*. The soluble chimeric forms of E-, L-, and P-selectin can be prepared by transfecting COS cells with pcDNA3 vector harboring selectin fused to Fc portion of IgG. Two days after transfection, culture supernatants of COS cells will be collected, passed through a Sepharose 4B column to remove non-specific binding to Sepharose, and then applied to a Protein A Sepharose column. After washing the protein A column with 20 mM phosphate buffer, pH 7.4, containing 0.2 M NaCl, the column-bound materials will be eluted with 0.2 M glycine-HCl buffer, pH 2.4. Thus in each fraction, 1 mL elution will be collected and neutralized by 0.2 mL of 1 M Tris-HCl buffer (pH 8.0). By absorbance at 280 nm of elution, positive fractions will be pooled and dialyzed against 20 mM phosphate buffer, pH 7.4, at 4°C overnight. Purified selectin: IgG chimeric protein will be aliquoted and stored at –80°C for several months. By this method, 500-mL culture supernatant from 1.0×10^8 transfected COS cells yielded 1.5 mg E-selectin : IgG chimeric protein. Purity of the preparation should be ascertained by sodium dodecyl sulfate-polyacrylamide gel electrophoresis (SDS-PAGE) followed by Coomassie blue staining.
2. Biotinylated PAA-sLe^x and biotinylated PAA-sLe^a (Glycotech, Rockville, MD) *(10)*.
3. Enzyme-linked immunosorbent assay (ELISA) plate (ICN Biomedicals INC, Aurora, OH).
4. ABTS peroxidase substrate (Pierce, Rockford, IL).

3. Methods

3.1. Selectin-Carbohydrate Ligand Binding Assay

1. A 96-well ELISA microtiter plate will be coated with 100 µL of E-, L-, or P-selectins (Calbiochem) at the concentration of 0.1~10 µg/mL in water at 4°C overnight.
2. Wash wells with tris-buffered saline (TBS) (20 mM Tris-HCl, pH 7.4, containing 0.2 M NaCl) three times.
3. Block wells with 3% bovine serum albumin (BSA) in TBS containing 1 mM CaCl$_2$ for 2 h.
4. Add biotinylated PAA-sLe^x (Glycotech), diluted to 0.5–5000 ng/100 µL with TBS containing 1 mM CaCl$_2$ to selectin coated well, and incubate at room temperature for 1 h.
5. Wash wells with TBS containing 1 mM CaCl$_2$.
6. Add 100 µL of peroxidase-conjugated avidin (Organon Teknika, West Chester, PA) (1 : 1000 diluted with TBS containing 1 mM CaCl$_2$) and incubate at room temperature for 30 min.
7. Wash plate with TBS containing 1 mM CaCl$_2$.
8. Add 100 µL of peroxidase substrate ABTS (Pierce, Rockford, IL).
9. Incubate at 37°C for 15–30 min to develop a green color.
10. Measure OD$_{405}$ by an ELISA reader.

3.2. Ligand Inhibition Assay

The potential selectin ligand can be tested. An example using synthetic peptides as inhibitor is described below.

1. Coat an ELISA plate with E-selectin IgG at 10 µg/mL (optimum condition determined above) at 4°C overnight.
2. Wash unbound E-selectin with TBS.
3. Block wells with 3% BSA TBS containing 1 mM CaCl$_2$ at room temperature for 2 h.
4. Add various amount of inhibitor together with 500 ng/100 µL (*see* **Note 1**) biotin-PAA-sLe^a (*see* **Note 2**) in TBS containing 1 mM CaCl$_2$. Incubate at room temperature for 1 h.
5. Wash plate with TBS containing 1 mM CaCl$_2$.
6. Add 100 µL of peroxidase-conjugated avidin (1 : 1000 diluted with TBS containing 1 mM CaCl$_2$) and incubate at room temperature for 30 min.
7. Wash plate with TBS containing 1 mM CaCl$_2$.
8. Add ABTS 100 µL to each well.
9. Incubate at 37°C for 15–30 min until green color develops.
10. Measure OD$_{405}$ in an ELISA reader.

See **Fig. 1** for an example.

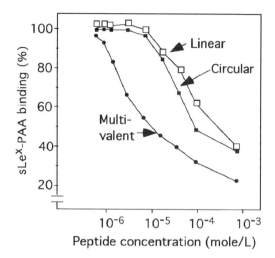

Fig. 1. Inhibition of PAA-sLe^x- biotin to E-selectin:IgG chimera in the presence of inhibitor, IELLQAR peptides. Linear, monomeris IELLQAR peptide; circular, C-IELLQAR-C with disulfide bond; multivalent, [IELLQAR]$_8$ linked to multivalent (8 branches) peptide core.

4. Notes

1. Titration of E-selectin and PAA-oligosaccharide is necessary for optimizing the inhibition assay. Choose the concentration of PAA-sLe^a which does not saturate selectin but high enough to see the inhibition. The sensitivity differs among the different lot of commercial PAA-oligosaccharides. Sialic acid is easily hydrolyzed by acid. If PAA-sLe^a or PAA-sLe^x are stored in –20°C freezer in solution, the pH should be checked by spotting the solution on pH paper.
2. In the above described assay, sLe^a was found to be a better ligand for E-selectin than sLe^x (*10*). Therefore the inhibition assays for E-selectin was carried out using PAA-sLe^a (*11*).

References

1. Lowe, J. B. (1997) Selectin ligands, leukocyte trafficking, and fucosyltransferase genes. *Kidney Int.* **51**, 1418–1426.
2. Frenette, P. S., Mayadas, T. N., Rayburn, H., Hynes, R. O., and Wagner, D. D. (1996) Susceptibility to infection and altered hematopoiesis in mice deficient in both P- and E-selectins. *Cell* **84**, 563–574.
3. McEver, R. P. (1989) GMP-140, a platelet a-granule membrane protein is also synthesized by vascular endothelial cells and is localized in Weibel-Palade bodies. *J. Clin. Invest.* **84**, 92–99.
4. Fukuda, M. and Hiraoka. N. (1999) C-type lectins and sialyl Lewis X oligosaccharides. Versatile roles in cell-cell interaction. *J. Cell Biol.* **147**, 467–470.

5. Kannagi, R. (1997) Carbohydrate-mediated cell adhesion involved in hematogenous metastasis of cancer. *Glycoconj. J.* **14,** 577–584.

6. Irimura, T., Nakamori, S., Matsushita, Y., et al. (1993) Colorectal cancer metastasis determined by carbohydrate-mediated cell adhesion: role of sialyl-Lex antigens. *Sem. Cancer Biol.* **4,** 319–324.

7. Lasky, L. A., Singer, M. S., Dowbenko, D., et al. (1992) An endothelial ligand for L-selectin in a novel mucin-like molecule. *Cell* **69,** 927–938.

8. Baumhueter, S., Singer, M. D., Henzel, W., et al. (1993) Binding of L-selectin to the vascular sialo mucin CD34. *Science* **262,** 436–438.

9. Weitz-Schmidt, G., Stokmaier, D., Scheel, G., Nifant'ev, N. E., Tuzikov, A. B., and Bovin, N. (1996) An E-selectin binding assay based on a polyacrylamide-type glycoconjugate. *Anal. Biochem.* **238,** 184–190.

10. Fukuda, M. N., Ohyama, C., Lowitz, K., et al. (2000) A peptide mimic of E-selectin ligand inhibits sialyl Lewis X-dependent lung colonization of tumor cells. *Cancer Res.* **60,** 450–456.

11. Sawada, R., Tsuboi, S., and Fukuda, M. (1994) Differential E-selectin-dependent adhesion efficiency in sublines of a human colon cancer exhibiting distinct metastatic potentials. *J. Biol. Chem.* **269,** 1425–1431.

11

Determination of Peak Serum Levels and Immune Response to the Humanized Anti-Ganglioside Antibody–Interleukin-2 Immunocytokine

Jacquelyn A. Hank, Jean E. Surfus, Jacek Gan, Amy Ostendorf, Stephen D. Gillies, and Paul M. Sondel

1. Introduction

Tumor reactive monoclonal antibodies (mAb) have been developed and tested as anti-tumor therapy. Some mAb have shown efficacy and are now approved as clinical cancer therapy. The mechanism of action for the antitumor effect includes tumor cell destruction by effector cells with Fc receptors such as natural killer (NK) cells and macrophages. These cells recognize the mAb binding to the tumor cells and mediate antibody-dependent cellular cytotoxicity (ADCC). Enhanced ADCC is mediated by effector cells that have been activated by exposure to the cytokine IL-2 (1). Thus, in murine models, enhanced tumor destruction is produced when tumor bearing animals are treated with a combination of antitumor mAb and IL-2 (2). Clinical testing of mAb and IL-2 is underway.

A more recent approach is attempting to improve on the efficacy of this combination by creating genetically engineered fusion proteins. A fusion protein linking an intact anti-tumor Ab and the cytokine IL-2 was designed in order to target the cytokine directly to the tumor in vivo (3). The hu14.18-IL-2 immunocytokine (IC) directly targets IL-2 to tumors expressing the disialoganglioside GD2. This ganglioside is expressed on neuroblastoma and melanoma cells. The humanized IC has a circulating half-life that is significantly longer than the half-life of IL-2, yet significantly shorter than

From: *Methods in Molecular Medicine, vol. 85: Novel Anticancer Drug Protocols*
Edited by: J. K. Buolamwini and A. A. Adjei © Humana Press Inc., Totowa, NJ

the half-life of the original humanized antibody *(4,5)*. This IC has substantial antitumor activity in animal models and is more effective than antibody or cytokine alone, and also more effective than the combination of antibody and cytokine as separate molecules *(6)*. Clinical testing of these humanized fusion proteins requires sensitive assays able to quantitate the intact Ab-IL-2 molecule in human serum. We have developed a sensitive enzyme-linked immunosorbent assay (ELISA) for quantitation of hu14.18-IL-2 *(7)*. In addition to the in vivo immune activation induced by the IC, it may be influenced by the antibody response made by the treated patient against the IC. To evaluate this, we have developed an ELISA to detect the generation of a specific immune response that blocks the ability of the IC to bind to its specific antigen, GD2. This assay, which detects the patient's antibody response to the IC will be used to determine if the generation of an immune response against the IC affects the half-life of the IC or affects the in vivo function, such as in vivo binding or activation of NK cells. The following protocols provide the detailed methods used for these two assays.

2. Materials
2.1. Detection of hu14.18-IL-2 Immunocytokine

1. Antibody-IL-2 immunocytokine, hu14.18-IL-2 (Lexigen Pharmaceuticals, Lexington, MA).
2. Murine anti-idiotypic antibody 1A7 (IgG1) specific for the 14.18 idiotype, obtained from K. Foon and M. Chatterjee, University of Cincinnati and Titan Pharmaceuticals, Inc (Scottsdale, AZ).
3. ELISA micro plates- C8 Maxisorp Nunc Immunomodules (Nunc, Roskilde, Denmark).
4. Sodium Bicarbonate Buffer: 0.795 g sodium carbonate (Na_2CO_3 - MW 105.99), 1.465 g sodium bicarbonate ($NaHCO_3$ - MW 84.01), 0.100 g sodium azide (NaN_3 - MW 65.01), 400 mL double distilled water, Adjust pH to 9.6 and bring up to 500 mL volume. May be stored indefinitely at +4°C.
5. Phosphate Buffered Saline (PBS, Sorensen's formula, 10X stock): 2.00 g potassium chloride (KCl - MW 74.56), 2.00 g potassium phosphate monobasic (KH_2PO_4 - MW 136.09), 80 g sodium chloride (NaCl - MW 58.44), 11.44 g sodium phosphate dibasic (Na_2HPO_4 - MW 142.0), 2.00 g sodium azide (NaN_3 - MW 65.01), Add double distilled H_2O up to 1000 mL. Stir and adjust pH to 7.2.
6. Washing buffer (1X PBS/0.05% Tween20): 200 mL 10X PBS stock, 1700 mL doubled distilled water, 1 mL Tween-20 (Sigma St. Louis, MO), Stir and adjust pH to 7.2, then bring up the volume to 2000 mL with double distilled water.
7. Blocking Buffer: Dissolve 5 g of nonfat dried milk (Carnation or other store brand) in 100 mL of 1X PBS (without Tween20) and mix thoroughly.
8. Sample Buffer: 2 g of nonfat dried milk mixed into 100 mL of washing buffer.

9. 100 mM Tris-HCl (10X stock): 121.14 g Tris (TRIZMA) base (MW 121.14), 2.00 g sodium azide (NaN$_3$ - MW 65.01), Add 900 mL double distilled water and after dissolving adjust pH to 7.4 with concentrated HCl. Bring volume up to 1000 mL with double distilled water.
10. Tris-Tween: 0.1 M Tris-HCl containing 0.05% Tween 20.
11. Goat anti-human IL-2 antibody coupled to biotin diluted to a concentration of 0.035 µg/mL in Tris-Tween (R and D Systems, Minneapolis, MN).
12. ExtrAvidin-alkaline phosphatase (Sigma, St. Louis, MO) diluted according to manufacturers specifications (1/5000) in Tris-Tween.
13. p-Nitrophenylphosphate (1 mg/mL in diethanolamine buffer, Sigma, St. Louis, MO).
14. Diethanolamine buffer (Alkaline phosphatase substrate buffer): Dissolve 245 mg of magnesium chloride (MgCl$_2$ - MW 95.21) in 400 mL of double distilled water. Add 48 mL of diethanolamine (C$_4$H$_{11}$NO$_2$ - MW 105.1), stir and adjust pH to 9.8 with concentrated HCl. Bring to a final volume of 500 mL with double distilled water. Store at +4°C in the dark.

2.2. Detection of Anti-Idiotypic Antibodies

1. ELISA micro plates, 96-well Falcon #3915 flat bottom polystyrene plates.
2. Disialoganglioside, GD2 (Advanced ImmunoChemical Inc, Long Beach CA) suspended in 100% ethanol at 2.5 ng/mL.
3. GD2 blocking buffer: (PBS with 3% human serum albumin and 0.05% thimerosal).
4. GD2 washing buffer: (PBS with 0.1% human serum albumin, 0.1% Tween 20 and 0.05% thimerosal).
5. Goat anti-human IL-2 antibody coupled to biotin diluted to a concentration of 0.0083 µg/mL in GD2 washing buffer (R and D Systems, Minneapolis, MN).
6. ExtrAvidin-HRP conjugate (Sigma-Aldrich Chemicals, St. Louis MO) diluted to 2 µg/mL, according to manufacturer's specifications.
7. TMB (Dako Chemicals, Carpinteria, CA) used according to manufacturers specifications.
8. Stop Solution: 2 M H$_2$SO$_4$.

3. Methods

3.1. Assay for Detection of hu14.18-IL-2 Immunocytokine (see Fig. 1)

3.1.1. Preparation of Plates

1. Coat ELISA micro plates overnight at 4°C with 120 µL per well of the anti-idiotypic antibody 1A7 (2 µg/mL) in sodium carbonate buffer (15 mM).
2. Wash the plates 3× with washing buffer.
3. Block the plates with 200 µL/well blocking buffer for 3 h at room temperature.
4. Wash the plates 3× with washing buffer.
5. Store blocked plates filled with washing buffer up to 1 mo.
6. Prior to use remove washing buffer from the microwells.

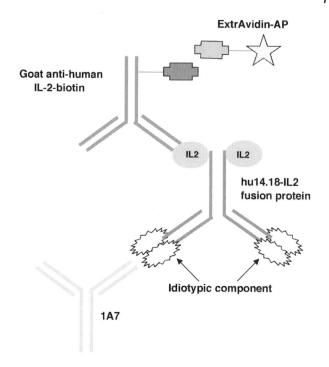

Fig. 1. Assay to detect hu14.18-IL-2 Immunocytokine: Antibody 1A7, specific for the idiotypic determinants of the 14.18 antibody, is used as the capture antibody in this sandwich ELISA. Immunocytokine bound to 1A7 is detected using a biotinylated goat anti-human IL-2 antibody, developed by ExtrAvidin-alkaline phosphatase.

3.1.2. Sample Collection and Preparation

1. Blood samples collected from patients are kept on ice until serum separation.
2. The blood collection tubes are spun in a centrifuge at $800-1500g$.
3. Separated serum is aliquoted at 0.5 mL/cryovial and stored at −20 to −80°C until use.

3.1.3. Preparation of Standards

1. Hu14.18-IL-2 fusion protein is thawed and diluted to 25 ng/mL (the highest standard) in Tris/Tween.
2. Prepare 5 serial twofold dilutions of the 25 ng/mL preparation in sample buffer containing 5% human serum.

3.1.4. Assay Procedure

1. Remove washing buffer from the microwells.
2. Add 100 μL of standards and experimental samples to duplicate wells.
3. Incubate the plates overnight at 4°C in a moist chamber.

4. Wash the plates 5× with washing buffer.
5. Add 100 µL of goat anti-human IL-2 antibody coupled to biotin.
6. Incubate plate for 3 h at room temperature in a moist chamber on an orbital shaker.
7. Wash the plates 5× with Tris-Tween.
8. Add 100 µL ExtrAvidin-alkaline phosphatase.
9. Incubate for 1 h at room temperature on the orbital shaker.
10. Wash the plates 5× with Tris-Tween.
11. Add 100 µL of *p*-nitrophenyl-phosphate as substrate to stain the plate.
12. Incubate the plate at room temperature in the dark for approximately 30 min.
13. Measure optical density (OD) at 405 nm with a 492 nm reference wavelength (OD 405/492) using an ELISA microplate reader.
14. Plot OD vs concentration for the standard curve.
15. Determine the concentration of intact immunocytokine in serum samples using linear regression or other curve fitting techniques (*see* **Note 2**).

3.2. Assay for the Detection of Anti-Idiotypic Antibodies (see Fig. 2)

1. Absorb 100 µL GD2 onto each well of the 96-well Falcon #3915 flat-bottom polystyrene plate (100 µL/well of a 2.5 ng/mL suspension for a final concentration of 250 pmol/well.)
2. Dry the plate overnight at room temperature under vacuum.
3. Block the plate with 200 µL of GD2 blocking buffer for 3.5 h at 37°C.
4. Wash the plate 4 times with GD2 wash buffer.
5. Mix hu14.18-IL-2 (250 ng/mL) with an equal volume of patient pre- and post-treatment serum as collected above (*see* **Note 1**).
6. Incubate the serum-hu14.18-IL-2 mixture at room temperature for 30 min.
7. Add 100 µL/well of the mixture to duplicate wells.
8. Incubate the plate for 2 h at 37°C.
9. Wash the plate 4× with GD2 washing buffer.
10. Add 100 µL/well biotinylated goat-anti-human-IL-2 antibody.
11. Incubate the plate for 2 h at 37°C.
12. Wash the plate 4× with GD2 washing buffer.
13. Add 100 µL/well of ExtrAvidin-HRP conjugate.
14. Incubate the plate for 1 h at 37°C.
15. Add 100 µL/well of TMB.
16. Incubate the plate for 10 min in the dark at room temperature with shaking.
17. Stop the reaction by adding 50 µL/well of STOP solution.
18. Read absorbance at a wavelength of 450 nm/570 nm reference wavelength (OD450/470) using an ELISA plate reader.
19. Determine % inhibition using the following formula

$$\% \text{ inhibition} = \frac{\text{OD pretreatment} - \text{OD posttreatment}}{\text{OD pretreatment sample}} \times 100$$

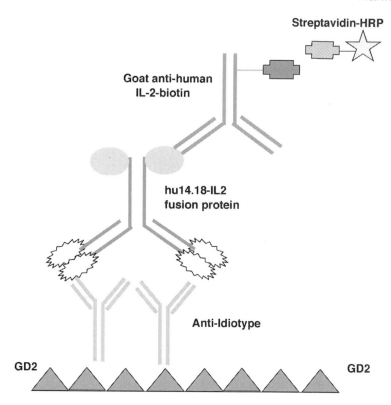

Fig. 2. Assay to detect anti-idiotypic antibody: Disialoganglioside GD2 antigen is used as the capture reagent in this sandwich ELISA. Patient serum is combined with a limiting concentration of hu14.18-IL-2 prior to addition to the antigen-coated plate. Anti-idiotypic antibodies in the serum block the antigen specific binding site of the hu14.18-IL-2 and inhibit the binding of the IC to GD2. Immunocytokine bound to GD2 is detected using a biotinylated goat anti-human IL-2 antibody, developed by Streptavidin-HRP. To ensure a specific anti-idiotypic response the level of binding achieved with a patient sample obtained following treatment must be compared to the binding seen with a baseline pretreatment sample.

4. Notes

1. Serum Sampling: A baseline serum sample obtained prior to any administration of hu14.18-IL-2 ("pre") is used for a negative control in the assay to detect hu14.18-IL-2. It is also used to determine the background level in the assay to detect anti-idiotypic antibody. We have found that intact IC is detectable in serum for up to 12–14 h following a 4-h continuous infusion of hu14.18-IL-2. Peak levels of IC are seen in samples obtained during a 4-h continuous infusion. When assaying to detect anti-idiotypic antibody, it is best to use serum specimens obtained at times when the patient should not have detectable hu14.18-IL-2

circulating in the serum. Sufficient time should be allowed for the patient to mount an antibody response. We have seen significant levels of anti-idiotypic antibodies in the serum obtained from some patients at one, two and three weeks following an initial course of treatment. We have also seen antibody responses develop following a second course of therapy that were not seen following the initial course.

2. Data Analysis: In the hu14.18-IL-2 detection assay above, the quantity of hu14.18-IL-2 can be accurately determined in absolute amounts. The standard curve can be constructed by plotting the OD vs the concentration and performing linear regression. In some ELISA assays, this standard method may not be the most appropriate method. There are currently a number of computer software packages that offer a range of curve fitting techniques for handling ELISA data. The software we are currently using is Magellan, available from Tecan in Salzburg Austria.

3. Interpreting the data from the second assay, the binding inhibition assay, which detects antibodies specifically able to block the binding of the immunocytokine to GD2 coated plates is more complex. The initial results are reported in OD values. The OD value obtained with a serum sample obtained prior to treatment with the immunocytokine is compared with the OD values obtained with a serum sample obtained following treatment. The serum is mixed with a limiting amount of the IC (125 ng/mL final concentration). Serum obtained prior to treatment should not inhibit or block the ability of the IC to bind to GD2, while serum containing anti-idiotypic antibodies will specifically inhibit the ability of the IC to bind to the GD2 coating the plate. This assay must be accurately calibrated so that the quantity of hu14.18-IL-2 used in **step 5** of **Subheading 3.2.** is not in excess, but results in an OD reading within the mid to high end of the linear portion of the regression line obtained with serial dilutions of hu14.18-IL-2 IC binding to GD2 coated plates. Patient pretreatment serum should not have pre-existing anti-IC antibody, and thus should not be able to specifically block binding of hu14.18 to GD2. Thus, the level of 14.18-IL-2 binding noted with pretreatment serum is considered 100%. As an assay control, it is helpful to monitor antibody known to block the specific binding. **Fig. 3** shows the concentration dependent specific inhibition of IC binding to GD2 using samples containing increasing concentrations of the murine anti-idiotypic antibody 1A7.

4. In this assay used to detect antibodies to the IC, the serum sample is diluted 1:2 with the suspension of hu14.18-IL-2. Once antibodies are detected, the serum can be diluted further to determine how far the sample can be diluted and still facilitate effective blocking, or the level of inhibition can be compared to a known concentration of 1A7 achieving the same level of inhibition.

5. Assay specificity: The high specificity of these assays and the very low background levels are attributed to the use of an anti-IL-2 reagent to detect the hu14.18-IL-2 IC. This system also ensures that both the antibody component and the IL-2 component of the "fusion protein" are present. In the process of developing these assays, we initially tested a goat anti-human IgG1 reagent as

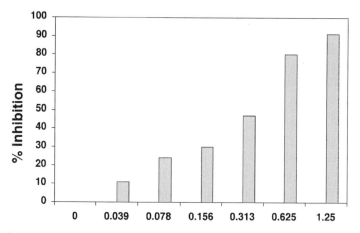

Concentration of Mouse Monoclonal Anti-Idiotype Antibody (µg/mL)

Fig. 3. Concentration dependent specific inhibition of hu14.18-IL-2 binding to GD2 by the murine monoclonal 1A7 antibody: The assay described in **Fig. 2** was run using increasing concentrations of the 1A7 anti-idiotypic antibody as a blocking reagent. 100 percent binding of hu14.18-IL-2 (in the absence of any 1A7) gave an OD reading of 1.83. The percent inhibition achieved was determined using the following formula.

$$1 - \frac{\text{OD with 1A7}}{\text{OD without 1A7}} \times 100$$

the secondary reagent of this "sandwich" ELISA to detect the IgG1 component of the hu14.18-IL-2 bound to 1A7 or GD2 on the plate. Under these conditions, some patients' pretreatment serum showed high background levels. It has been reported that the prevalence of anti-mouse antibodies in serum from healthy individuals may be as high as 40% *(8)*. These anti-mouse antibodies may bind to the 1A7 used to capture the IC and contribute to a high background level if the assay is developed with an antibody to human Ig.

References

1. Hank, J. A., Robinson, R. R., Surfus, J., et al. (1990) Augmentation of antibody dependent cell mediated cytotoxicity following in vivo therapy with recombinant Interleukin-2. *Cancer Res.* **50,** 5234–5239.
2. Reisfeld, R. A. (1992) Monoclonal antibodies in cancer immunotherapy. *Clin. Lab. Med.* **12,** 201–216.
3. Lode, H. N. Xiang, R., Becker, J. C., Gillies, S. D., and Reisfeld, R. A. (1998) Immunocytokines: a promising approach to cancer immunotherapy. *Pharmacol. Ther.* **80,** 277–292.

4. Gillies, S. D., Young, D., Lo, K. M., and Roberts, S. (1993) Biological activity and in vivo clearance of antitumor antibody/cytokine fusion proteins. *Bioconj. Chem.* **4,** 230–235.

5. Kendra, K., Gan, J., Ricci, M., et al. (1999) Pharmacokinetics and stability of the ch14.18-interleukin-2 fusion protein in mice. *Cancer Immunol. Immunother.* **48,** 219–229.

6. Lode, H. N., Xiang, R., Dreier, T., Varki, N. M., Gillies, S. D., and Reisfeld, R. A. (1998) Natural killer cell-mediated eradication of neuroblastoma metastases to bone marrow by targeted interleukin-2 therapy. *Blood* **91,** 1706–1715

7. Gan, J., Kendra, K., Ricci, M., Hank, J. A., Gillies. S. D., and Sondel, P. M. (1999) Specific enzyme-linked immunosorbent assays for quantitation of antibody-cytokine fusion proteins. *Clin. Diagnost. Lab. Immunol.* **6,** 236–342.

8. Carpenter, B. A. (1992) Enzyme-Linked Immunoassays, in *Manual of Clinical Laboratory Immunology*, 4th Ed. (Rose, N., deMacario, E. C., Fahey, J. L., Friedman, H., and Penn, G. M., eds.) American Society for Microbiology Press, Washington, DC, pp. 2–9.

IV

IMMUNOHISTOCHEMICAL ASSAYS IN THE CLINICAL SETTING

12

Immunohistochemical Determination of EGFR-Tyrosine Kinase Inhibition in Clinical Samples

Shazli N. Malik, Roble G. Bedolla, Manuel Hidalgo, Michael G. Brattain, and Jeffrey I. Kreisberg

1. Introduction

The epidermal growth factor receptor (EGFR) family consists of four closely related transmembrane receptors including the EGFR (erbB1), erbB2 (HER2), erbB3 (HER3), and erbB4 (HER4). EGFR (erbB1) was the first member to be described and sequenced (*1*). The EGFR is a 170 kDa plasma membrane glycoprotein composed of a single polypeptide chain of 1186 amino acids (*2,3*). The receptor consists of an extracellular ligand-binding domain, a transmembrane lipophilic segment, and an intracellular tyrosine-kinase (TK) domain (*4*). Binding of the ligands such as epidermal growth factor (EGF) and transforming growth factor α (TGFα) to the extracellular ligand-binding domain results in receptor dimerization, activation of its intrinsic TK activity and autophosphorylation of the receptor (*2*). These effects lead to activation of a signal transduction cascade of biochemical and physiological changes that culminate in DNA synthesis, cell division, and inhibition of apoptosis (*2*).

EGFR is expressed in all epithelial and many mesenchymal cells. It has a wide range of functions depending on the tissue's origin and state of differentiation (*3*). Dysregulation of the EGFR and EGFR-family signal transduction pathways has been implicated to play a critical role in the pathogenesis of multiple human tumors (*5–7*), including non-small cell lung, breast, prostate, gastrointestinal, pancreatic, and ovarian carcinomas. Increased expression of EGFR is generally associated with invasion, metastasis, late stage disease,

From: *Methods in Molecular Medicine, vol. 85: Novel Anticancer Drug Protocols*
Edited by: J. K. Buolamwini and A. A. Adjei © Humana Press Inc., Totowa, NJ

chemotherapy and hormone therapy resistance, and poor outcome *(7,8)*. Because of the involvement of EGFR tyrosine kinase (EGFR-TK) signal transduction pathways in a variety of tumors, this pathway has become a key target for anti-cancer drug design *(9–13)*. Currently, there are several compounds in clinical and pre-clinical development that specifically target tyrosine kinase phosphorylation. These compounds fall into several categories: (a) small molecule kinase inhibitors, (b) monoclonal antibodies, (c) bi-specific and single chain antibodies, (d) immunotoxin conjugates, and (e) antisense oligonucleotides.

The effect of these therapies can be assessed in target tissues by obtaining consecutive pre- and post-treatment biopsy specimens from the patients treated with the above agents. Levels of total and phosphorylated EGFR expression are determined in both specimens by immunohistochemistry. Expression of phosphorylated EGFR is determined with an antibody to phosphorylated EGFR (Y1173). The degree of EGFR-TK phosphorylation inhibition is assessed by comparing the baseline level of expression of total EGFR and phosphorylated EGFR in the pre-treatment biopsy specimen versus the level of expression in the post-treatment specimen.

2. Materials

1. Oven.
2. Plus coated slides (Fisher Scientific).
3. Xylene.
4. Graded alcohols 100%, 95%, 80%.
5. Distilled water.
6. Humidified chamber.
7. Gauze, 4×4.
8. Coplin jars.
9. Proteinase K (DAKO).
10. 1X TBS-T: 0.05 M Tris-HCl, pH 7.6, 0.15 M NaCl, 0.1% Tween20.
11. Quench solution: 0.1% sodium azide (NaN_3) in 3% H_2O_2 in 1X TBS-T.
12. 10% bovine serum albumin (BSA).
13. 1% BSA.
14. Primary diluent: 1X TBS-T, 10X BSA, 0.1% NaN_3.
15. LSAB2 system, Peroxidase (DAKO).
16. DAB (Diaminobenzidine substrate chromogen).
17. DAB enhancer (Signet).
18. Hematoxylin.
19. Polymount, xylene based.
20. Cover slips.
21. Total EGFR antibody (Zymed) dilution 1:40.

22. Catalyzed Signal Amplification kit, Peroxidase (DAKO).
23. Catalyzed Signal Amplification ancillary kit (DAKO): (a) Target retrieval solution, (b) Avidin-biotin block, (c) Antibody diluent with background reducing components, (d) 10X TBS-T: 0.05 M Tris HCl, 0.3 M NaCl, 0.1% Tween 20.
23. Phosphorylated EGFR antibody Y1173 (Calbiochem) dilution 1:50.

3. Methods

3.1. Specimen Processing

1. Fix fresh biopsy specimens in 10% neutral buffered formalin for 24 h.
2. Process in tissue processor and embed in paraffin.
3. Cut 2-µm thick sections and place on plus coated slides.

3.2. Immunohistochemistry for Total EGFR

1. Heat sections to 60°C for 30 min.
2. Rehydrate in xylene and graded alcohols.
3. Perform antigen retrieval by incubating slides in Proteinase K for 5 min.
4. Rinse slides sequentially in PBS and TBS-T.
5. Quench endogenous peroxidase activity by incubating in TBS-T containing 0.1% sodium azide and 0.3% hydrogen peroxide for 15 min.
6. Rinse slides 3× with TBS-T.
7. Incubate with primary antibody (EGFR 1:40) diluted in primary diluent for 90 min in a humidified chamber.
8. Rinse slides 3× with TBS-T.
9. Incubate with biotinylated secondary antibody from LSAB2 kit for 15 min.
10. Rinse slides 3× with TBS-T.
11. Incubate with streptavidin from LSAB2 kit for 15 min.
12. Rinse slides 3× with TBS-T.
13. Incubate with diaminobenzidine (DAB) chromogen substrate containing DAB enhancer for 10 min.
14. Counter stain slides with hematoxylin.
15. Rinse once in tap water followed by one rinse in TBS-T, followed by another rinse in tap water.
16. Dehydrate in graded alcohols, clear with xylene and mount with xylene-based permanent mounting medium.

3.3. Immunohistochemistry for Phosphorylated EGFR

A specialized staining system from DAKO called catalyzed signal amplification (CSA) system is required for staining with the anti-phospho-EGFR (Y1173) antibody. This system is an extremely sensitive immunohistochemical staining procedure incorporating a signal amplification method based on the peroxidase catalyzed deposition of a biotinylated phenolic compound, followed by a secondary reaction with streptavidin peroxidase.

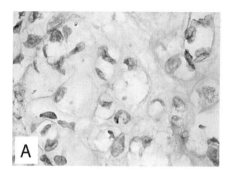 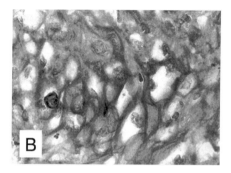

Fig. 1. Immunoperoxidase staining for total EGFR in squamous cell carcimona of the skin. **(A)** Tissue treated with isotypic negative control showing no staining. **(B)** Same tissue treated with anti-EGFR antibody showing strong membrane staining.

1. Follow **Subheading 3.2., steps 1** and **2**.
2. Perform antigen retrieval by placing slides in a coplin jar containing target retrieval solution (DAKO) in a water bath previously heated to 95°C. Incubate for 20 min.
3. Allow slides to cool for 20 min.
4. Rinse 3× with TBS-T.
5. Perform avidin-biotin block: (a) Incubate slides in avidin for 10 min. Rinse 3× in TBS-T, (b) Incubate slides in biotin for 10 min. Rinse 3× in TBS-T.
6. Start staining procedure following instructions from CSA kit.

3.4. Quantitation of Staining

The total EGFR and phosphorylated EGFR can be semi-quantitatively assessed by scoring the intensity of staining from 0 (no staining), 1+ (weakly-positive staining of tumor cells), 2+ (moderately positive staining of tumor cells), and 3+ (strongly positive staining of tumor cells). In addition, percent of tumor cell staining can be recorded by counting the total number of cells staining in a particular field vs the total number of cells present in that field. The ratio is described as percentage. Positive staining for total EGFR is defined as membrane, and phospho-EGFR as membrane, cytoplasmic, and nuclear staining of tumor cells (*see* **Fig. 1** and **2**). Computerized software is also available for quantitation of the above staining.

4. Notes

1. Sections should be air dried for 24 h prior to starting the immunohistochemistry procedure.
2. At any step, sections should not be allowed to dry out. This results in nonspecific staining.

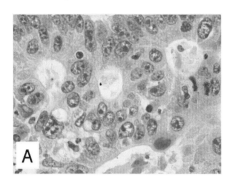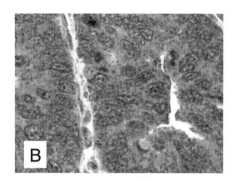

Fig. 2. Immunoperoxidase staining for phosphorylated EGFR in human colon cancer. (**A**) Tissue treated with isotypic negative control showing no staining. (**B**) Same tissue treated with anti-phosphorylated EGFR antibody showing membrane and cytoplasmic staining.

References

1. Ullrich, A., Conssens, L., Hayflick, J. S., et al. (1984) Human epidermal growth factor receptor cDNA sequence and aberrant expression of the amplified gene in A431 epidermoid carcinoma cells. *Nature* **309,** 418–425.
2. Carpenter, G. and Cohen, S. (1990) Epidermal growth factor. *J. Biol. Chem.* **265,** 7709–7712.
3. Wells, A. (1999) EGF receptor. *Int. J. Biochem. Cell Biol.* **31,** 637–643.
4. Ullrich, A. and Schlessinger, J. (1990) Signal transduction by receptors with tyrosine kinase activity. *Cell* **61,** 203–212.
5. Wells, A. (2000) Tumor invasion: role of growth factor-induced cell motility. *Adv. Cancer Res.* **78,** 31–101.
6. Khazaie, K., Schirrmacher, V., and Lichtner, R. B. (1993) EGF receptor in neoplasia and metastasis. *Cancer Metastasis Rev.* **12,** 255–274.
7. Salomon D. S., Brandt R, Ciardiello F., and Normanno, N. (1995) Epidermal growth factor-related peptides and their receptors in human malignancies. *Crit. Rev. Oncol. Hematol.* **19,** 183–232.
8. Ebert, A., Wechselberger, C., Martinez-Lacaci, I., Bianco, C., Weitzel, H. K., and Salomon, D. S. (2000) Expression and function of EGF-related peptides and their receptors in gynecological cancer—from basic science to therapy. *J. Recept. Signal Transduct. Res.* **20,** 1–46.
9. Wikstrand, C. and Bigner, D. (1998) Prognostic applications of the epidermal growth factor receptor and its ligand, transfroming growth factor-alfa. *J. Natl. Cancer Inst.* **90,** 799–800.
10. He, Y., Zeng, Q., Drenning, S. D., Melhem, M. F., et al. (1998) Inhibition of human squamous cell carcinoma growth in vivo by epidermal growth factor receptor antisense RNA transcribed from the U6 promoter. *J. Natl. Cancer Inst.* **90,** 1080–1087.

11. Redemann, N., Holzmann, B., von Ruden, T., Wagner, E. F., Schlessinger, J., and Ullrich, A. (1992) Anti-oncogenic activity of signalling-defective epidermal growth receptor mutants. *Mol. Cell. Biol.* **12,** 491–498.
12. Mendelsohn, J. (1997) Epidermal growth factor receptor inhibition by a monoclonal antibody as anticancer therapy. *Clin. Cancer Res.* **3,** 2703–2707.
13. Bos, M., Mendelsohn, J., Kim, Y. M., Albanell, J., Fry, D. W., and Baselga, J. (1997) PD153035, a tyrosine kinase inhibitor, prevents epidermal growth factor receptor activation and inhibits growth of cancer cells in a receptor number-dependent manner. *Clin. Cancer Res.* **3,** 2099–2106.
14. Noonberg, S. and Benz, C. (2000) Tyrosine kinase inhibitors targeted to the epidermal growth factor receptor subfamily: role as anticancer agents. *Drugs* **59,** 753–767.
15. Lawrence, D. and Niu, J. (1998) Protein kinase inhibitors: the tyrosine-specific protein kinases. *Pharmacol. Ther.* **77,** 81–114.

13

Immunohistochemical Assays of Farnesyltransferase Inhibition in Patient Samples

Alex A. Adjei

1. Introduction

As a result of early reports indicating that farnesylation was required for maturation of Ras proteins, there has been extensive interest in farnesyl-transferase (FT) as a potential target of antineoplastic therapy *(1–3)*. At the present time, three different FT inhibitors (FTIs), SCH66336, R115777, and BMS-214662, are undergoing clinical testing. Phase III studies with R115777 in pancreatic and colorectal cancer have completed accrual. Because the FTIs are among the first potential anticancer drugs that inhibit aberrantly activated signal transduction pathways in neoplastic cells, there is considerable interest in assessing their cellular effects in the clinical setting. A variety of assays have been proposed for this purpose.

Conceptually, the simplest assay for FT inhibition involves preparing extracts from FTI-treated cells and measuring the remaining ability of FT to farnesylate a substrate polypeptide. These assays are being performed in conjunction with some FTI trials. However, they are relatively cumbersome and difficult to implement in the setting of large multi-institutional clinical trials.

Other potential assays evaluate the inhibition of processing of other FT substrates. Of the numerous farnesylated polypeptides, the co-chaperone protein HDJ-2 *(4)* and the intranuclear intermediate filament protein lamin A *(5)* are known to undergo mobility shifts when FT is inhibited *(6,7)*, and have been shown to be appropriate markers of FT inhibition *(8)*. The evaluation of the accumulation of prelamin A in buccal mucosa cells by immunohistochemistry represents a simple assay that can be performed in conjunction with large

From: *Methods in Molecular Medicine, vol. 85: Novel Anticancer Drug Protocols*
Edited by: J. K. Buolamwini and A. A. Adjei © Humana Press Inc., Totowa, NJ

clinical trials. This assay can also be utilized to examine fresh tumor cells. Prelamin A is not expressed in all tissue types. Thus, it is absent from peripheral blood mononuclear cells and a number of leucocyte precursors. Prelamin A is also variably expressed in leukemic blasts. In these instances, evaluation of HDJ-2 by Western blotting *(8)* can be performed. In summary, mobility shifts in the co-chaperone protein HDJ-2 is universally applicable to all tissues. Prelamin A accumulation by immunohistochemistry is simple and more convenient for use in large clinical trials, provided the tissue type being examined contains lamin A.

2. Materials

1. Primary antibodies: (i) Monoclonal anti-human lamin A *(9)*, (ii) Polyclonal anti-human prelamin A antibody. This antibody was generated in our laboratories as follows: A high titer polyclonal serum that recognizes the carboxyl terminal domain of human prelamin A was raised by immunizing rabbits with the peptide CLLGNSSPRTQSPQN coupled to keyhole limpit hemocyanin as described by Sinensky et al. *(10)*.
2. Secondary antibodies: Affinity-purified Rhodamine-conjugated anti-mouse IgG, Fluorescein-conjugated anti-rabbit IgG. From Kirkegaard & Perry (Gaithersburg, MD).
3. Tongue depressors.
4. Microscope slides (Superfrost,™ Fischer Scientific).
5. Phosphate Buffered Saline (PBS).
6. Acetone.
7. Buffer A: (10% (w/v) powdered milk in 150 mM NaCl, 10 mM Tris-HCl, pH 7.4, at 21°C, 100 U/mL penicillin G, 100 µg/mL streptomycin, and 1 mM sodium azide.
8. Zeiss LSM 310 confocal microscope (Carl Zeiss, Inc., New York, NY).
9. Digital camera.

3. Methods

3.1. Buccal Mucosa Sampling

The patient has no food for approximately 15 min prior to this procedure.

1. On the day of FTI treatment, patients should gently swish and spit approximately 100 mL of saline, and repeat. This is done to clear the mouth of food debris and proteases.
2. Firmly scrape the inside of the patient's mouth with a clean wooden tongue depressor (*see* **Note 1**).
3. Spread the scraped cells on a clean charged microscope slide (Superfrost+, Fischer Scientific). Using a fresh tongue depressor each time, the scraping and deposition is repeated until a total of four slides are obtained.

4. Air dry these buccal smears for 30 min, and fix in acetone (−20°C for 15 min) (*see* **Note 2**). Samples can then be stored in buffer A until immunohistochemistry is performed.

5. Repeat this procedure after the patient has been on an FTI for the appropriate number of days.

3.2. Immunohistochemistry

1. Treat cells with a mixture of murine monoclonal anti-lamin A (1:3000) and rabbit anti-prelamin A (1:750) in buffer A at 4°C for 12–16 h.

2. Remove the primary antibodies, and wash the samples 6× with PBS over a 20-min period.

3. Incubate for 30 min with a mixture of affinity-purified rhodamine-conjugated anti-mouse IgG and fluorescein-conjugated anti-rabbit IgG (20 µg/mL each).

4. Wash 6× with PBS over a 20-min period.

5. Mount in Vectashield (Vector Laboratories, Burlingame, CA) and seal with clear nail polish, and examined on a Zeiss LSM 310 confocal microscope (Carl Zeiss, Inc., New York, NY).

6. With each batch of buccal mucosa cells, A549 cells treated with FTI or diluent are included as positive and negative controls, respectively. Sensitivity of the photomultiplier tubes on the confocal microscope should be adjusted so that the signal for prelamin A in diluent-treated A549 cells is just below the limit of detection, a result consistent with the appearance of the specimens by conventional fluorescence microscopy. With the sensitivity of the confocal microscope fixed at this level (*see* **Note 3**), all other specimens can then be examined in the conventional and laser scanning modes. Images can subsequently be imported into Adobe Photoshop or appropriate software for processing. Any adjustments to brightness or contrast should be applied identically to paired samples harvested prior to and after therapy with FTIs (*see* **Figs. 1** and **2**).

4. Notes

1. Buccal mucosa should be scraped firmly, otherwise there is a chance of not obtaining any cells on the slide.

2. Once air-dried, the slide with buccal mucosa cells should be fixed in acetone within 3 h, to prevent proteolytic degradation of prelamin A.

3. Because of the nature of computer-image analysis, the importance of maintaining the same microscopic settings throughout the entire experiment cannot be overemphasized. In particular, the amount of illumination should be standardized for the entire experiment. The microvessels are thin and transparent and thus appear bright in the photomicrograph.

4. This method can be applied to the evaluation of inhibition of other protein targets such as epidermal growth factor receptor, with one caveat: the protein of interest should be known to be expressed consistently in buccal mucosa cells.

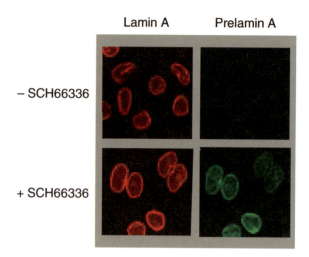

Fig. 1. Evaluation of prelamin A processing in cultured cells. One week after reaching confluence, A549 cells were incubated for 24 h with diluent (top row) or 200 nM SCH66336 (bottom row). After the cells were fixed in acetone, double label indirect immunofluorescence was performed using monoclonal anti-lamin A (left) and polyclonal antiserum that recognizes the precursor peptide at the carboxyl terminus of lamin A (right). The incubation with primary antibodies was performed in the absence (top two rows) or presence (bottom row) of 10 µg/mL CLLGNSSPRTQSPQN, the peptide that was utilized to raise the prelamin A-specific serum. In each row, the same field was imaged using excitation wavelengths of 568 nm (left) or 488 nm (right).

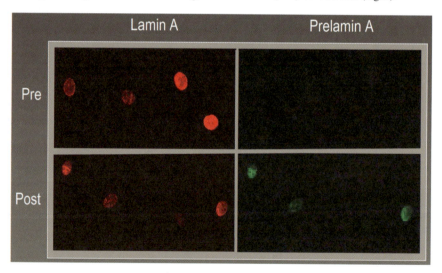

Fig. 2. Detection of prelamin A in buccal mucosa cells from an SCH66336-treated patient. Buccal smears were double labeled with mouse anti-lamin A (left) and rabbit anti-prelamin A (right) followed by fluorochrome-labeled secondary antibodies. Corresponding fields were photographed. The patient was treated with 200 mg b.i.d. of SCH66336 for 7 d. Top panel, pretreatment sample; Bottom panel, sample taken on morning of d 8.

5. This method should not be applied to the evaluation of prelamin A accumulation in lymphocytes or leukemic cells, since these cells do not consistently possess any lamins. In these situations other methods of assessing FT inhibition such as evaluation of the accumulation of unfarnesylated HDJ-2 *(8)* or the evaluation of FT enzyme inhibition *(11)*, should be utilized.
6. When tumor tissues from biopsy material are utilized, prelamin A accumulation can be evaluated by Western blotting. Unfarnesylated HDJ-2 can also be evaluated by Western blotting in tumor tissues or peripheral blood mononuclear cells *(8)*.

Acknowledgment

The author is a Research Scholar of the American Cancer Society.

References

1. Cox, A. D. and Der, C. J. (1997) Farnesyltransferase inhibitors and cancer treatment: targeting simply Ras? *Biochim. Biophys. Acta* **1333,** F51–F71.
2. Gibbs, J. B. and Oliff, A. (1997) The potential of farnesyltransferase inhibitors as cancer chemotherapeutics. *Ann. Rev. Pharmacol. Toxicol.* **37,** 143–166.
3. Gelb, M. H., Scholten, J. D., and Sebolt-Leopold, J. S. (1998) Protein prenylation: from discovery to prospects for cancer treatment. *Curr. Opin. Chem. Biol.* **2,** 40–48.
4. Neckers, L., Mimnaugh, E., and Schulte, T. W. (1999) Hsp90 as an anti-cancer target. *Drug Resist. Updat.* **2,** 165–172.
5. Sinesky, M., Fantle, K., Trujillo, M. A., et al. (1994) The processing pathway of prelamin A. *J. Cell Sci.* **107,** 61–67.
6. Sinensky, M., Fantle, K., and Dalton, M. (1994) An antibody which specifically recognizes prelamin A but not mature lamin A: application to detection of blocks in farnesylation-dependent protein processing. *Cancer Res.* **54,** 3229–3232.
7. Britten, C. D., Rowinsky, E., Yao, S.-L., et al. (1999) The farnesyl protein transferase (FPTase) inhibitor L-778,123 in patients with solid cancers. *Proc. Am. Soc. Clin. Oncol.* **18,** 155A.
8. Adjei, A. A., Davis, J. N., Erlichman, C., Cutler, D., Svingen, P. A., and Kaufmann, S. H. (2000) Comparison of potential markers of farnesyltransferase inhibition. *Clin. Cancer Res.* **6,** 2318–2325.
9. Loewinger, L. and McKeon, F. (1988) Mutations in the nuclear lamin proteins resulting in their aberrant assembly in the cytoplasm. *EMBO J.* **7,** 2301–2309.
10. Sinensky, M., Fantle, K., and Dalton, M. (1994) An antibody which specifically recognizes prelamin a but not mature lamin A: application to detection of blocks in farnesylation-dependent protein processing. *Cancer Res.* **54,** 3229–3232.
11. Karp, J. E., Lancet, J. E., Kaufmann, S. H., et al. (2001) Clinical and biologic activity of the farnesyltransferase inhibitor R115777 in adults with refractory and relapsed acute leukemias: a phase I clinical-laboratory correlative trial. *Blood* **97,** 3361–3369.

V

Protein Chaperoning/Degradation Protocols

14

Assays for HSP90 and Inhibitors

Wynne Aherne, Alison Maloney, Chris Prodromou,
Martin G. Rowlands, Anthea Hardcastle, Katherine Boxall,
Paul Clarke, Michael I. Walton, Laurence Pearl, and Paul Workman

1. Introduction

The molecular chaperone HSP90 is currently under investigation as a promising target for anticancer drug discovery. It constitutes 1–2% of total cellular protein and is present in the cell as a dimer in association with a number of other proteins *(1)*. HSP90 is involved in ensuring adequate protein folding and preventing non-specific aggregation of proteins following chemical mutation or stress *(2)*. Under physiological conditions, together with its endoplasmic reticulum homolog GRP94, HSP90 plays a housekeeping role in the cell, maintaining the conformational stability and maturation of several key client proteins, including oncogenic kinases (e.g., ERBB2, RAF-1, CDK4, and LCK), steroid receptors, and mutant TP53 *(3)*. A number of HSP90 inhibitors have already been identified. These include the benzoquinone ansamycin natural product geldanamycin and its analog, 17-allylamino-17-demethoxy-geldanamycin (17AAG), together with the chemically dissimilar natural product radicicol. The predominant mechanism of action of these agents involves binding to HSP90 at the ATP binding site in the N-terminal domain of the protein, leading to inhibition of the intrinsic ATPase activity of HSP90 *(4–6)*. Inhibition of HSP90 ATPase activity prevents recruitment of co-chaperones and encourages the formation of a type of HSP90 heterocomplex from which these client proteins are targeted for degradation via the ubiquitin proteosome pathway *(3,7)*. Treatment with HSP90 inhibitors leads to selective degradation of important proteins involved in cell proliferation, cell cycle regulation, and apoptosis, processes which are fundamentally important in cancer *(8)*. It is

From: *Methods in Molecular Medicine, vol. 85: Novel Anticancer Drug Protocols*
Edited by: J. K. Buolamwini and A. A. Adjei © Humana Press Inc., Totowa, NJ

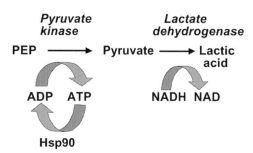

Fig. 1. The pyruvate kinase/lactate dehydrogenase linked assay for the measurement of HSP90 ATPase activity

these events following HSP90 inhibition that are believed to be responsible for the antitumor activity of HSP90 inhibitors in cell culture and animal models *(7,9)*. Currently, 17AAG is in Phase I clinical trial jointly in our Center and the Royal Marsden Hospital (in association with Cancer Research Campaign UK and the United States National Cancer Institute), and also at other centers in the United States.

In this chapter, a number of procedures to assess HSP90 function and its inhibition are described. Two methods that have been developed to measure the intrinsic ATPase activity of HSP90 are detailed, using yeast HSP90 as a model system. The first method utilizes a regenerating coupled enzyme assay and the second assay, based on the use of malachite green for the measurement of inorganic phosphate, was designed for high throughput screening (HTS) to identify novel HSP90 inhibitor drug candidates. Molecular markers indicative of HSP90 inhibition have been identified by us and other groups *(10,11)*, and these can be readily measured using Western blotting techniques. A cell-based ELISA (enzyme-linked immunosorbent assay), similar to those described for other proteins and post-translational modifications *(12,13)*, has also been developed in our laboratory. This technique provides an alternative higher throughput assay for determining pharmacodynamic endpoints during the evaluation of novel HSP90 inhibitors synthesized at the lead optimization stage of the drug development process. The assay may also prove useful as a cell-based primary screen for the identification of compounds that inhibit HSP90 by a non-ATPase directed mechanism.

1.1. Coupled Enzyme Assay

The ATPase assay is performed using the pyruvate kinase/lactate dehydrogenase linked assay described by Ali et al. *(14)*, the basis of which is shown in **Fig. 1**. The ADP that is generated by HSP90 is phosphorylated by pyruvate kinase, utilizing phosphoenol pyruvate as substrate, to produce ATP and pyruvate as products (*see* **Notes 1–4**). Pyruvate is then converted to lactic acid by lactate dehydrogenase utilizing NADH. This consumption of NADH leads to a decrease in UV absorbance at 340 nm, monitored spectrophotometrically. Thus for every mole of ADP that is generated by the ATPase activity of HSP90, one mole of NADH is utilized. It should be noted that prior to the addition of HSP90, the enzyme system converts any contaminating ADP present in the ATP substrate to ATP. This is important for enzymes such as HSP90 that show a stronger affinity for the binding of ADP than ATP.

1.2. Malachite Green Assay

Colorimetric assays for the determination of phosphate, based on the formation of a phosphomolybdate complex, can be carried out in a few steps with inexpensive reagents, and are well suited to the automation required for high throughput screening *(15)*. Enzymes that release inorganic phosphate are assayed using the reaction of the cationic dye, malachite green, with the phosphomolybdate complex to generate a blue-green color with an absorbance maximum at 610 nm *(16–18)*. The method has been used in both high throughput *(19)* and ultra-high throughput screening formats *(20)*. However, this method is complicated by the non-enzymatic hydrolysis of ATP in the presence of acidic malachite green reagent, causing an increase in color *(21,22)*. This process is mediated by molybdate and can be overcome by the addition of sodium citrate immediately after adding the reagent *(23–25)*. We have used this modification to the 96-well microtiter plate assay previously described for other ATPases *(23)* to produce the following protocol for HSP90 ATPase, which we employ for high throughput screening.

1.3. Assessment of Molecular Markers of HSP90 Inhibition Using Western Blotting

The cellular effects of HSP90 inhibitors can be measured using a number of molecular markers. As already mentioned, HSP90 inhibition leads to the depletion of several important cellular signalling proteins. RAF-1 is readily detectable by Western blotting and has been shown to be depleted in a number of human tumor cell lines following exposure to HSP90 inhibitors *(7–9,11)*. Depletion is normally observed by 6 h, with maximum depletion occurring at 24 h (*see* **Fig. 2**). In addition to RAF-1, depletion of several other HSP90 client proteins can be measured by immunoblotting, e.g., CDK4 and ERBB2. However, it is important to note that some of these proteins are cell line specific, e.g., ERBB2, is expressed mainly in breast, thyroid, kidney, and some ovarian

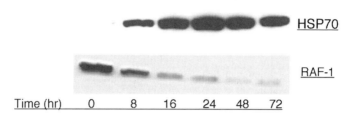

Fig. 2. RAF-1 depletion and HSP70 induction following 17AAG treatment (60 n*M*, equivalent to 5× IC$_{50}$) of A2780 human ovarian cancer cells

tumor cell lines. Another very important marker of HSP90 inhibition is heat shock protein 70 (HSP70). A HSF-1 (heat shock factor 1) dependent increase in HSP70 levels has been reported by us and other groups *(10,11)*, and this effect can serve as a positive indicator of HSP90 inhibitor action (*see* **Fig. 2**). The immunoblotting method described is based on standard techniques but is described in detail for ease of reference.

1.4. Assessment of Molecular Markers of HSP90 Inhibition Using ELISA

Although Western blotting has become a universally used technique for evaluating the level of protein expression in cell lines and tissue lysates, the number of samples that can be included on each gel is limited. In addition, relatively large numbers of cells are required to detect proteins expressed at a low level and precise quantitation is difficult. Cell-based ELISA methods *(12,13)* offer several advantages for evaluating the pharmacodynamic effects of novel mechanism-based inhibitors and may be the method of choice for comparing inhibitors identified during the iterative process of lead identification and optimization. The technique can be used to rapidly rank the effectiveness of compounds as well as to investigate the molecular mechanisms of their action. The increased sample throughput possible with ELISA means that compounds can be simultaneously studied in multiple replicates at different doses and exposure times. Also, the number of cells required per observation can be greatly reduced compared to those required for immunoblotting. The assays are carried out directly on cells grown and treated in microtiter plates, thereby removing the necessity for preparing cell lysates. ELISA techniques can in theory be applied to any cellular protein or post-translational modification for which an antibody is available and results are at least semi-quantitative. The ELISA protocol we use for assessing HSP70 expression following exposure of cells to HSP90 inhibitors is described in **Subheading 3.4.**

2. Materials

2.1. Coupled Enzyme Assay

Materials are of the highest purity available commercially.

1. 1 M Tris-HCl buffer, pH 7.5.
2. 100 mM KCl.
3. 100 mM MgCl$_2$.
4. 10 mg/mL phosphenol pyruvate (PEP, Roche, 108 294) stored at 4°C.
5. 4 mg/mL ATP (Sigma, A-9187) stored at –20°C.
6. 35.5 mg/mL NADH (Roche, 837 075) stored at 4°C.
7. 10 mg/mL pyruvate kinase (Roche, 109 045) stored at 4°C.
8. 10 mg/mL lactate dehydrogenase (Roche, 127 221) stored at 4°C.
9. 15 mM geldanamycin (in 100% DMSO), freshly prepared.

2.2. Malachite Green Assay

Chemicals are of the highest purity commercially available and all aqueous solutions are made up in analytical reagent grade (AR) water. Because of the need to minimize contamination with inorganic phosphate, precautions should be taken with solutions and apparatus used in the assays. Glassware and pH meters are rinsed with double distilled or deionized water before use and, wherever possible, plasticware should be used. Gloves are worn for all procedures.

1. Immulon 96-well (Thermo Labsystems) or Cliniplate 384-well flat-bottomed polystyrene multiwell plates (Thermo Labsystems).
2. Assay buffer: 100 mM Tris-HCl, pH 7.4, 20 mM KCl, 6 mM MgCl$_2$, stored at 4°C.
3. Malachite green (0.0812% w/v) (Sigma M 9636), stored at room temperature.
4. Polyvinyl alcohol USP (2.32% w/v) (Sigma P 1097) in boiling water (*see* **Note 5**), allowed to cool and stored at room temperature.
5. Ammonium molybdate (5.72% w/v) in 6 M hydrochloric acid, stored at room temperature.
6. Sodium citrate (34% w/v), stored at room temperature.
7. ATP, disodium salt, special quality (Boehringer Mannheim 519979), stored at 4°C.
8. HSP90 protein purified to >95% purity (6) and stored at –80°C as 10 μL aliquots containing 0.5 mg of protein.

2.3. Assessment of Molecular Markers of HSP90 Inhibition Using Western Blotting

1. 17AAG, geldanamycin and radicicol are stored as 2 mM stocks in DMSO at –20°C.
2. Human tumor cell lines grown in Dulbecco's modified Eagle's medium (DMEM) supplemented with 4500 mg/mL glucose, 10% fetal bovine serum (FBS), 200 mM

L-glutamine and 5 mL non-essential amino acids in a humidified atmosphere of 5% CO_2 at 37°C.

3. Lysis buffer: 150 mM NaCl, 50 mM Tris-HCl (pH 7.5), 1% NP40, 0.2% w/v sodium dodecyl sulphate (SDS), 2 mM phenylmethylsulfonyl fluoride (PMSF), 10 µg/L aprotinin, 10 µg/L leupeptin, 1 mM sodium orthovanadate, 0.5 mM dithiothreitol (DTT), 0.5 mM NaF, 0.5 mM β-glycerophosphate. Prepare as required and store at –20°C.

4. Bicinchoninic acid (BCA) protein assay reagents (PerBio Science UK, Ltd).

5. Casein blocking buffer: 0.5% casein, 0.02% thiomersal in phosphate buffered saline (PBS). Store at 4°C up to 2 wk.

6. Wash buffer: phosphate buffered saline (PBS) containing 0.05% Tween 20.

7. Tris-glycine gradient polyacrylamide precast gels (4–20%) (1 mm thick) (Novex).

8. Nitrocellulose membrane (0.2 µm pore size) (InVitrogen).

9. Ponceau Red stain: 2% w/v in 30% trichloroacetic acid (TCA)/30% bovine serum albumin (BSA) (Sigma).

10. Enhanced chemiluminescence (SuperSignal) reagents (PerBio Science UK, Ltd).

11. Photographic film (Hyperfilm ECL, Amersham Pharmacia Biotech).

2.4. Assessment of Molecular Markers of HSP90 Inhibition Using ELISA

1. Human tumor cell lines (e.g., HCT116 and HT29 colon carcinoma cells) cultured as described above (*see* **Subheading 2.3.**).

2. 96-well clear microtiter tissue culture plates (Falcon).

3. DMSO diluted in dH_2O (8% v/w).

4. HSP90 inhibitors at required concentration dissolved in DMSO.

5. Fixing solution: 0.25% glutaraldehyde, 3% paraformaldehyde and 0.25% Triton-X 100.

6. Blocking solution: 5% dried milk (Marvel) in PBS, prepared daily.

7. Anti-HSP70 monoclonal antibody (Stressgen, SPA 810).

8. DELFIA® wash buffer, enhancement solution, assay buffer and Europium labelled anti-mouse IgG (1244–1330) from PerkinElmer Life Sciences.

9. BCA protein assay reagents (Perbio Science UK Ltd.).

3. Methods

3.1. Coupled Enzyme Assay

1. Mix together 10 mL of 1 M Tris buffer, pH 7.5, 20 mL of 100 mM KCl and 6 mL of 100 mM $MgCl_2$. This is buffer A, and is kept at 37°C for the duration of the assay and then discarded at the end of each day.

2. Maintain some distilled water (dH_2O) at 37°C.

3. Dissolve 12.8 mg of ATP in 2 mL of buffer A and place on ice.

4. Dissolve 10 mg of PEP in 1 mL of buffer A and place on ice.

5. Add 0.25 mL of buffer A to 8.9 mg of NADH and place on ice.

6. Place the pyruvate kinase and lactate dehydrogenase on ice.
7. To the reference cuvet add 360 µL of buffer A, 520 µL of dH$_2$O, 80 µL of ATP, and 40 µL of PEP solution.
8. To the test cuvets add 360 µL of buffer A, 490 µL of dH$_2$O, 80 µL of ATP, 40 µL of PEP, 20 µL of pyruvate kinase, and 2 µL of lactate dehydrogenase solutions.
9. Mix the contents of the cuvets and zero the absorbance at 340 nm. Then add 2 µL of the NADH, and the absorbance should increase. Follow the reaction at 37°C until a stable baseline is obtained.
10. Add the HSP90 to the test cuvets and adjust the volume of the cuvets to 1 mL with dH$_2$O and follow the decrease in the absorbance at 340 nm using a suitable spectrophotometer, e.g., Shimadzu UV-240.
11. Add 2 µL of geldanamycin and follow the decrease in the absorbance at 340 nm (*see* **Note 1**). The HSP90 ATPase activity is given by the difference between the rates in **steps 9** and **10** (*see* **Note 2**).
12. The rate of the reaction (moles/min/mL) is derived from $\Delta OD/(1000 \times 6200\,M^{-1}\,cm^{-1})$, where the value 6200 is the extinction coefficient of NADH. This can be converted to specific activity (mole ATP/min/mg) or turnover (moles/min/mole) by dividing the rate by the mg or molar amount of HSP90 used in the reaction.

3.2. Malachite Green Assay

1. On the day of use, prepare the malachite green reagent from the stock solution. Mix two parts of malachite green with one part each of polyvinyl alcohol and ammonium molybdate and two parts of water. Initially, the reagent is a dark brown color, but after standing at room temperature for about 2 h, it attains a golden yellow color and is ready for use.
2. For the high throughput screening assays, the test compounds are dissolved at 200 µM in 2.0% DMSO, and contained in daughter plates derived from the chemical libraries. Transfer 5 µL of each sample from the daughter plate to each well of the assay plate using automated equipment (*see* **Note 7**). This represents a final concentration in the well of 40 µM. The first and last rows of the 96-well plate contain solvent only and represent the control and background values, respectively.
3. In order to determine an IC$_{50}$ value, prepare a range of stock concentrations of the compound in DMSO. Five appropriate concentrations are used depending on the relative potency of each compound. Transfer a 1 µL aliquot of each concentration to the wells of the assay plate and add 4 µL of the assay buffer.
4. Dissolve the ATP in the assay buffer to give a stock concentration of 2.5 mM and store at room temperature.
5. Add a 10 µL aliquot to each well to give a final assay concentration of 1 mM.
6. Just before use, thaw the HSP90 protein on ice and suspend in chilled assay buffer to a stock concentration of 0.25 mg/mL and keep on ice. Start the incubation by adding 10 µL of stock HSP90 to each well, except for the background wells, which receive 10 µL of assay buffer, giving a final assay volume of 25 µL.

7. Shake the plates (approx 2 min) using a plate shaker (e.g., Wellmixx, Thermo Labsystems) or MTS4 (IKA-Schuttler), seal them with plastic film and incubate for 3 h at 37°C.

8. To stop the incubation, add 80 µL of the malachite green reagent to each well and shake the plate again.

9. Add 10 µL of 34% sodium citrate (*see* **Note 6**) to each well and shake again. This leads to the development of the blue-green color in the controls, while the backgrounds are yellowish.

10. Measure the absorbance at 620 nm using a suitable plate reader (e.g., Victor[2], Perkin Elmer Life Sciences). Under the above conditions, the control absorbance value is 0.7–1.0, while the background is 0.15–0.20, signal to noise ratio of ~30. The Z′ factor *(26)* calculated from data obtained using these conditions was 0.8, indicating an assay highly suitable for screening purposes.

3.3. Assessment of Molecular Markers of HSP90 Inhibition Using Western Blotting

1. Lyse cells (approx 4×10^6 cells) in 100 µL of lysis buffer for 30 min on ice. When adding the lysis buffer, shear cells by pipetting up and down using a Gilson P200 pipet.

2. Spin lysates for 1 min at 13, 000g at 4°C, retrieve supernatant and store at –70°C.

3. Determine protein concentration using BCA protein assay reagents.

4. Load samples of cell lysates (50 µg protein/lane) onto gel and separate proteins by SDS-polyacrylamide gel electrophoresis (SDS-PAGE) using a 4–20% Tris-glycine gel.

5. Transfer proteins to nitrocellulose membrane using optimum conditions for the equipment available. In our laboratory we use 150 mA for 2 h and the Mighty Small transfer system (Hoeffer). At this stage, the membrane is usually stained with Ponceau Red solution for 5 min to visualize protein bands and to check for equal loading.

6. Block the blotted nitrocellulose membrane in casein blocking buffer for at least 1 h at room temperature with constant agitation (e.g., using a Gyro-Rocker STR9, Stuart).

7. Dilute all primary antibodies to the recommended dilution (*see* **Table 1**) in the casein blocking buffer and incubate with the nitrocellulose membrane overnight at room temperature with agitation.

8. Wash the nitrocellulose membrane twice for 10 min each with wash solution and incubate in the appropriate enzyme-labelled secondary antibody (*see* **Table 1**) for 1 h at room temperature with agitation. Both anti-mouse and anti-rabbit secondary antibodies were diluted 1:1000 in casein blocking buffer.

9. Wash the nitrocellulose membrane 4× for 10 min each with wash solution.

10. Visualize the protein bands using enhanced chemiluminescence reagents as described by the manufacturer and expose to photographic film (usually requires 1–5 min exposure).

Table 1
Sources and Dilutions of Antibodies Used for Western Blotting

Marker protein	Company	Primary antibody dilution	Secondary Antibody (all from Amersham Pharmacia Biotech)
Polyclonal rabbit RAF-1 (C-19)	Santa Cruz	1 : 500	Anti-rabbit-IgG-HRP
Polyclonal rabbit LCK	UpState Biotechnology	1 : 5000	Anti-rabbit-IgG-HRP
Monoclonal mouse HSP70 SPA-840	Stressgen	1 : 1000	Anti-mouse-IgG-HRP

3.4. Assessment of Molecular Markers of HSP90 Inhibition Using ELISA

1. Plate 190 µL of cells (42,000 cells/mL; 8000 cells/190 µL/well) manually or using a Multidrop dispenser (Thermo Labsystems).
2. Incubate the cells for 36 h at 37°C in a 5% CO_2 air mixture.
3. Add 10 µL of 8% DMSO (control) or compound dissolved in 8% DMSO to each well (this results in a final concentration of 0.4% DMSO in each well).
4. Incubate the cells in the presence of DMSO or compound for up to 48 h.
5. 'Flick out' the medium by hand and fix and permeabilize the cells by the addition of 100 µL fixing solution. Incubate at 37°C for 30 min.
6. Wash the plates twice in PBS using an automated washer (Wellwash 5000 ten plate stacker-washer or Wellwash Ascent single plate washer, Thermo Labsystems).
7. Block the plates by addition of blocking solution (100 µL) and incubate for 30 min.
8. Add 100 µL of primary antibody diluted to 0.95 µg/mL in PBS to each well and incubate the plate for 1.5 h. Wash the plates once with DELFIA® wash solution.
9. Add 100 µL of Europium labelled anti-mouse IgG diluted in DELFIA® assay buffer to 75 ng/mL and incubate for 1 h. Wash plates once with DELFIA® wash solution as before.
10. Add 100 µL of DELFIA® enhancement solution to each well.
11. Measure the fluorescence (615 nm) in Victor[2] 1420 multilabel counter (Perkin-Elmer Life Sciences) using the time-resolved measurement mode.
12. Wash the plates once with PBS, and measure protein concentration by the addition of 200 µL of BCA reagent to each well, shake for 1–2 min and incubate for 30 min at 37°C. Read absorption at 570 nm.
13. Express the ELISA results by normalizing to protein in the well (Eu counts (cpm) divided by OD_{570}). Compare the effect of HSP90 inhibitors on HSP70 expression with DMSO treated controls.

4. Notes
4.1. Coupled Enzyme Assay

1. Details of the purification of the yeast HSP90 protein have previously been described *(6)*. The ATPase activity of the yeast HSP90 at 37°C is ~0.7 moles ATP/min/mg protein. Relative to other ATPases, this activity is very low and consequently HSP90 preparations must be highly purified.
2. To show that the ATPase activity that is measured is because of HSP90 rather than background contaminating ATPase activity, the activity must be shown to be geldanamycin sensitive.
3. All assays are conducted in triplicate with a HSP90 concentration of 2 µ*M*.
4. This assay is relatively time consuming and throughput is consequently low. Each assay takes around 60 min to complete.

4.2. Malachite Green Assay

5. The polyvinyl alcohol dissolves in boiling water with difficulty, and stirring for 2–3 h is required.
6. The time interval between addition of the malachite green reagent and the sodium citrate should be kept as short as possible in order to reduce the non-enzymatic hydrolysis of ATP. Once the sodium citrate is added, the colour is stable for up to 4 h at room temperature.
7. Compounds can be added to the assay plates using a Rapidplate 96/384 (Zymark). A Multidrop 384 dispenser (Thermo Labsystems) can be conveniently used to add reagents to the plate.
8. The assay conditions were optimized with respect to time, protein, and substrate concentration in order to achieve linearity of enzyme activity under the described protocol.
9. The above assay protocol is used with 96-well plates, but a reduction in volumes readily allows the use of 384-well plates.
10. To determine specific activity of HSP90, a range of inorganic phosphate concentrations (0–10 µ*M*) are prepared and the absorbance at 620 nm measured as described. Specific activity is calculated from the resulting calibration curve.

4.3. Assessment of Molecular Markers of HSP90 Inhibition Using Western Blotting

11. The protein bands are normally evaluated visually. Densitometry has proved to be an unreliable method for the evaluation of HSP70 expression as the intensity of the band can exceed the linear range of the photographic film.
12. It is important to note when choosing the time points for the experiment that in some cell lines RAF-1 protein levels recover after 24 h.
13. Western blotting is currently being utilized in a 17AAG Phase I clinical trial to analyze these pharmacodynamic markers in peripheral blood lymphocytes and tumor tissue to determine whether the compound is acting via its proposed mechanism of action.

14. RAF-1 is not expressed in all peripheral blood lymphocytes and shows inter-patient variation (unpublished observations). We have found that the best marker for examining client protein depletion in peripheral blood lymphocytes is the tyrosine kinase, LCK.

15. Increased expression of HSP70 following HSP90 inhibition can also be measured at the messenger RNA level. We have published methodology for determining the affects of HSP90 inhibitors on the expression of HSP70 and other genes using microarray analysis *(11)*.

4.4. Assessment of Molecular Markers of HSP90 Inhibition Using ELISA

16. Cells plated in 96-well plates are incubated in a plastic box to reduce evaporation from the outside wells. In addition, ELISA incubation steps are carried out in a 37°C laboratory incubator and in a moist environment, e.g., plastic box lined with damp tissue paper.

17. All additions to the microtitre plate can be achieved using a multichannel pipette or for larger numbers of plates an automated dispenser such as a Multidrop (Labsytems).

18. For convenience, if the effects of compounds are being studied at several time points the ELISA can be carried out in batches, plates being stored (in a container) at 4°C following the fixation step. In this case the plates are washed only once following fixation and again immediately before the first ELISA step (*see* **Subheading 3.4., step 6**). In addition all the plates can be stored for subsequent protein determination.

19. In our hands, reproducibility of both the measured Europium counts and the protein measurements is between 10–15% (CV).

20. We have routinely used DELFIA® reagents *(27)* in our cell-based ELISAs. This endpoint provides high sensitivity and the time-resolved measurements reduce interference from non-specific fluorescence. However, it is also possible to use a horse radish peroxidase secondary antibody conjugate and either a colorimetric (e.g., tetramethylbenzidine) or chemiluminescent reagent (e.g., ECL reagent, Amersham Pharmacia Biotech) for endpoint measurement.

21. It is recommended that a blank consisting of secondary antibody only (i.e., no primary antibody) together with an appropriate primary antibody control (e.g., isotype matched IgG) are included in assays during the process of optimizing reagent concentrations.

References

1. Pratt, W. B. (1997) The role of the Hsp90-based chaperone system in signal transduction by nuclear receptors and receptors signalling via MAP kinase. *Annu. Rev. Pharmacol. Toxicol.* **37**, 297–326.

2. Smith, D. F., Whitesell, L., and Katsanis, E. (1998) Molecular chaperones: biology and prospects for pharmacological intervention. *Pharmacol. Revs.* **50**, 493–513.

3. Neckers, L., Schulte, T. W., and Momnaaugh, E. (1999) Geldanamycin as a potential anti-cancer agent: its molecular target and biochemical activity. *Invest. New Drugs* **17,** 361–373.

4. Prodromou, C., Roe, S. M., O'Brien, R., Ladbury, J. E., Piper, P. W., and Pearl, L. H. (1997) Identification and structural characterization of the ATP/ADP-binding site in the Hsp90 molecular chaperone. *Cell* **90,** 65–75.

5. Stebbins, C. E., Russo, A., Schneider, C., Rosen, N., Hartl, F. U., and Pavletich, N. P. (1997) Crystal structure of an Hsp90-geldanamcyin complex: targeting of a protein chaperone by an antitumor agent. *Cell* **89,** 239–250.

6. Panaretou, B. Prodromou, C., Roe, S. M., et al. (1998) ATP binding and hydrolysis are essential to the function of the HSP90 molecular chaperone in vivo. *EMBO J.* **17,** 4829–4836.

7. Kelland, L. R., Sharp, S. Y., Rogers, P. M., Myers, T. G., and Workman, P. (1999) DT-diaphorase expression and tumour cell sensitivity to allylamino-17-demethoxygeldanamycin, an inhibitor of heat shock protein 90. *J. Natl. Cancer Inst.* **91,** 1940–1949.

8. Hostein, I., Robertson, D., Di Stefano, F., Workman, P., and Clarke, P.A. (2001) Inhibition of signal transduction by the Hsp90 inhibitor 17-allylamino-17-demethoxygeldanamycin results in cytostasis and apoptosis. *Cancer Res.* **61,** 4003–4009.

9. Schulte, T. W. and Neckers, L. M. (1998) The benzoquinone ansamycin 17-allylamino-17-demethoxy-geldanamycin binds to Hsp90 and shares important biologic activities with geldanamycin. *Cancer Chemother. Pharmacol.* **42,** 273–279.

10. Whitesell, L., Mimnaugh, E. G., De Costa, B., Myers, C. E. and Neckers, L. M. (1994) Inhibition of heat shock protein HSP90-pp60v-src heteroprotein complex formation by benzoquinone ansamycins: essential role for stress proteins in oncogenic transformation. *Proc. Natl. Acad. Sci. USA* **91,** 8324–8328.

11. Clarke, P. A., Hostein, I., Banerji, U., Stefano, F. D., Maloney, A., Walton, M., Judson, I. and Workman, P. (2000) Gene expression profiling of human colon cancer cells following inhibition of signal transduction by 17-allylamino-17-demethoxygeldanamycin, an inhibitor of the Hsp90 molecular chaperone. *Oncogene* **19,** 4125–4133.

12. Stockwell, B. R., Haggarty, S. J. and Schreiber, S. L. (1999) High-throughput screening of small molecules in miniaturized mammalian cell-based assays involving post-translational modifications. *Chem. Biol.* **6,** 71–83.

13. Versteeg, H. H., Nijhuis, E., Van Den Brink, G. R., Evertzen, M., Pynaert, G.N., Van deventer J. H., Coffer, P. J. and Peppelenbosch, M. P. (2000) A new phosphospecific cell-based ELISA for p42/p44 mitogen-activated protein kinase (MAPK), p38 MAPK, protein kinase B and cAMP-response-element-binding protein. *Biochem. J.* **350,** 717–722.

14. Ali, J. A., Jackson, A. P., Howells, A. J. and Maxwell, A. (1993) The 43-kilodalton N-terminal fragment of the DNA gyrase β protein hydrolyses ATP and binds coumarin drugs. *Biochemistry* **32,** 2717–2724.

15. Cogan, E. B., Birrell, G. B. and Griffith, O. H. (1999) A robotics-based automated assay for inorganic and organic phosphates. *Anal. Biochem.* **271,** 29–35.

16. Baykov, A. A., Evtushenko, O. A. and Avaeva, S. M. (1988) A malachite green procedure for orthophosphate determination and its use in alkaline phosphatase-based enzyme immunoassay. *Anal. Biochem.* **171,** 266–270.

17. Harder, K. W., Owen, P., Wong, L. K. H., Aebersold, R., Clark-Lewis, I. and Jirik, F. R. (1994) Characterization and kinetic analysis of the intracellular domain of human protein tyrosine phosphatase β (HPTPβ) using synthetic phosphopeptides. *Biochem. J.* **298,** 395–401.

18. Maehama, T., Taylor, G. S., Slama, J. T. and Dixon, J. E. (2000) A sensitive assay for phosphoinositide phosphatases. *Anal. Biochem.* **279,** 248–250.

19. Rumsfeld, J., Ziegelbauer, K. and Spaltmann, F. (2000) High-throughput assay for inorganic pyrophosphatases using the cytosolic enzymes of *Saccharomyces cerevisiae* and human as an example. *Protein Expr. Purif.* **18,** 303–309.

20. Lavery, P., Brown, M. J. B. and Pope, A. J. (2001) Simple absorbance-based assays for ultra-high throughput screening. *J. Biomol. Screen.* **6,** 3–9.

21. Chan, K.-M., Delfert, D. and Junger, K. D. (1986) A direct colorimetric assay for Ca^{2+} stimulated ATPase activity. *Anal. Biochem.* **157,** 375–380.

22. Henkel, R. D., Vandeberg, J. L. and Walsh, R. A. (1988) A microassay for ATPase. *Anal. Biochem.* **169,** 312–318.

23. Lanzetta, P. H., Alvarez, L. J., Reinach, P. S. and Candia, O. A. (1979) An improved assay for nanomole amounts of inorganic phosphate. *Anal. Biochem.* **100,** 95–97.

24. Schirmer, E. C., Queitsch, C., Kowal, A. S., Parsell, D. A. and Lindquist, S. (1998) The ATPase activity of hsp104, effects of environmental conditions and mutations. *J. Biol. Chem.* **273,** 15,546–15,552.

25. Baginski, E. S. Epstein, E. and Zak, B. (1975) Review of phosphate methodologies. *Ann. Clin. Lab. Sci.* **5,** 399–416.

26. Zhang J. H., Chung T. D. and Oldenburg K. R. (1999) A simple statistical parameter for use in evaluation and validation of high throughput screening assays. *J. Biomol. Screen.* **4,** 67–73.

27. Hemmila, I. and Webb, S. (1997) Time-resolved fluorometry: an overview of the labels and core technologies for drug screening applications. *Drug Discovery Today* **2,** 373–381.

15

Assays for Proteasome Inhibition

Peter J. Elliott, Teresa A. Soucy, Christine S. Pien, Julian Adams, and Eric S. Lightcap

1. Introduction

The ubiquitin-proteasome pathway has an essential role in the regulation of numerous cellular proteins, including those mediating inflammatory conditions and cancer *(1–6)*. Intracellular proteins destined for proteolysis are first tagged with polyubiquitin chains through a cascade of enzyme-catalyzed events. These 'marked' proteins are then degraded via the 26S proteasome in an ATP-dependent manner *(7)*. The 26S proteasome (EC 3.4.99.46) is a large, multisubunit enzyme (MW=2000 kDa) found in high concentration in all mammalian cells. The ATP hydrolytic activity and the specific subunits that bind ubiquitin in the 26S are located within a protein complex known as the 19S subunit which caps either end of the 20S core. The ATP-independent proteolytic activity of the proteasome is contained within this central 20S core (MW = 730 kDa), a multicatalytic protease that has three well character-ized peptidase activities. The three peptidases: chymotryptic, tryptic, and postglutamyl peptide hydrolytic activities, are associated with three distinct subunits: $\beta5^*$, $\beta2^*$, and $\beta1^*$, respectively *(8)*. Each site is defined by its ability to hydrolyze peptide substrates in vitro, with hydrophobic, basic or acidic amino acids in the P_1 position.

Multiple inhibitors of the proteasome have been designed based upon either the natural product, lactacystin *(9)*, or synthetic peptidyl derivatives *(10)*. PS-341, a synthetic and potent peptidyl boronic acid, is a novel inhibitor of the chymotryptic site within the 20S proteasome *(11)*. This molecule shows at least 500-fold selectivity for the proteasome over other enzymes and receptors and exhibits substantial potency in cell-free and in vitro cell-based assays.

From: *Methods in Molecular Medicine, vol. 85: Novel Anticancer Drug Protocols*
Edited by: J. K. Buolamwini and A. A. Adjei © Humana Press Inc., Totowa, NJ

PS-341 has shown significant activity in preclinical murine tumor models *(3)* where the anti-tumor activity was positively correlated with the degree of proteasome inhibition measured both in white blood cell and tumor biopsy material.

PS-341 is currently under evaluation as an anti-cancer agent in multiple Phase I and Phase II clinical trials in which blood levels of the drug are being measured by LC/MS/MS to determine standard pharmacokinetic parameters. Based on animal models (including nonhuman primates), the drug is rapidly distributed throughout the body and plasma levels fall to near detection limits within minutes of intravenous dosing. The pharmacodynamic profile of the drug has also been evaluated to assess the activity of PS-341 at its target site, the proteasome. As such, it is possible not only to evaluate blood levels of PS-341 but also to record the level of enzyme inhibition over time.

To explore the possibility that the proteasome activity assay could be used in future preclinical studies and in clinical trials, the present series of experiments were undertaken. The ex vivo assays reported here were developed utilizing the current knowledge of the catalytic activities within the 20S proteasome *(12,13)*. The focus of the method development was to obtain a simple rapid and reproducible assay that could be used to determine accurately the level of proteasome activity in rodent blood samples treated with PS-341. To confirm that the tryptic and chymotryptic activities were only owing to the proteasome, a proteasome inhibitor from a second structurally unrelated class was also employed, *clasto*-lactacystin-β-lactone (lactacystin). Using multiple assays it was possible to cross-validate each format and determine the optimal assay methodology.

Herein, we describe the development of these pharmacodynamic assays to record proteasome activity present within biological material. This unique method of measuring proteasome activity is sensitive, accurate, and reproducible. This assay not only determines basal proteasome activity in naïve biological material, but can also be utilized to evaluate the effects of drugs that modify such activity. Assay variations were developed for use in whole blood samples or sub-populations of blood cells. As such, this method will allow the determination of the activity of inhibitors at their biological target, the proteasome, and provide a method for studying their pharmacodynamics as an alternative, or an additional procedure, to pharmacokinetic measurements.

In summary, a novel approach to determining the degree of inhibition has been applied to the proteasome in blood. The assay consists of measuring proteasome activity at two sites (chymotryptic and tryptic) within the 20S core of the proteasome and determining the degree of inhibition conferred by PS-341. Variations of the assay allow similar data sets to be calculated in sub-populations of blood cells.

Currently, the assays are being explored in clinical trials to validate the methods and to determine the optimum conditions for collection, storage and preparation of samples. To date, the assays provide a source of real-time pharmacodynamics on individual patients dosed with PS-341. In the future, these results will be invaluable for correlation with drug blood levels, safety and clinical activity data. In addition, the resolution of issues around measuring blood cell proteasome inhibition should be applicable to other biological material (e.g., tissue biopsy). Finally, the current cuvet-based version of the assay should be readily adaptable to a high-throughput 96-well plate format.

2. Materials

Chemicals should be the purest grade commercially available. All aqueous solutions should be prepared with water purified by reverse osmosis or ion exchange further treated with a Millipore MilliQ Plus UF water purifying system (or equivalent system) resulting in water with a resistivity greater than 16 MΩ•cm.

1. Pierce Coomassie Plus Protein Assay kit (or equivalent).
2. Phosphate buffered saline (PBS): 10 mM phosphate, 2.7 mM KCl, 137 mM NaCl, pH 7.4 ± 0.1.
3. 1 M HEPES, pH 8.2 ± 0.1.
4. 0.5 M ethylene diamine tetraacetic acid (EDTA), pH 8.0 ± 0.1.
5. Chymotryptic substrate (Bachem): Dissolve Suc-LLVY-AMC in DMSO (25 mg/ 5.45 mL) and store resultant 6 mM substrate in 100 µL aliquots at –20°C (–25 to –10°C).
6. Tryptic substrate (Bachem): Dissolve Bz-VGR-AMC in DMSO (50 mg/8.46 mL) and store resultant 10 mM substrate in 100 µL aliquots at –20°C (–25 to –10°C).
7. 2% sodium dodecyl sulfate (SDS): Prepare 2% SDS in water (2 g/100 mL) in a glass bottle. Store in 1 mL aliquots at –20°C (–25 to –10°C). Do not use Corning polystyrene filter system flasks for SDS preparation or storage.
8. AMC Stock Solution: AMC is dried under vacuum for 3 d, then dissolved in DMF (0.114 mg/mL). Store the 20 mM AMC stock solution in 1 mL aliquots at –20°C (–25 to –10°C) in screw-top vials.
9. Blood collection tubes containing sodium heparin.
10. Becton Dickinson Vacutainer CPT Cell Preparation Tubes.
11. Microcentrifuge capable of 6600g.
12. Microfuge tubes (1.5 mL).
13. Conical centrifuge tubes (15 and 50 mL).
14. Visible range 96-well microplate reader.
15. Fluorometer (e.g., Hitachi F-4500 fluorometer) with temperature control.
16. 3-mL disposable polystyrene fluorescence cuvets.
17. Magnetic cuvet stir bars.
18. Chymotryptic Substrate Buffer: 20 mM HEPES, pH 8.2, 0.5 mM EDTA, 0.05% SDS, 1% DMSO, 60 µM LLVY-AMC. To a clean 50 mL glass bottle (rinsed with

methanol and air-dried), add 600 µL 1 *M* HEPES, pH 8.2, 30 µL 0.5 *M* EDTA, pH 8.0, 750 µL 2% SDS, 300 µL 6 m*M* LLVY-AMC, and bring to volume (30 mL) with water. Chymotryptic substrate buffer (30 mL; typical batch) is prepared and can be stored at 4°C for up to 1 mo. This is sufficient for testing 15 samples (2 mL/ sample). Larger batches may be prepared if stored at 4°C. Only the amount of chymotryptic substrate buffer to be used within 24 h should be brought to 37°C ± 2°C.

19. Chymotryptic Substrate Buffer for maximal activity from white blood cells: (20 m*M* HEPES, 0.5 m*M* EDTA, 0.035% SDS, 1% DMSO, 60 µ*M* LLVY-AMC). To a clean 50 mL glass bottle (rinsed with methanol and air-dried), add 600 µL 1 *M* HEPES, pH 8.2, 30 µL 0.5 *M* EDTA, pH 8.0, 525 µL 2% SDS, 300 µL 6 m*M* LLVY-AMC, and bring to volume (30 mL) with water. Proteasome activity from white blood cells can be measured accurately using the assay buffer listed in **step 18**, but this assay buffer will give better activity with white blood cell samples of relatively low activity. To determine inhibition by specific activity, samples must be compared using the same assay buffer. Whole blood cell samples require 0.05% SDS to give accurate results.

20. Tryptic Substrate Buffer (20 m*M* HEPES, 0.5 m*M* EDTA, 0.6% DMSO and 60 µ*M* VGR-AMC). To a clean 50 mL glass bottle (rinsed with methanol and air-dried), add 600 µL 1 *M* HEPES, pH 8.2, 30 µL 0.5 *M* EDTA, pH 8.0, 180 µL 10 m*M* VGR-AMC, and bring to volume (30 mL) with water. Tryptic substrate buffer (30 mL; typical batch) is prepared and can be stored at 4°C for up to 1 mo. This is sufficient for testing 15 samples (2 mL/sample). Larger batches may be prepared if stored at 4°C. Only the amount of tryptic substrate buffer to be used within 24 h should be brought to 37°C ± 2°C.

3. Methods

This protocol describes the ex vivo assay method for measurement of proteasome activity in peripheral whole blood or white blood cells. The assay is based upon the chymotryptic and the tryptic activities of the proteasome. It uses fluorometry to measure the rate at which the proteasome hydrolyzes an amide bond in a small peptide substrate. Measurement of these rates in the absence and presence of an inhibitor allows a determination of what proportion of the proteasome is bound by an inhibitor. For tightly bound inhibitors, this assay can be correlated with the amount of inhibition of the proteasome in vivo. In addition, since some inhibitors of proteasome activity completely inhibit the chymotryptic activity but do not inhibit the tryptic activity, the percent of proteasome bound by such an inhibitor can be directly determined by the ratio of the chymotryptic and tryptic activities. This assay has been used to measure proteasome activity in peripheral whole blood or white blood cells in humans, Cynomolgus monkeys, dogs, rats, and mice. There are several steps involved in the measurement of 20S proteasome activity in blood cells. These include preparation of the blood sample, protein assay of the sample, fluorometer calibration, fluorometric assay of both chymotryptic and tryptic activities, and calculation of results.

3.1. Preparation of Peripheral Whole Blood (PWB) Sample

1. Collect the required amount of blood into a tube containing anticoagulant (e.g., heparin).
2. The blood is then treated using the sample transfer protocols (*see* **Notes** for other protocols).
3. Sample Transfer Protocol: The cells from the collected blood (PWB) may be prepared as follows: (a) Transfer whole blood (10–1000 µL) to a 1.5 mL microfuge tube; (b) Centrifuge at 6600*g* for approx 10 min at 4 ± 3°C; (c) Aspirate off supernatant; (d) Pellet may be frozen at –70 ± 10°C or on dry ice. These frozen pellets may be shipped to the site of analysis on dry ice. Pellets should stored at –70 ± 10°C for no more than 2 yr.
4. Whole Blood Lysates are prepared by the following procedure: (a) If samples are frozen, quick thaw samples by placing them in a 37 ± 2°C bath for a couple of minutes; (b) Place blood samples on ice; (c) Transfer 10 µL sample to a clean 1.5-mL microfuge tube; (d) Lyse the cells by adding 300 µL 5 m*M* EDTA to each sample (0.5 mL 0.5 *M* EDTA in 50 mL water). Let the samples stand on ice at least 15 min. Red blood cells that have been frozen will be substantially lysed but all procedures should still be followed; (e) Centrifuge at 6600*g* for approx 10 min at 4 ± 3°C; (f) Carefully collect the supernatant (~250 µL) into a clean 1.5 mL microfuge tube; (g) Add an equal volume of 40 m*M* HEPES, 1.0 m*M* EDTA, 20% glycerol, pH 7.6 to the supernatant. Mix by tapping the microfuge tube; (h) Store the lysate sample frozen at –70 ± 10°C for no more than 2 yr. Lysate samples may be shipped on dry ice.
5. Samples may be thawed and refrozen up to 10×.

3.2. Preparation of Peripheral White Blood Cell (WBC) Samples

Peripheral white blood cells are separated from blood samples upon collection and lysed for storage at –70°C until tested. To prevent interference with the assay it is important that the sample preparation remove all red blood cells. If the sample is contaminated with red blood cells, chymotryptic assays should be done at 0.05% SDS. Separation is done in Becton Dickinson Vacutainer CPT Cell Preparation Tubes.

1. Draw 8 mL of blood into CPT tubes and invert 5×, gently.
2. Within 10 min of blood draw, spin for 30 min at 1500*g* at 25°C.
3. Discard the upper half of the plasma layer.
4. Transfer the remaining plasma layer above the plug to a 15-mL polypropylene conical tube. Be careful not to include any red blood cells (RBCs). If RBCs are inadvertently collected, put all plasma back into CPT tubes and respin.
5. Wash with PBS and respin at 600*g* for 10 min at 25°C.

6. Carefully pour off the supernatant and allow the tubes to drain for 3 min. A cotton swab may be used to remove any other drops that may have remained in the tubes.
7. Store WBC pellets at –70°C until ready for lysis or shipment on dry ice.
8. Pour off the supernatant and resuspend the pellet in ~1 mL cold PBS.
9. Transfer the suspension to a 1.5-mL microfuge tube.
10. Centrifuge at 6600g for 10 min at 4°C.
11. Aspirate off the supernatant.
12. Lyse the cells by adding 200 µL 0.5 mM EDTA to each sample. Let the samples stand on ice for at least 15 min.
13. Centrifuge at 6600g for 10 min at 4°C.
14. Carefully collect the supernatant (~200 µL) into a clean 1.5 mL microfuge tube.
15. Store lysate sample frozen at –70 ± 10°C.

3.3. Coomassie Protein Assay

1. Perform the Coomassie (Bradford) protein assay in duplicate in accordance with manufacturer's instructions.
2. Dilute the BSA protein standard (2 mg/mL) 1:1 with water. This 1000 µg/mL stock solution is further diluted to 500, 250, 125, and 62.5 µg/mL. These standards may be stored at –20°C (–10 to –25°C) and reused.
3. Transfer 10 µL of each standard dilution to wells in duplicate.
4. Transfer 10 µL of sample supernatant into a 96-well microplate with 90 µL water (1:10 dilution).
5. Add 10 µL of the 1:10 diluted sample to new wells in duplicate.
6. Add 300 µL Coomassie Plus to wells containing standards and diluted samples.
7. Read on the microplate reader at 595 nm.
8. Prepare a standard curve and calculate sample concentrations.
9. The duplicate protein results must differ by no more than 10%, otherwise repeat the assay.

3.4. Fluorometer Calibration

1. Thaw a vial containing 20 mM AMC stock solution and prepare a 50 µM AMC solution (5 µL 20 mM AMC stock solution into 2 mL DMF). Refreeze 20 mM AMC stock solution.
2. Prepare 2 µM AMC by 1:25 dilution of 50 µM AMC stock solution in DMSO.
3. Record the zero value for chymotryptic substrate buffer under assay settings (λ_{ex} = 380 nm; λ_{em} = 440 nm; excitation band width = 10 nm; emission band width = 20 nm). Add 5 µL of 2 µM AMC into 2 mL of chymotryptic substrate buffer approx every 30 s for a total of five times to produce a calibration curve for 0–50 pmol AMC. Record the fluorometer calibration values.

3.5. Fluorometric 20S Proteasome Assay

1. Make sure that the chymotryptic or tryptic substrate buffer has equilibrated to 37 ± 2°C before running samples.

2. Rinse a magnetic cuvette stir bar and 3 mL polystyrene fluorometric cuvet with deionized water and methanol.
3. Place the magnetic cuvette stir bar in the 3 mL polystyrene fluorometric cuvet.
4. Add 2 mL of chymotryptic or tryptic substrate buffer (at $37 \pm 2°C$) to the cuvet.
5. Check that the baseline is stable with minimal noise (*see* **Notes 3–5**).
6. Add 10–100 μg of test sample to the cuvette and let the reaction run for 5–10 min ($\lambda_{ex} = 380$ nm; $\lambda_{em} = 440$ nm).
7. Measure the maximum linear slope (for at least 1 min of data, *see* **Note 7**).
8. If the rate is less than 1 pmol AMC/min, repeat the measurement using twice the amount of test sample used in **step 6**.

3.6. Calculations

1. Specific Activity:

$$SpA_C = \{(m_C)/(0.000001 \times vol_C \times [pn])\}/m_{fluor})/60$$

where SpA_C is the chymotryptic specific activity of the blood sample (pmol AMC/s•mg protein), m_C is the slope from the chymotryptic assay (FU/min), vol_C is the volume of blood sample added to the chymotryptic assay (μL), [pn] is the concentration of protein in the sample added to the chymotryptic assay (μg/mL), and m_{fluor} is the slope from the fluorometer calibration (FU/pmol AMC).

2. Chymotryptic to tryptic activity ratio:

$$v_C/v_T = (m_C \times vol_T)/(m_T \times vol_C)$$

where v_C/v_T is the ratio of the chymotryptic activity to the tryptic activity in a blood sample, m_C is the slope from the chymotryptic assay (FU/min), vol_T is the volume of blood sample added to the tryptic assay (μL), m_T is the slope from the tryptic assay (FU/min), and vol_C is the volume of blood sample added to the chymotryptic assay (μL).

3. Percent inhibition by specific activity:

$$\%I(SpA) = 100 \times (1 - SpA_{Ci}/SpA_{Cu})$$

where $\%I(SpA)$ is the percent inhibition of chymotryptic proteasome activity calculated using specific activity, SpA_{Ci} is the specific activity from the chymotryptic assay in the inhibited sample, and SpA_{Cu} is the specific activity from the chymotryptic assay in the uninhibited sample.

4. Percent inhibition by chymotryptic to tryptic ratio:

$$\%I(C:T) = 100 \times (k_C/k_T - v_C/v_T)/(k_C/k_T - v_C/v_T + 1.35 \times v_C/v_T)$$

where $\%I(C:T)$ is the percent inhibition of the chymotryptic proteasome activity calculated using the ratio of chymotryptic to tryptic proteasome activities from a blood sample, k_C/k_T is the ratio of chymotryptic to tryptic activities in the uninhibited blood sample, and v_C/v_T is the ratio of chymotryptic to tryptic activities in the inhibited sample.

3.7. Assay Validity

The following assay results are typical of clinical results for whole blood assays evaluated thus far. Although significant variation occurs in values from multiple individuals, variation within an individual is not a problem.

1. The sample protein concentration is 500–6000 µg/mL.
2. The ratio of the chymotryptic to tryptic activities (in pmol AMC/s × mg protein) prior to treatment is 0.9–3.5.
3. The chymotryptic specific activity prior to treatment is 0.4–1.3 pmol AMC/s × mg protein.
4. The tryptic specific activity before or after treatment is 0.2–0.8 pmol AMC/s × mg protein.
5. The chymotryptic specific activity for white blood cells prior to treatment is 25–35 pmol AMC/s × mg protein.

4. Notes
4.1. Sample Transfer Protocols

1. The collected blood may be frozen on dry ice immediately after collection. These samples should be transferred to the analytical site on dry ice. These samples should be stored at −70 ± 10°C for no more than 2 yr.
2. The collected blood may be stored and shipped on ice. These samples should be received and processed no more than 48 h after collection.

4.2. Fluorometric Assays

3. Dust in the cuvet will create significant noise. Rewash the stir bar and cuvet, if necessary.
4. High noise may result from a fast stir bar.
5. A rolling baseline indicates a stopped stir bar.
6. Complete activation of the 20S proteasome in the presence of SDS is achieved within 10 min. Consistent results for the chymotryptic assay are obtained for readings taken after 4 min and up to 10 min.
7. Activation of the proteasome is not seen in the absence of SDS. Therefore the maximum slope for the tryptic assay may occur anywhere within the 10 min reaction curve. In general, the maximum slope has been observed between 1.5 and 3 min.

4.3. Modifications for 96-Well Plate Format

This assay has been modified for 96-well plate format. A Packard Instruments Multiprobe 104DT workstation was used to format plates and a BioTek FL600 microplate spectrofluorometer was used to follow the kinetics at 37°C (λ_{ex} = 380 nm (20 nm bandwidth), λ_{em} = 450 nm (50 nm bandwidth)).

8. The assay is linear for 1–10 µg protein/well. Dilute the blood sample, if necessary, in 10 m*M* HEPES, 1 m*M* EDTA, 10% glycerol, pH 8.0 to obtain 30–300 µg protein/mL.

9. Change the final volume for both assay buffers from 30 mL to 23 mL (1.3X concentrated) and heat to 37°C.

10. Pipet 30 µL blood sample/well into a black 96-well fluorometric plate (Corning/Costar plate #3915) in triplicate.

11. Pipet 100 µL chymotryptic assay buffer/well and place plate on plate carrier and begin assay. Read the change in fluorescence every 40 s for 25 min with a 4 s shaking at setting 2 between each time the plate is read.

12. The average slope from 8–25 min is determined to calculate the rate in the chymotryptic assay.

13. Pipet 30 µL blood sample (30–300 µg protein/mL)/well into a black 96-well fluorometric plate (Corning/Costar plate #3915) in triplicate.

14. Pipet 100 µL tryptic assay buffer/well and place plate on plate carrier and begin assay. Read the change in fluorescence for 25 min using the same protocol as for the chymotryptic assay.

15. The average slope from 1–18 min is determined to calculate the rate in the tryptic assay.

16. Calculations are done as with the cuvet-based assay.

References

1. Ciechanover, A. (1998) The ubiquitin-proteasome pathway: on protein death and cell life. *EMBO J.* **17,** 7151–7160.

2. Palombella, V. J., Conner, E. M., Fuseler, J. W., et al. (1998) Role of the proteasome and NF-kB in streptococcal cell wall-induced polyarthritis. *Proc. Natl. Acad. Sci. USA* **95,** 15,671–15,676.

3. Adams, J., Palombella, V. J., Sausville, E. A., et al. (1999) Proteasome inhibitors: a novel class of potent and effective anti-tumor agents. *Cancer Res.* **59,** 2615–2622.

4. Campbell, B., Adams, J., Shin, Y. K., and Lefer, A. M. (1999) Cardioprotective effects of a novel proteasome inhibitor following ischemia and reperfusion in the isolated perfused rat heart. *J. Mol. Cell Cardiol.* **31,** 467–476.

5. Elliott, P. J., Pien, C. S., McCormack, T. A., Chapman, I. D., and Adams J. (1999) Proteasome inhibition: a novel mechanism to combat asthma. *J. Allergy Clin. Immunol.* **104,** 294–300.

6. Phillips, J. B., Williams, A. J., Adams, J., Elliott, P. J., and Tortella, F. C. (2000) The proteasome inhibitor, PS-519, reduces infarction and attenuates leukocyte infiltration in a rat model of focal cerebral ischemia. *Stroke* **31,** 1686–1693.

7. DeMartino, G. N. and Slaughter, C. A. (1999) The proteasome, a novel protease regulated by multiple mechanisms. *J. Biol. Chem.* **274,** 22,123–22,126.

8. Lupas, A. and Baumeister, W. (1998) The 20S proteasome, in *Ubiquitin and the Biology of the Cell* (Peters, J. M., Harris, J. R., and Finley, D., eds.), Plenum Press, New York, pp. 127–146.

9. Fenteany, G. and Schreiber, S. L. (1998) Lactacystin, proteasome function, and cell fate. *J. Biol. Chem.* **273,** 8545–8548.

10. Elliott, P. J. and Adams, J. (1999) Recent advances in understanding proteasome function. *Curr. Opin. Drug Disc. Dev.* **2,** 484–490.

11. Adams, J., Behnke, M., Chen, S., et al. (1998) Potent and selective inhibitors of the proteasome: dipeptidyl boronic acids. *Bioorg. Med. Chem. Lett.* **8,** 333–338.

12. Lightcap, E. S., McCormack, T. A., Pien, C. S., Chau, V., Adams, J., and Elliott, P. J. (2000) Proteasome inhibition measurements: clinical applications. *Clin. Chem.* **46,** 673–683.

13. Stein, R. L., Melandri, F., and Dick, L. (1996) Kinetic characterization of the chymotryptic activity of the 20S proteasome. *Biochemistry* **35,** 3899–3908.

VI

PROTEIN–PROTEIN AND PROTEIN–DNA INTERACTIONS

16

The Mammalian Two-Hybrid Assay for Detection of Coactivator-Nuclear Receptor Interactions

Curtis M. Tyree and Kay Klausing

1. Introduction

The two-hybrid assay was described in 1989 as a method to determine protein-protein interactions in living cells (*1*). The principle of the assay relies on the fact that the DNA binding and transactivation domains are separable and can operate in heterologous contexts in most transcription factors (*2*). The two-hybrid assay exploits this fact by detecting the interaction between two chimeric proteins, each containing one part (either the DNA-binding domain or the transactivation domain) of a transcription factor. A protein-protein interaction between the other parts of the chimeras will bring the two parts of the transcription factor together, producing an increase in transcription from a reporter gene. The first chimera is composed of a DNA binding domain that recognizes the DNA elements in the promoter to be used and one interaction target protein. The yeast activator proteins GAL4 and Lex A have been commonly used as sources of these domains. The second chimera is a fusion of the second interaction target protein with a strong activation domain (for example, the herpes simplex virus activator protein VP16). A complete transactivator protein will be restored only if the two test proteins interact: the GAL4 DNA binding domain of the fusion protein will specifically bind to the multimerized GAL4 binding sites in the luciferase reporter, but cannot activate unless this fusion protein brings the VP16 activation domain into the vicinity of the promoter through a protein-protein interaction between the chimeric proteins (*see* **Fig. 1**). The two-hybrid assay has been used most extensively for two purposes: 1) The structural and functional analysis of the interaction between two cloned proteins; and 2) The discovery of novel proteins that associate with a target protein

From: *Methods in Molecular Medicine, vol. 85: Novel Anticancer Drug Protocols*
Edited by: J. K. Buolamwini and A. A. Adjei © Humana Press Inc., Totowa, NJ

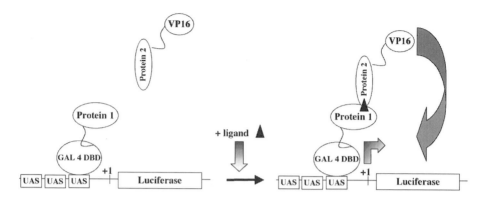

Fig. 1. Schematic representation of the mammalian two-hybrid assay. Transcription of a reporter gene, luciferase, is activated upon interaction of protein 1 with protein 2 due to proximity of the strong VP16 activation domain to the promoter. For assays with nuclear hormone receptors, the coactivator is usually protein 1 and the interaction with protein 2 (the receptor) is induced by ligand.

of interest, using a library of cDNAs fused to VP16 and the "bait" or target protein fused to a DNA binding domain. There are also many variations on the two-hybrid theme that have been described by Kolanus *(3)* and Drees *(4)*.

Most of the research with the two-hybrid assay has been performed in yeast cells. Yeast is especially well suited for the analysis and detection of novel interacting proteins. Yeast can be plated, selected, or screened using a variety of growth or colorimetric characteristics. The insertion of custom promoters in the genomic DNA of yeast to create custom selection or screening criteria is much more facile than in mammalian cells. These attributes combined, have made yeast a well-studied and successful model organism to identify and analyze protein-protein interactions.

The use of yeast cells for the two-hybrid approach, although very useful for screening for novel interacting proteins, has several drawbacks. First, screens in yeast have a high false positive rate; many interactions detected in yeast cannot be verified in mammalian cells. Second, many of the post-translational modifications that are important for proper folding and protein function for mammalian proteins do not occur in yeast. Third, yeast cells are less permeable to small molecules than mammalian cells and harbor active pumps homologous to multi-drug resistance pumps. These attributes have important implications for studying mammalian proteins, and the third issue is especially important in the arena of drug discovery.

We have applied this technology mainly in our nuclear receptor drug discovery programs. This review will describe our experience and techniques

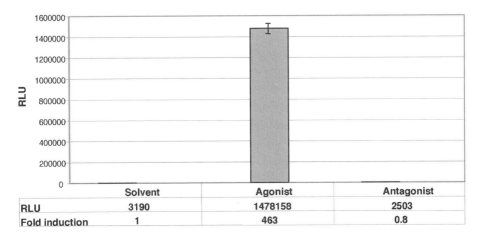

	Solvent	Agonist	Antagonist
RLU	3190	1478158	2503
Fold induction	1	463	0.8

Fig. 2. Agonist, but not antagonist, induces the interaction between the coactivator hRIP140 and the nuclear receptor hRXRα. 0.5 μg 5X GAL4-Luc was co-transfected with 0.1 μg of GAL4-RIP140 (350–530) vector and 0.1 μg VP16-hRXRα-LBD (220–462) using the calcium phosphate method. Twenty-four hours after the transfection 1 μ*M* of either agonist or antagonist or the equivalent volume of solvent (DMSO) was added to the well for another 24 h. The plates were harvested as described. The graph shows the luciferase value and the table shows the luciferase counts as well as the fold induction by ligand (solvent is set to 1).

as examples of possibilities for using the two-hybrid assay in mammalian cells for drug discovery. Nuclear receptors are ligand-regulated transcription factors capable of modulating gene expression in many physiological contexts including development, reproduction, inflammation, cardiovascular function, and many aspects of metabolism *(5)*. Ligand binding induces a conformational change in the receptor, which enables the nuclear receptor to interact with a group of proteins collectively called cofactors. These cofactors may be coactivators or corepressors *(6)*. Ligand-dependent interaction of receptors with coactivators can be studied with the mammalian two-hybrid assay. These experiments use transient transfection of cells with plasmids to express the appropriate chimeric proteins together with the appropriate reporter plasmid. The cells are then treated with appropriate ligands and the expression of the reporter gene determined.

Typical results are shown in **Figs. 2** and **3**. In **Fig. 2**, the central portion of the coactivator RIP140 (amino acids 350–530) was expressed as a fusion with the GAL4 DNA-binding domain. The second chimera composed of the ligand-binding domain of the nuclear retinoid-X-receptor (RXR, amino acids 220–462) and VP16. As expected, the agonist induces a strong interaction

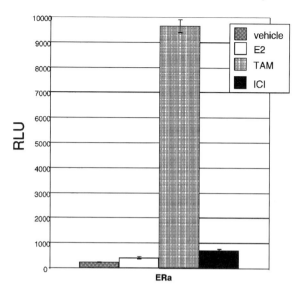

Fig. 3. Interaction of ERα and ERβ with a peptide. 0.5 μg 5X GAL4-Luc was co-transfected with 0.1 μg GAL4-α/β III-peptide vector and 0.1 μg VP16-hERα LBD (amino acids 252–595) using the Fugene Method. Twenty-four hours after the transfection, 100 n*M* of the indicated ligands or the equivalent volume of solvent (DMSO) was added to the cells and incubated for 24 h. The plates were harvested as described. The graph shows the reporter activity as luciferase values. This peptide associates only with tamoxifen-liganded ERα.

between the two proteins, while the antagonist does not promote this interaction. Partial agonists would still promote this interaction, although not to the extent of a full agonist.

2. Materials

1. Reporter plasmid containing multimerized GAL4 binding sites upstream of a minimal promoter driving the expression of a luciferase reporter gene are currently not commercially available. However, a construct driving CAT expression is commercially available as part of the "Matchmaker" kit (Clontech cat. no. K1602-1, pG5CAT) in which case the luciferase assay needs to be substituted by a CAT assay (non-radioactive CAT assay kits are available from Molecular Probes cat. no. F-2900). Alternatively, the CAT gene can be replaced by the luciferase gene by standard molecular cloning techniques.
2. First partner fused to the GAL4 DNA binding domain (using the Clontech vector pM or equivalent).
3. Second partner fused to the VP16 transactivation domain (using the Clontech vector pVP16 or equivalent).

4. β-gal control plasmid (pβ-gal-Control from Clontech, cat. no. 6047-1 or 6177-1 or equivalent).
5. Tissue-culture treated 12-well plates (Costar cat. no. 3513 or equivalent).
6. White 96-well plates (Dynex Microlite 1).
7. Dulbecco's Modified Eagle's Medium (DMEM, Bio-Whittaker or equivalent).
8. Charcoal-absorbed fetal calf serum (HyClone or equivalent).
9. Phosphate-buffered saline (PBS).
10. 2.5 M $CaCl_2$ (sterile filtered).
11. 2X HEPES buffer: 50 mM HEPES, 300 mM NaCl, 1.5 mM Na_2HPO_4, pH 6.93, sterile filtered.
12. FuGENE 6 (Roche, cat. no. 1814443).
13. Buffer A: 20 mM Tricine-KOH, pH 7.8, 20 mM KCl, 5 mM $MgSO_4$, 1 mM ethylene diamine tetraacetic acid (EDTA), 1 mM ethylene glycol tetraacetic acid (EGTA).
14. 250 mM Tris-HCl, pH 7.8.
15. [³H]Acetyl CoA (ICN, 1 mCi/mL) (or [³H]Chloramphenicol if the Promega kit is used).
16. 5 mM chloramphenicol (Roche).
17. 5 mM acetyl CoA (Amersham-Pharmacia).
18. Scintillation cocktail (PPO/Toluene or equivalent).
19. 7 M Urea.
20. ONPG (ortho-nitrophenylphosphate) stock: 30 mg/mL in 0.1 M phosphate buffer.
21. β-mercaptoethanol (stock 14.3 M).
22. Plate reader (Wallac Victor or equivalent).
23. Scintillation counter (for CAT assays).
24. Calcium phosphate.

All chemicals where the supplier is not mentioned are from Sigma.

3. Methods
3.1. Tissue Culture

1. Plate approx cells 60,000 cells/well (for CV-1 cells, adjust according to proliferation rate, wells should be confluent at harvest on d 3) for a 12-well plate on d 1 in 1 mL medium.
2. On d 2, perform the transfection as following: (a) Calcium phosphate method: The calcium phosphate-DNA-precipitate should contain a maximum of 20 µg DNA/mL precipitate, and a maximum of 1/10 of the DNA precipitate (by volume) should be added to the medium. As an example for 1 well in a 12-well dish: the maximal total amount of DNA is 2 µg, which should be diluted in 45 µL of H_2O, to which 5 µL of 2.5 M $CaCl_2$ is added and mixed. Then an equal volume of 2X Hepes buffer (50 µL) is slowly added drop-by-drop while gently vortexing. The total volume is 100 µL, which is 0.1 mL medium. The precipitate is allowed to form for 20 min at room temperature (22°C). Add the precipitate to cells and incubate overnight; (b) FuGENE 6 -method: This follows the general guidelines

as supplied by the manufacturer (Roche). As an example for 1 well in a 12-well dish, add 6 μL of FuGENE 6 to 100 μL of plain medium (no serum) and incubate for 5 min at room temperature. Add the mix to the DNA mix, 2 μg total DNA maximum, and incubate for 30 min at room temperature. Add the complex to the plated cells. The 2 μg DNA should consist of 0.5 μg reporter and 0.1 μg GAL4 and VP16 fusions each; optionally 0.5 μg β-gal control vector, and a filler plasmid (pGEM, pUC) to 2 μg total.

4. On d 3, wash the cells once with PBS, add 1 mL of fresh medium per well including the test compound, incubate the cells for at least 24 h.

5. On day 4, harvest the cells: wash once with 1 mL PBS, aspirate completely. For luciferase and β-galactosidase assays, add 100 μL lysis buffer per well of a 12-well plate, incubate 20 min at room temperature, do NOT shake. Transfer 50 μL to a 96-well plate. The lysate can be stored at –80°C if necessary. For CAT assays scrape cells off the plate, transfer into Eppendorf tubes, spin and resuspend in 100 μL of 250 mM Tris buffer, pH 7.8. Lyse the cells by three freeze-thaw cycles. Alternatively the cells can be lysed in the reporter lysis buffer from Promega, which permits analysis of all three reporter systems.

3.2. Assays

1. Luciferase assay: Commercially available kits can be used, Clontech cat. no. K2039-1, Promega cat. no. 4030 or Tropix cat. no. LS200. Using a multichannel pipettor, transfer 20 μL of the above lysate to a white 96-well plate, add 100 μL of assay buffer, read the plate immediately in a suitable reader (Wallac Victor or equivalent, 0.2–1 s (possibly longer) per well).

2. β-Galactosidase assay: (alternative commercially available kits can be used, Clontech cat. no. K20348-1 or Tropix cat. no. BM100S): Add 200 μL of reaction buffer (0.1 M Na$_3$PO$_4$, pH 7.5, 50 mM β-mercaptoethanol, 1 mM MgSO$_4$, 0.6 mg/mL ONPG) to the residual 30 μL lysate, incubate at 37°C until a light yellow color appears (generally within 15–40 min). Stop the reaction with 100 μL of 1 M Na$_2$CO$_3$, read OD at 420 nm.

3. CAT assay: (Promega offers a kit (cat. no. E1000) which contains all reagents except [^{14}C] chloramphenicol): Treat extracts to be tested in the CAT assay for 10 min at 60°C to inactivate endogenous CAT activity. Transfer 25 μL of the extract to a 96-well plate, add 35 μL of 250 mM Tris-HCl, pH 7.8, 20 μL of 5 mM chloramphenicol (in 250 mM Tris-HCl, pH 7.8) and 20 μL of acetyl-CoA mix (0.6 μL 5 mM Acetyl-CoA, 0.4 μL [^{3}H] Acetyl-CoA, 19.0 μL 75 μM HCl). For background control wells, leave out the chloramphenicol. Incubate for 1 h at 37°C. Stop the reaction by adding 100 μL 7 M urea, spin down precipitate in microfuge. Transfer entire reaction into a scintillation vial containing 800 μL 7 M Urea, add 4.5 mL scintillation cocktail and vigorously shake for 5–10 min on a shaker. Let sit for 5 min to separate phases. Count in a scintillation counter. Subtract background (– chloramphenicol wells) from all samples.

4. Notes

1. Constructs: (a) Reporter: Currently there is no luciferase reporter construct commercially available that uses multimerized GAL4 binding sites and a minimal promoter driving luciferase expression. Therefore, these vectors have to be made by using commercially available promoterless luciferase constructs (like pGL3 basic, Promega cat. no. E 1751). Alternatively, the commercially available CAT vectors can be used and a CAT assay can be substituted for the luciferase assay; (b) Fusion vectors: It is obvious that the genes of interest have to be cloned into the correct frame and orientation without introducing stop codons. It is therefore easiest to subclone PCR products of the protein genes by designing primers with the appropriate restriction sites and the correct frame. Since nuclear receptors have a strong intrinsic activation function, they are usually not expressed as the GAL4 fusion as this would result in high basal levels of activity and therefore a loss in sensitivity. This applies to any protein with a strong activation function. Expressing transactivating proteins as VP16 fusions will result in a more robust signal with less background. For proteins with unknown transactivation potential, it is wise to make both fusions with each partner to get the best possible signal (the vectors mentioned under "Materials" have identical multiple cloning sites making this easy).

   For our studies with nuclear receptors we either fuse the entire receptor coding region or just the ligand binding domain (beginning with the hinge region, *see* **ref. 1** for a general review of nuclear receptors) to the VP16 transactivation domain, creating a receptor protein with an N-terminal VP16 fusion.

   In our experience it is worth making several constructs, since subtle differences in the exact fusion site can make a big difference in how this assay performs. Generally, starting the fusion at the flexible hinge region gave best results.

   With coactivators, we generally use the part of the molecule that contains the receptor interaction domain (for a general review of co-activators see Xu et. al. *[6]*), usually consisting of several LXXLL interaction motifs, spread over a few hundred amino acids. It is however possible to express the entire protein or just a single LXXLL-motif as GAL4 fusion. For the experiment shown in **Fig. 2** we chose a fragment of the coactivator protein RIP140 (amino acids 350–530), which encompasses a cluster of 3 interaction motifs (out of a total of 9 motifs in this protein *[7]*). For the peptide construct shown in **Fig. 3** we directly fused the coding region for the 15-mer peptide *(8)* to the GAL4 coding region using no additional flanking sequences.

2. Transfections: It is easier to establish the transfection procedure using FuGENE 6 (Roche) rather than calcium phosphate. The manufacturer provides a detailed protocol and the transfection efficiencies achieved are generally higher and the reproducibility better than with calcium phosphate. The calcium phosphate procedure is more cost-effective, but requires more experience. For reproducible results and good transfection efficiencies, attention has to be paid to the correct

pH of the HEPES buffer, which will affect the consistency of the precipitate. It is best to initially prepare several batches of HEPES buffer in pH 0.05 increments (from pH 6.8 to 7.2) and test empirically which pH works best. As the temperature strongly affects the consistency of the precipitate, attention has to be paid that the procedures is always performed at the same temperature. We found that 22°C works best for the pH given above.

For both methods, the relative ratios for each interacting pair and the absolute amount of plasmids have to be titrated carefully for best results. A good starting point has been 0.5 µg reporter and 0.1 µg GAL4 and VP16 fusions each (per 2 µg DNA for 1 well of a 12-well plate). First, the reporter plasmid is titrated from 1 µg down to 0.1 µg. Next, the GAL4 and VP16 fusion protein vectors are titrated against each other (using 0.05, 0.1, and 0.2 µg). In case of nuclear receptors and their ligand dependent interaction with coactivators, the conditions, under which the greatest fold induction by ligand is observed, are chosen. If the measured interaction is constitutive, the GAL4 fusion protein can be compared to the GAL4 parent vector and the greatest differential is chosen.

It is a good idea to initially include 0.5 µg β-galactosidase control vector to normalize for well-to-well variability of the transfection. Once the conditions have been optimized there should be very little variability and the β-galactosidase control plasmid can be omitted.

3. Assays: (a) Luciferase: This assay has a wide dynamic range and therefore the amount of extract used is not very critical. Using the described protocol (the "glow" luciferase assay), the timing of reagent addition is not that critical as the signal is stable for several minutes; (b) β-Galactosidase: As this assay doesn't have the wide dynamic range and the sensitivity of the luciferase assay, both the amount of extract added and the incubation time are critical. The amount and incubation time given above are only guidelines and the color development has to be monitored during the incubation period to keep the assay in the linear range (generally, 0.2–0.8 OD); (c) CAT assay: The detergent (0.1% Triton X-100) used for extract preparation for luciferase and β-galactosidase assays interferes with the activity of the CAT enzyme. Therefore alternative lysis methods, like freeze-thaw cycles or Promega's reporter lysis buffer, have to be employed. Some cell lines naturally have high endogenous CAT activity, which has to be inactivated by a 10 min incubation step at 60°C. It is important that only the portion of the cell lysate destined to be used for the CAT assay is treated this way, as the heat will inactivate both luciferase and β-galactosidase. The CAT assay also does not have a wide dynamic range and care has to be taken to ensure that it is in the linear range. It is absolutely necessary to add cold acetyl-CoA to the [^{3}H]acetyl-CoA to ensure an adequate supply of substrate for the enzyme. The amount of extract used and the incubation time has to be determined empirically since they depend on the reporter activity (which in turn depends on the relative strength of the association of the two test proteins). The amount and time given above are a good starting point. If the CAT activity levels are low, more extract (up to 60 µL) and longer incubation times (up to 20 h) can be used to obtain a higher signal. It

is advisable to establish a standard curve with a CAT enzyme preparation using a range of 0.1–0.00625 Units/assay using a twofold serial dilution.

4. Data analysis: Since the transfection efficiency can vary greatly from well to well, the luciferase or CAT reporter activity should be normalized to the activity of the constitutive β-Galactosidase reporter, at least initially, until the transfection protocol has been optimized. Preferentially, the same amount of extract from each transfection experiment should be used to determine reporter activity. A typical normalization is (luciferase activity [CPS or light units per second] or CAT activity [units]/extract volume [μL])/(OD 420 nm/(extract volume [μL] × incubation time [min])).

References

1. Fields, S. and Song, O. (1989) A novel genetic system to detect protein-protein interactions. *Nature* **340**, 245–246.
2. Ma, J. and Ptashne, M. (1987) A new class of yeast transcriptional activators. *Cell* **51**, 113–119.
3. Kolanus, W. (1999) The two hybrid toolbox. *Curr. Top. Microbiol. Immunol.* **243**, 37–54.
4. Drees, B. L. (1999) Progress and variations in two-hybrid and three-hybrid technologies. *Curr. Opin. Chem. Biol.* **3**, 64–70.
5. Kumar, R. and Thompson, E. B. (1999) The structure of the nuclear hormone receptors. *Steroids* **64**, 310–319.
6. Xu, L., Glass, C. K., and Rosenfeld, M. G. (1999) Coactivator and corepressor complexes in nuclear receptor function. *Curr. Opin. Genet. Dev.* **9**, 140–147.
7. Cavailles, V., Dauvois, S., L'Horset, F., et al. (1995) Nuclear factor RIP140 modulates transcriptional activation by the estrogen receptor. *EMBO J.* **14**, 3741–3751.
8. Norris, J. D., Paige, L. A., Christensen, D. J., et al. (1999) Peptide antagonists of the human estrogen receptor. *Science* **285**, 744–746.

17

Preparation of DNA-Protein Complexes Suitable for Spectroscopic Analysis

Nouri Neamati, Manisha Murthy, and Yun-Xing Wang

1. Introduction

During the past several years, remarkable progress has been made in solving the structures of high molecular weight proteins using X-ray crystallography and multidimensional nuclear magnetic resonance (NMR) spectroscopy. As the structures of more proteins are being routinely solved, there is a growing need to solve the structures of many of such proteins in complex with DNA. Although a plethora of techniques is now available to study DNA-protein interaction, none provides detailed structural information at the molecular level *(1,2)*. DNA-protein interactions are important in gene regulation, recombination, repair, transcription, and translation, and understanding these interactions at the molecular level is of paramount importance, which in many cases are responsible for various abnormalities.

X-ray crystallography and NMR spectroscopy both have their advantages and limitations, however, a main thrust of both techniques is the quality of the sample being studied. Obtaining good quality DNA-protein complexes in solution or crystalline state requires exploring a variety of conditions and in many cases have proven futile. For crystallography, the major problems have been the precipitation of the complex and the difficulty in obtaining diffractable crystals, whereas for NMR, the major problem has been the obtaining of a sufficient quantity of a "well-behaved" complex in solution. In cases where proteins form stable complexes with short duplex DNA containing a bona fide DNA-binding domain, isolation and purification present less difficulty (see for example, **ref.** *3*). Unfortunately, obtaining tight or irreversible complexes are

From: *Methods in Molecular Medicine, vol. 85: Novel Anticancer Drug Protocols*
Edited by: J. K. Buolamwini and A. A. Adjei © Humana Press Inc., Totowa, NJ

often required to provide structural information. Herein, we review available technologies that could potentially be used to obtain sufficient quantities of samples for spectroscopic analyses.

Rapid expression of desired proteins in *Escherichia coli* followed by purification, as well as synthesis of DNA on a large scale is now very practical and economical. However, various pilot experiments are required to determine the efficiency and practicality of each methodology. For example, in some cases it is only sufficient to run an electrophoretic mobility shift assay (EMSA) to obtain a crosslinked product or to check the efficiency of the product. DNA modification techniques are potentially required when complexes are reversible, unstable, or difficult to isolate. In some cases, fluorescent techniques may be used to characterize these complexes and to provide confirmatory or complementary information. Fluorescent techniques allow for minimal perturbation of the native equilibria and may incorporate either an extrinsic or an intrinsic fluorescent probe. Detailed analyses of such techniques have been reviewed previously and are not elaborated here.

1.1. Band-Shift Assays

Bandshift, also known as gel retardation or EMSA assays, is simple, efficient, convenient, and highly sensitive for detecting DNA-protein complex formation on a polyacrylamide gel. A radiolabeled DNA is normally used as a probe and reacted with a desired protein or protein mixtures in a suitable reaction buffer. The mixture is electrophoresed under non-denaturing conditions on a polyacrylamide gel. The DNA-protein complexes will migrate as a distinct band, much slower than the free DNA. This method can be used to detect DNA-binding proteins in vivo as well as in vitro for both sequence-specific and non-specific proteins. The band-shift assay can be used for quantitative estimation of the dissociation constants for protein-DNA complexes, as well as visualization of protein-protein interactions between a DNA-binding protein and other non-DNA-binding proteins. A second protein may also bind to the DNA-protein complex, which migrates even slower as a distinct band and is referred to as a super-shift. The material and methods described below are for quantitation and visualization of the product, and a side-by-side experiment is run on a larger scale to isolate sufficient quantity of samples. Based on the extent of crosslinking, the unreacted material should be removed by HPLC prior to spectroscopic analysis.

1.2. Site-Specific DNA-Protein Crosslinking via DNA Modifications

By incorporating a reactive group on a DNA and placing it at various positions and reacting that with the protein of interest, it is possible to map the molecular interaction between these macromolecules (*see* **Table 1**). It is

Table 1
Examples of Oligonucleotides Containing Modified Sequence

Sequence[a,b]
5′-nnnnnnnnnnnnnnnnnnnnMnn-3′
5′-nnnnnnnnnnnnnnnnnnMnnn-3′
5′-nnnnnnnnnnnnnnnnnMnnnn-3′
5′-nnnnnnnnnnnnnnnnMnnnnn-3′
5′-nnnnnnnnnnnnnnnMnnnnn-3′
5′-nnnnnnnnnnnnMnnnnnnnn-3′
5′-nnnnnnnnnnnnMnnnnnnnnn-3′
5′-nnnnnnnnnnMnnnnnnnnnn-3′

[a]For each duplex oligonucleotide only the top strand is shown.
[b]n can be any base and M represents the modified base.

easier to modify DNA than protein, hence a variety of modifications and/or photoactivatable reagents have been devised to crosslink DNA with protein. In addition, DNA modified with a reactive group is stable and can be easily incorporated on all bases or the phosphate backbone of DNA. DNA fragments are easily radiolabeled or fluorescent-labeled.

Two techniques, ultraviolet (UV) and chemical crosslinking, are routinely being used to complex DNA to proteins. In the first technique, a reactive moiety is attached to the bases or the phosphate group of DNA and requires UV light for activation. In the second method, the modified base is reactive and does not require UV or an exogenous crosslinking reagent to complex DNA and protein.

Numerous chemical and enzymatic reactions are employed to prepare a DNA fragment containing a photoactivatable crosslinking group (see for example **refs. 6–8**). The crosslinking moiety can be incorporated at a single, defined site to better map out the interaction between DNA and protein. The protein-DNA complex of interest is bombarded by ultraviolet radiation, initiating covalent crosslinking with proteins in direct physical proximity to the photoactivatible crosslinking group.

1.3. Application of Photocrosslinking Reagents

The best examples of photoactivatable crosslinking reagents are the aromatic azides (*see* **Fig. 1**). They form highly reactive nitrenes upon irradiation, which react indiscriminately with all surrounding groups by process of addition, abstraction of proton, nucleophilic attack, insertion, or coupling *(9–11)*. The advantages of photoaffinity labeling compared with affinity labeling, or chemical modification with group specific reagents, is that photoactivatible

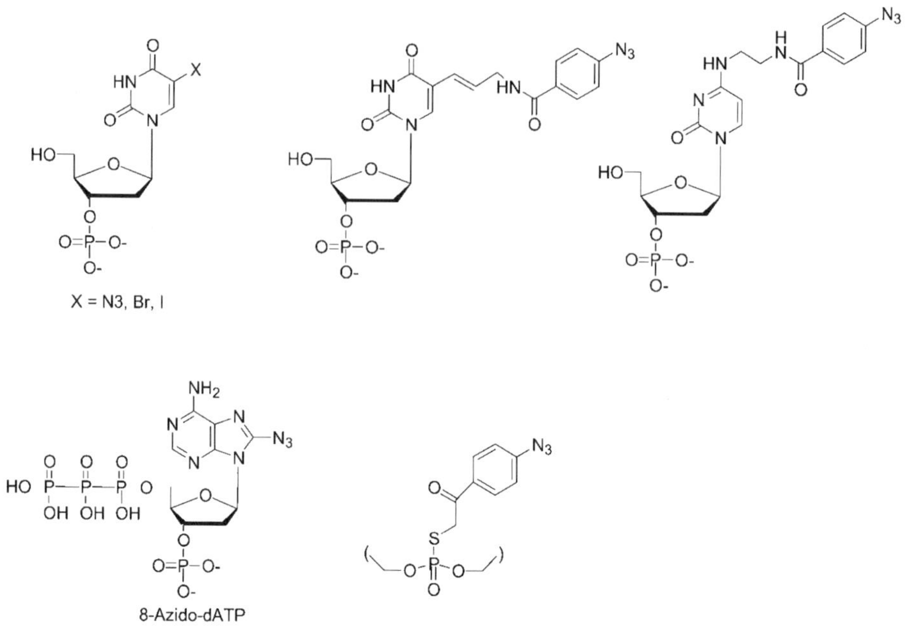

Fig. 1. Examples of photoactivatable deoxynucleotides.

nonreactive precursors can be activated at will by irradiation. These reagents do not link to the protein unless activated. Disadvantages of this method and many other crosslinking protocols are the low efficiency of the reaction and extensive damage to both DNA and protein that occurs during the reaction. To increase the yield, various laser techniques can be used. For example, the two-wavelength femtosecond laser can be used to obtain high yields of crosslinked DNA-protein complex without much DNA damage by the UV photons.

1.4. DNA-Protein Crosslinking via Schiff Base Formation of Abasic Site Residue and a Lysine

A facile approach of producing sufficient quantity of DNA-protein complexes is by reacting an abasic site-containing oligonucleotide with a protein. Lysine is a common amino acid in many proteins and reacts with the aldehyde to yield a Schiff base (*see* **Fig. 2**). This reaction is reversible. However, upon addition of borohydride, an irreversible complex is formed that is stable and can be purified in sufficient quantity for spectroscopic analysis.

1.5. DNA-Protein Crosslinking via Oxidation of 8-Oxoguanosine

Guanine is highly susceptible to oxidative damage and forms very reactive 8-oxo-guanine both in vitro and in vivo. Placing an 8-oxo-G:C pair into a

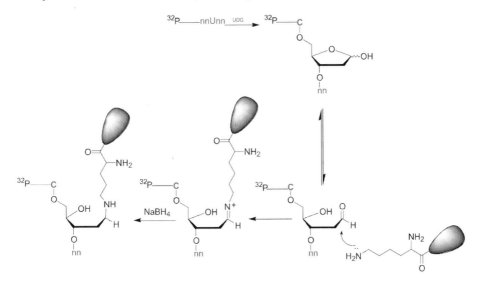

Fig. 2. Chemical crosslinking of DNA with protein. Uracil is incorporated at a designated site on a duplex oligonucleotide and radiolabeled with ^{32}P. Following addition of uracil DNA glycosylase and purification an abasic DNA is formed, which is reacted with desired protein to form a Schiff base. Upon addition of borohydride, an irreversible product is formed, which is stable and can be purified. Only the top strand of a DNA radiolabeled at 5′-end is shown.

DNA duplex produces little perturbation of DNA structure, but significantly enhances DNA reactivity. The fate of 8-oxo-G appears to follow the urate oxidation pathway leading, via 5-hydroxy-8-oxo-G, to a guanidinohydantoin moiety *(13)* (*see* **Fig. 3**). In the presence of a bound protein, it is thought that an active-site nucleophile might participate instead, leading to a covalent DNA-protein crosslink analogous to 5-hydroxy-8-oxoguanosine.

1.6. Chemical Modification of Lysine by Reductive Methylation

It is well established that the basic side chain of lysine participates strongly in DNA-protein recognition. In addition to interaction through non-specific charge-charge interactions with the phosphate backbone and by forming direct hydrogen bonds with functional groups of the bases, lysine's positive charge can also interact with the aromatic residues, similar to those between divalent metal-π interactions of aromatic amino acids. Modification of lysines via Schiff base formation as explained above or by reductive alkylation provides a powerful way to study DNA-protein interaction. A particularly useful reaction is the reductive methylation using ^{13}C or ^{3}H labeled formaldehyde and the reducing agent sodium cyanoborohydride. This is because under mild solution conditions, the accessible lysine residues on proteins are completely converted

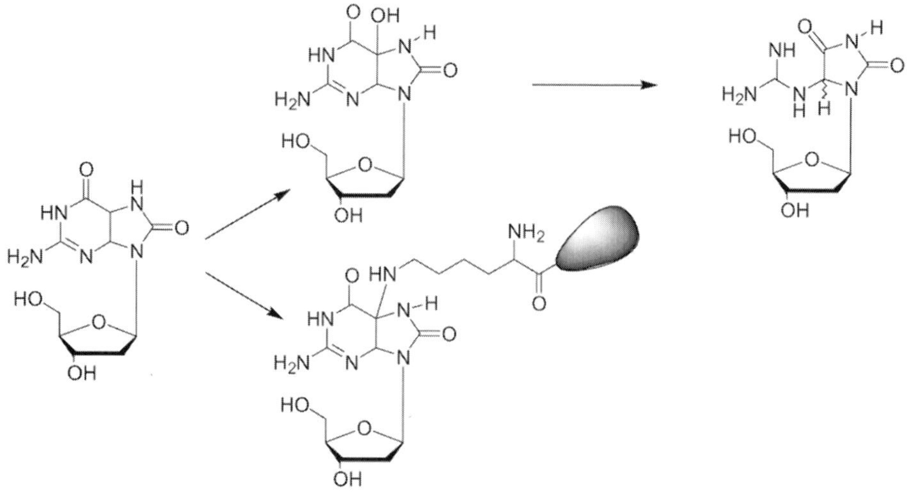

Fig. 3. Reactions of 8-oxoguanine. Nucleophilic attack by a water molecule yields 5-OH-8-oxoguanine, followed by hydrolysis and release of CO_2 to give guanidinohydantoin (top) or by the ε-amino group of a lysine in a protein to form a DNA-protein crosslink.

to the ε-N,N-dimethyl derivatives. The reaction occurs in two phases. First, the ε-amino group of the lysine forms an adduct with the formaldehyde to produce a Schiff base. This will then undergo reduction by sodium cyanoborohydride to the monomethylamine derivative. A further round of the reaction will produce the dimethyl derivative (14) (see Fig. 4).

Dimethylation of the lysine side chain is a small chemical change. It maintains its ionization and interaction properties comparable to the unmodified protein with slight loss of hydrogen bonding capacity. Reductive methylation experiments may incorporate ^{13}C and this is used as a probe to study the environment of lysine side chains in proteins using NMR spectroscopy (15,16). Such an incorporation of radiolabels into the proteins enables the number of accessible lysines to be determined.

1.7. Crosslinking Activity of Bifunctional Aldehydes

Aldehydes form a very important class of highly reactive organic compounds. The effect of a variety of saturated and unsaturated aldehydes was examined for their efficiency as DNA-protein crosslinking agents, and it was found that formaldehyde, glutaraldehyde, and acrolein were the most potent crosslinkers (17,18). Herein, we briefly discuss two of these reagents for in vitro studies because of their efficiency and accessibility.

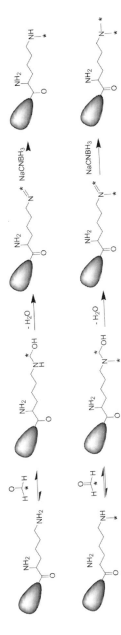

Fig. 4. Reductive methylation of lysine. A ^{13}C labeled formaldehyde is reacted with the ε-amino group of the lysine to generate a Schiff base, which is reduced with sodium cyanoborohydride to the ε-*N*-monomethyl-lysine. In the second step, the final product, ^{13}C labeled ε-*N*, *N*-dimethyl-lysine is formed by addition of formaldehyde.

1.7.1. Formaldehyde-Mediated DNA-Protein Crosslinking

Formaldehyde is a highly reactive agent that will produce protein-DNA crosslinks and protein-protein crosslinks between macromolecules in close contact *(19,20)*. Formaldehyde will react with amino groups of cytosines, guanines, and adenines, and the imino groups of thymines and probably guanines. In proteins, potential candidates for crosslinking are lysine, arginine, tryptophan, and histidine residues. The first stage involves the reaction with amino or imino groups and results in the formation of unstable methylol derivatives, which react with the adjacent second reacting group *(21)* (*see* **Fig. 5**).

1.7.2. Malondialdehyde-Mediated DNA-Protein Crosslinking

Malondialdehyde is a bifunctional DNA-protein crosslinking agent. It has been shown that only those proteins that can bind to DNA are capable of forming crosslinks *(22,23)*. For example, when bovine serum albumin (BSA) is used in the reaction mixture, there were no nonspecific DNA-protein interactions observed *(24)*, even though BSA contains several lysine residues. Crosslinking of proteins to DNA normally proceeds through the initial formation of protein adduct, followed by reaction with DNA. The crosslink formed is relatively stable and a NMR solution structure of malondialdehyde with DNA was recently solved *(25)*.

1.8. Fluorescence Spectroscopy

Fluorescence spectroscopy is a very sensitive technique to investigate the interaction of a protein with DNA in solution *(26)*. Either the intrinsic fluorescence of the aromatic amino acids (e.g., tyrosine or tryptophan) of the proteins or an extrinsic fluorophore can be used as a probe. In the absence of bona fide aromatic residue near the DNA-binding site, it is best to introduce tyrosine or tryptophan into the putative DNA-binding sites, or the bases in the DNA molecule may be modified with fluorescent reagents. Among the DNA modified fluorescent probes, 2-aminopurine (2AP), a highly fluorescent isomer of adenine, is one of the most widely used. It possesses several qualities that make it extremely desirable as a fluorescent probe: The structure of DNA is minimally perturbed by replacement of an adenine by 2AP, which forms a normal Watson-Crick base pair with thymine. Also, the fluorescence of this probe can be selectively excited in the presence of DNA, RNA, and protein, because it absorbs at a much longer wavelength than aromatic amino acids or the nucleic acid bases *(27–31)*. For mapping DNA-protein interaction, 2AP can be incorporated at various sites on the DNA as explained above for Schiff-base assays.

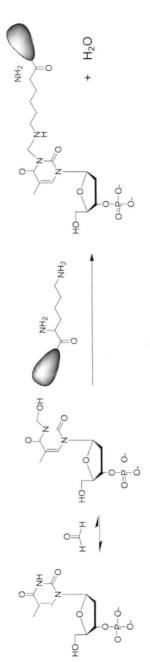

Fig. 5. Formaldehyde-mediated cross linking of DNA and protein. Formaldehyde reacts with a base to generate methylol derivatives, which forms a stable crosslinked product with a protein via a ε-amino group of the lysine.

Extrinsic fluorescent probes are also known to interact with or compete with a ligand for the binding of the protein. A variety of fluorescence probes have been employed for this purpose and the review of such probes is beyond the scope of this chapter.

1.9. Solution NMR Spectroscopy

Solution NMR spectroscopy is one of the important methods in studying DNA-protein complexes, not only in structural determination, but also in rapidly mapping the out-of-contact interface between protein and DNA molecules when structural determination is neither the goal nor attainable. However, in almost every case, obtaining a well-behaved NMR sample of a protein/DNA complex takes a major effort. It requires skills in molecular biology, protein/DNA biochemistry, as well as perseverance and pure luck.

1.9.1. Isotope-Labeled DNA Oligomers

To make use of multi-dimensional heteronuclear NMR spectroscopy to study protein-DNA complexes in solution, one requires $^{13}C/^{15}N$ isotope-labeled protein as well as DNA samples. Starting from the early 1990s, when $^{13}C/^{15}N$ isotope-enriched protein samples became available *(32,33)*, researchers have been able to determine high-resolution structures of proteins complexed with DNA oligomers in solution. In many cases, the proteins in context of complexes are relatively well defined, because isotope-labeled protein samples are used in studies, whereas the DNA molecules of the complexes are not because of a lack of $^{13}C/^{15}N$-labeled DNA samples and unique structural nature of nucleic acids.

Practical protocols to prepare isotope-labeled DNA samples for NMR spectroscopic studies became available only in recent years. They are solid-phase synthesis *(34)*, PCR-based synthesis using labeled dNTPs *(35)*, and enzyme-based synthesis *(36,37)*. These protocols lead to application of heteronuclear NMR, as well as most recent techniques such as Transverse Relaxation-Optimized Spectroscopy (TROSY) *(38)* and dipolar coupling measurements *(39)* in DNA. Among the protocols, solid-phase synthesis of DNA oligomers is far more versatile than other methods *(34)*. It can be used to synthesize virtually any DNA oligomer with any labeling scheme provided that phosphoamidite precursors are available.

1.9.2. NMR Sample Conditioning

Like any other sample for NMR studies, samples of protein/DNA complex studies also require extensive preliminary testing, or "conditioning," in order to find out the best condition under which the complexes behave well enough for studies. Not all protein-DNA complexes are suitable for study with NMR spectroscopy at the first trial. There are several criteria that determine if a protein-DNA complex is NMR-friendly: association constants between the protein and DNA molecule, solubility, thermal stability, and molecular size. To achieve a workable NMR sample, one often needs to conduct various titrations, such as pH, salt, and detergent at several temperatures while monitoring changes in chemical shift and linewidth of peaks using NMR experiments such as ^{15}N two-dimensional heteronuclear single quantum correlation spectroscopy (HSQC) to record the chemical shift perturbation of protein amides, or simple one-dimensional imino spectra of DNA base pairing.

The HSQC spectra not only can be used as a means to monitor optimization of solution conditions, but also are powerful tools to quickly derive a list of key residues in direct contact with DNA without necessarily knowing the 3D structure of the protein or complex. As an example, changes in ^{15}N and ^{1}H amide chemical shifts of MAP30, a protein extract from plant *Momordinca charatia* (bitter melon), titrated with HIV-1 long terminal repeat (LTR) DNA, was monitored with ^{15}N HSQC spectra and the results are depicted in **Fig. 6**. The residues whose chemical shifts are perturbed strongly are those located at the interface between the protein and DNA and in immediate contact to the DNA.

The association constant between protein and DNA is an important parameter in evaluating feasibility of preparing a non-covalent protein/DNA complex for studies. The association constant is obtained from various biophysical experiments, ranging from gel mobility shift (gel retardation) or filter-binding assay, to spectroscopic means including NMR. The protein-DNA interaction can be divided into three categories based on their association constant. They are weakly ($K_d > 10^{-6}$ M), intermediate ($10^{-9} < K_d < 10^{-6}$), and tightly ($K_d < 10^{-9}$) bound. NMR spectrocopists usually prefer either weakly associated or tightly bound complexes because of simplicity in interpretation of the spectrum. For the intermediately bound complexes, the spectra are more complicated to interpret because the complex, unbound DNA, and protein co-exist in solution and all give rise to distinct signals, depending on their chemical shift dispersion. To obtain a simple and interpretable spectrum, one often needs to make mutants, either of DNA, protein, or both to obtain a well-behaved complex.

The complex should be soluble at least above ~0.7 mM if the conventional triple resonance probe is used for detection (note that this concentration is several magnitudes higher than the physiological concentration). At this or higher concentration, the complex should be free from aggregation/self-association unless they are biologically relevant. Often mixing protein with DNA oligomer solutions of millimolar concentration produces a white precipitate. The white precipitate can be either because of non-specific aggregation as a result of interactions between DNA and protein, or insolubility of the

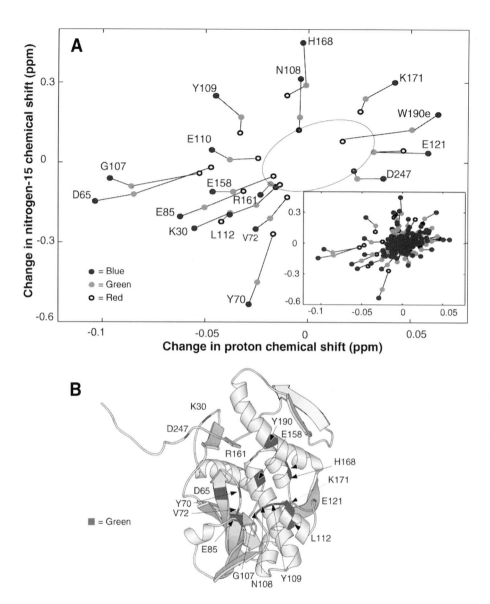

Fig. 6. MAP30 chemical shift perturbation by LTR DNA. MAP30/LTR DNA forms a complex that is insoluble under low salt and the complex dissociates at high salt concentration. Nevertheless, NMR spectroscopy still can be used to map out the interation surface on protein. (A) Changes in ^{15}N (y-axis) and ^{1}H (x-axis) amide chemical shifts of a 100 μM MAP30 solution, depicted by colored disks at DNA concentrations of 50 μM (white circle), 100 μM (gray circle), and 150 μM (black circle). Note that the sidechain of Trp190 was perturbed and that the vast majority of amide remained within the oval were not strongly perturbed (all data is shown in the lower right inset). (B) Ribbon diagram of MAP30 colored green to indicate residues whose chemical shifts were most sensitive and whose chemical shift perturbation are greater than ~37 and ~25 Hz in ^{1}H and ^{15}N dimensions, respectively to the addition of the LTR DNA.

complex itself. Increasing salt concentration may enhance the solubility of protein/DNA complexes, but often at the expense of possible weakening of the ionic interaction between protein and DNA, and may in turn lead to dissociation of the complex at high salt.

High thermal stability is very much desired for recording a good quality spectrum, but may not necessarily be suitable for the certain samples because fast exchange and thermal denaturation/degrdation that may incur to the samples. Even for samples that are stable at high temperature, for example, 40°C, the fast exchange of amide protons with water may also deteriorate sensitivity of NMR experiments even with techniques to preserve water magnetization at equilibrium.

The most noticeable limitation of the current NMR technology, in contrast to x-ray crystallography, is size. NMR spectroscopy detects a signal that is an average of different bond vectors of molecules tumbling in solution. These bond vectors undergo rotational diffusion that is best characterized by a correlation time. The correlation time increases as molecular size increases, leading to a less efficient averaging and faster decaying of NMR signals. Current NMR technology is capable of determining high resolution structures of singular molecules up to 30 kDa, although the newly developed NMR experiments may extend it to a higher molecular weight range in the future *(40,41)*. At the present time, in order to obtain workable NMR samples of complexes, NMR spectroscopists mainly rely on making smaller complexes in which protein fragments structurally mimic the intact protein and retain full or near full biological activity of the native protein. Almost all structures of protein/DNA complexes determined by solution NMR are protein domain fragments complexed with DNA oligomers.

2. Materials

2.1. Band-Shift Assays

1. ^{32}P radiolabled DNA.
2. Purified protein.
3. Electrophoresis apparatus and buffer.
4. Polyacrylamide gels.
5. Bovine serum albumin (BSA).

2.2. DNA-Protein Crosslinking via Schiff Base Formation of Abasic Site Residue and a Lysine

1. Uracil containing oligonucleotide.
2. Uracil DNA glycosylase.
3. γ-^{32}P[ATP].
4. Sodium borohydride.

2.3. DNA-Protein Crosslinking
via Oxidation of 8-Oxoguanosine

1. ^{32}P labeled DNA containing 8-oxoguanine modification.
2. Purified protein.
3. Na_2IrCl_6.
4. Reaction buffer: 100 mM sodium pyrophosphate (NaPi), pH 7.0, 1 M NaCl, 20 mM Tris-HCl, pH 7.5, 20% glycerol.
5. Stopping reaction: 250 mM EDTA, 50 mM HEPES, pH 7.0, sodium dodecyl sulfate-polyacrylamide gel electrophoresis (SDS-PAGE) loading buffer.

2.4. Malondialdehyde-Mediated DNA-Protein Crosslinking

1. Formaldehyde or Malondialdehyde.
2. DNA.
3. Protein.
4. Crosslinking reaction mixture—phosphate buffer, pH 7.4, NaCl.
5. Crosslinking termination mixture—Stop solution contains: 0.5% SDS.

3. Methods
3.1. Band-Shift Assays

Mix DNA and protein in a ratio of 10:1 protein to DNA in an appropriate buffer with or without BSA in a microfuge tube. Although reactions can be carried out at 37°C for 30 min, it is recommended to run a kinetic titration at various concentrations and time, to optimize the reaction. It is important to note that the size, PI, and aggregation state of the DNA-protein complex and ionic strength of the buffers influence the mobility of complexes and dictate the choice of gel matrix to be used for the assay. When larger DNA is used, agarose is preferred over polyacrylamide. The electrophoresis buffer (generally, TBE) should be the same as the binding buffer and for metal-binding proteins buffers without ethylene diamine tetraacetic acid (EDTA) should be used (for recent reviews, *see* **refs. [4,5]**).

3.2. DNA-Protein Crosslinking via Schiff Base
Formation of Abasic Site Residue and a Lysine

Incubate protein and oligonucleotide containing an abasic site (*see* **Table 1**) in reaction buffer recommended by the supplier. Add freshly prepared solution of sodium borohydride (0.1 M final concentration) and continue the reaction for an additional two minutes. For analysis on gel, add an equal volume (16 μL) of 2X SDS-PAGE buffer (100 mM Tris-HCl, pH 6.8, 4% 2-mercaptoethanol, 4% SDS, 0.2% bromophenol blue, 20% glycerol) to each reaction, and heat the reaction at 95°C for 3 min prior to loading a 20 µL aliquot on a 12% SDS-polyacrylamide gel. Run the gel at 120 V for 1.5 h, dry, and expose in a PhosphorImager cassette or autoradiography film *(12)*.

3.3. DNA-Protein Crosslinking via Oxidation of 8-Oxoguanosine

DNA and protein (1:10) are mixed in a reaction buffer and incubated for 15 min at 37°C. 500 µM of Na_2IrCl_6 is added to initiate the crosslinking reaction and incubated for an additional 15 min. An equal volume of stopping buffer is added and loaded on a 16 or 20% acrylamide gel for electrophoresis.

3.4. Malondialdehyde-Mediated DNA-Protein Crosslinking

DNA-protein crosslinks are routinely carried out at room temperature in a solution containing phosphate buffer, DNA and protein. The ionic strength of the solution is adjusted with NaCl. Crosslinking reactions are terminated by addition of a stop solution that has SDS.

4. Notes

1. In preparing DNA-protein complexes, it is important to take several precautions. First of all, when a protein contains cysteine residues, maintaining their native oxidation states is very important. If there is a disulfide bond between cysteines, one should not add a large excess of dithiothreitol (DTT) in the buffer, as it would disrupt the disulfide bond. On the other hand, if cysteines are not engaged in disulfide bond formation, one should add excess DTT to prevent either oxidation of the thiol groups in cysteines or the formation of non-biologically relevant intermolecular disulfide bonds. Second, generally speaking, ionic interaction is the major contributor to the DNA-protein complex formation. The presence of a large concentration (~300 mM) of salt reduces the ionic interaction between DNA and protein, and eventually leads to dissociation of the complex. This explains why it is sometimes difficult to make DNA-protein complexes when the proteins require several hundred millimolar of salt in order to solubilize in aqueous solution.
2. For a long DNA duplex, one might anneal the two strands by following heating and slow cooling steps to insure the duplex formation.

References

1. Moss, T. (2001) *DNA-Protein Interaction: Principles and Protocols*, 2nd ed., Humana Press, Totowa, NJ.
2. Travers, A. and Buckle, M. (2000) *DNA-Protein Interaction.* Oxford University Press, Oxford, UK.

3. Conlin, R. M. and Brown. R. S. (2001) Reconstitution of protein-DNA complexes for crystallization, in *DNA-Protein Interaction: Principles and Protocols*, 2nd ed. (Moss, T., ed.), Humana Press, Totowa, NJ, pp. 547–556.

4. Fairall, L., Buttinelli, M. and Panetta, G. (2000) *Bandshift, Gel Retardation Or Electrophoretic Mobility Shift Assays*. Oxford University Press, Oxford, UK.

5. Laniel, M. A., Beliveau, A., and Guerin, S. L. (2001) Electrophoretic mobility shift assays for the analysis of DNA-protein interactions, in *DNA-Protein Interaction: Principles and Protocols*, 2nd ed. (Moss, T., ed.), Humana Press, Totowa, NJ, pp. 13–30.

6. Gao, M., Cui, H. R., Loe, D. W., et al. (2000) Comparison of the functional characteristics of the nucleotide binding domains of multidrug resistance protein. *J. Biol. Chem.* **275**, 13,098–13,108.

7. Persinger, J. and Bartholomew, B. (2001) Site-directed DNA photoaffinity labeling of RNA polymerase III transcription complexes, in *DNA-Protein Interaction: Principles and Protocols*, 2nd ed. (Moss, T., ed.), Humana Press, Totowa, NJ, pp. 363–381.

8. Zofall, M. and Bartholomew, B. (2000) Two novel dATP analogs for DNA photoaffinity labeling. *Nucl. Acids Res.* **28**, 4382–4390.

9. Meffert, R., Dose, K., Rathgeber, G. and Schafer, H. J. (2001) Ultraviolet crosslinking of DNA-protein complexes via 8-azidoadenine, in *DNA-Protein Interaction: Principles and Protocols*, 2nd ed. (Moss, T., ed.), Humana Press, Totowa, NJ, pp. 323–335.

10. Naryshkin, N., Kim, Y., Dong, Q., and Ebright, R. H. (2001) Site-specific protein-DNA photocrosslinking. Analysis of bacterial transcription initiation complexes, in *DNA-Protein Interaction: Principles and Protocols*, 2nd ed. (Moss, T., ed.), Humana Press, Totowa, NJ, pp. 337–361.

11. Naryshkin, N., Revyakin, A., Kim, Y. Mekler, V., and Ebright, R. H. (2000) Structural organization of the RNA polymerase-promoter open complex. *Cell* **101**, 601–611.

12. Mazumder, A., Neamati, N., Pilon, A. A., Sunder, S., and Pommier, Y. (1996) Chemical trapping of ternary complexes of human immunodeficiency virus type 1 integrase, divalent metal, and DNA substrates containing an abasic site: Implications for the role of lysine 136 in DNA binding. *J. Biol. Chem.* **271**, 27,330–27,338.

13. Hickerson, R. P., Chepansoke, C. L., Williams, S. D., David, S. S., and Burrows C. J. (1999) Mechanism-based DNA-protein crosslinking of MutY via oxidation of 8-oxoguanosine. *J. Am. Chem. Soc.* **121**, 9901–9902.

14. Taylor, I. A. and Webb, M. (2001) Chemical modification of lysine by reductive methylation. A probe for residues involved in DNA binding, in *DNA-Protein Interaction: Principles and Protocols*, 2nd ed. (Moss, T., ed.), Humana Press, Totowa, NJ, pp. 301–314.

15. Zhang, M., Huque, E., and Vogel, H. J. (1994) Characterization of trimethyllysine 115 in calmodulin by ^{14}N and ^{13}C NMR spectroscopy. *J. Biol. Chem.* **269**, 5099–5105.

16. Zhang, M., Thulin, E., and Vogel, H. J. (1994) Reductive methylation and pKa determination of the lysine side chains in calbindin D9k. *J. Protein Chem.* **13,** 527–535.
17. Costa, M., Zhitkovich, M., Harris, A., Paustenbach, D., and Gargas, M. (1997) DNA-protein cross-links produced by various chemicals in cultured human lymphoma cells. *J. Toxicol. Environ. Health* **50,** 433–439.
18. Kuykendall, J. R. and Bogdanffy, M. S. (1992) Efficiency of DNA-histone crosslinking induced by saturated and unsaturated aldehydes in vitro. *Mutat. Res.* **283,** 131–136.
19. Strutt, H. and Paro, R. (1999) Mapping DNA target sites of chromatin proteins in vivo by formaldehyde crosslinking, in *Chromatin Protocols* (Becker, P. B., ed.), Humana Press, Totowa, NJ, pp. 455–467.
20. Toth, J. and Biggin, M. D. (2000) The specificity of protein-DNA Crosslinking by formaldehyde: in vitro and in drosophila embryos. *Nucl. Acids Res.* **28,** 4.
21. Brodolin, K. (2000) *Protein-DNA Crosslinking with Formaldehyde In Vitro.* Oxford University Press, Oxford, UK.
22. Nair, V., Cooper, C. S., Vietti, D. E., and Turner, G. A. (1986) The chemistry of lipid peroxidation metabolites: crosslinking reactions of malondialdehyde. *Lipids* **21,** 6–10.
23. Summerfield, F. W. and Tappel, A. L. (1984) Detection and measurement by high-performance liquid chromatography of malondialdehyde crosslinks in DNA. *Anal. Biochem.* **143,** 265–271.
24. Voitkun, V. and Zhitkovich, A. (1999) Analysis of DNA-protein prosslinking activity of malondialdehyde in vitro. *Mutat. Res.* **424,** 97–106.
25. Mao, H., Reddy, G. R., Marnett, L. J., and Stone, M. P. (1999) Solution structure of an oligodeoxynucleotide containing the malondialdehyde deoxyguanosine adduct N2-(3-oxo-1-propenyl)-dG (ring- opened M1G) positioned in a (CpG)3 frameshift hotspot of the Salmonella typhimurium hisD3052 gene. *Biochemistry* **38,** 13,491–13,501.
26. Fluorescence Correlation Spectroscopy and Related Methods. Proceedings of a workshop. Jena, Germany, March 2000. *Biol. Chem.* **382,** 353–504.
27. Jean, J. M. and Hall, K. B. (2001) 2-Aminopurine fluorescence quenching and lifetimes: role of base stacking. *Proc. Natl. Acad. Sci. USA* **98,** 37–41.
28. Larsen, O. F., van Stokkum, I. H., Gobets, B. van Grondelle, R., and van Amerongen, H. (2001) Probing the structure and dynamics of a DNA hairpin by ultrafast quenching and fluorescence depolarization. *Biophys. J.* **81,** 1115–1126.
29. Rachofsky, E. L., Osman, R., and Ross, J. B. (2001) Probing structure and dynamics of DNA with 2-aminopurine: effects of local environment on fluorescence. *Biochemistry* **40,** 946–956.
30. Rachofsky, E. L., Seibert, E., Stivers, J. T., Osman, R., and Ross, J. B. (2001) Conformation and dynamics of abasic sites in DNA investigated by time-resolved fluorescence of 2-aminopurine. *Biochemistry* **40,** 957–967.
31. Wennmalm, S., Blom, H., Wallerman, L., and Rigler, R. (2001) UV-Fluorescence correlation spectroscopy of 2-aminopurine. *Biol. Chem.* **382,** 393–397.

32. Bax, A., Ikura, M., Kay, L. E, Barbato, G., and Spera, S. (1991). Multi-dimensional triple resonance NMR-Spectroscopy of isotopically uniformly enriched proteins— a powerful new srategy for structure determination. *CIBA Foundation Symposia* **161,** 108–135.

33. Clore, G. M. and Gronenborn, A. M. (1991) Structures of larger proteins in solution: three- and four-dimensional heteronuclear NMR spectroscopy. *Science* **252,** 1390–1399.

34. Kojima, C., Ono, A. M., Ono, A., and Kainosho, M. (2001) Solid-phase synthesis of selectively-labeled DNA: applications for multidimensional nuclear magnetic resonance spectroscopy. In *Nuclear Magnetic Resonance of Biologica Macromolecules, Pt A* (James, T. L., ed.), Academic Press, Orlando, FL, pp. 261–283.

35. Louis, J. M., Martin, R. G., Clore, G. M., and Gronenborn, A. M. (1998) Preparation of uniformly isotope-labeled DNA oligonucleotides for NMR spectroscopy. *J. Biol. Chem.* **273,** 2374–2378.

36. Mer, G. and Chazin, W. J. (1998) Enzymatic synthesis of region-specific isotope-labeled DNA oligomers for NMR analysis. *J. Am. Chem. Soc.* **120,** 607–608.

37. Smith, D. E., Su, J. Y., and Jucker, F. M. (1997) Efficient enzymatic synthesis of ^{13}C, ^{15}N-labeled DNA for NMR studies. *J. Biomolec. NMR* **10,** 245–253.

38. Riek, R., Pervushin, K., Fernandez, C., Kainosho, M., Wuthrich, K. (2001) [(13)C, (13C]– and [(13)C, (1)H]–TROSY in a triple resonance experiment for ribose-base and intrabase correlations in nucleic acids. *J. Am. Chem. Soc.* **123,** 658–664.

39. Wu, Z., Ono, A., Kainosho, M., Bax, A. (2001) H…N hydrogen bond lengths in double stranded DNA from internucleotide dipolar couplings. *J. Biomol. NMR* **19,** 361–365.

40. Pervushin, K., Riek, R., Wider, G., and Wuthrich, K. (1997) Attenuated T2 relaxation by mutual cancellation of dipole-dipole coupling and chemical shift anisotropy indicates an avenue to NMR structures of very large biological macromolecules in solution. *Proc. Natl. Acad. Sci. USA* **94,** 12,366–12,371.

41. Riek, R., Pervushin, K., Wuthrich, K. (2000) TROSY and CRINEPT: NMR with large molecular and supremolecular structures in solution. *Trends Biochem. Sci.* **25,** 462–468.

VII

ANTISENSE

18

Antisense Oligonucleotide Inhibitors of MDM2 Oncogene Expression

Ruiwen Zhang and Hui Wang

1. Introduction

1.1. Antisense Therapeutics

Antisense therapy represents a novel genetic-based therapeutic approach, initiated by Zamecnik et al. about 20 years ago *(1)*. The rationale for antisense oligonucleotide therapeutics is straightforward: to identify a specific inhibitor of an mRNA of interest on the basis of the nucleotide sequence of the mRNA and design a complementary oligonucleotide (oligo). Thus, antisense approaches offer the possibility of specific, rational drugs. Over the years, although there have been many concerns that have limited enthusiasm for the development of these drugs from the preclinical to the clinical level *(2,3)*, significant advances have been made in this field of research. The development of improved synthetic methods yielding sufficient quantities of antisense oligos has allowed extensive preclinical and clinical pharmacologic and toxicologic studies. Advanced antisense chemistry providing various modifications of oligos has resulted in improved pharmacokinetic, pharmacodynamic, and toxicologic profiles of antisense oligos. Extensive studies examining both specific and non-specific effects of oligos have led to a better design of antisense sequences to target genes. More recently, several antisense oligos have entered clinical use or clinical trials, including those targeted to genes important in human cancers *(4–10)*, with the first antisense drug Vitravene being approved for the treatment of patients with cytomegalovirus-induced retinitis *(5)*. Research in the antisense field has been reviewed periodically *(3–9)*.

From: *Methods in Molecular Medicine, vol. 85: Novel Anticancer Drug Protocols*
Edited by: J. K. Buolamwini and A. A. Adjei © Humana Press Inc., Totowa, NJ

The effects of antisense oligos can be evaluated both in vitro and in vivo. As shown in many earlier published studies, the antisense effects are usually first examined in cell-free systems, confirming that antisense oligos selectively hybridize with their specific mRNA targets, resulting in decreased expression of the targeted proteins. Those antisense oligos that have been found effective are then further examined at cellular and molecular levels. While there is some variability on cellular uptake depending on the chemistry of antisense oligos, many oligos can apparently cross the cell membrane into the cytosol in sufficient quantities to cause the desired antisense effect. Cellular pharmacokinetic studies have also examined various approaches to increase cellular uptake of antisense oligos by using liposomes, phospholipids, and other means to increase membrane penetrability of these oligos.

The in vivo preclinical pharmacologic evaluation of antisense oligos has employed animal studies, predominantly in murine species. Pharmacokinetic studies examining the fate of antisense oligos in vivo, i.e., absorption, distribution, metabolism and excretion, have mainly been undertaken after administration of phosphorothioate oligonucleotides (PS-oligos), representing the first generation antisense oligos. PS-oligos have a short distribution half-life and a longer elimination half-life in plasma, and are distributed widely into and retained in all major tissues following intravenous, intraperitoneal, or subcutaneous administration *(10–16)*. Extensive metabolism of antisense oligos has been observed, although the mechanisms are not fully understood. PS-oligos are degraded primarily from the 3′-end, but degradation from the 5′-end or both the 3′- and 5′-ends has been observed as well *(15,16)*.

In the development of second generation antisense oligos, major efforts have been devoted to stabilizing PS-oligos by various modifications of their structure *(17–21)*. Increased biostability of antisense oligos has at least two advantages: an intact antisense oligo provides a longer duration of action; and fewer degradation products generated would avoid potential unwanted side effects from these metabolites. Plasma pharmacokinetics of PS-oligo are, in general, not associated with the length or primary sequence of oligo, but associated with the modification of the backbone and specific segments at the 3′ and/or 5′ end *(15–21)*.

Compared with preclinical studies, far fewer clinical studies of oligos have been reported. Most clinical studies thus far have used PS-oligos *(4–11)*. Examples of clinical trials currently underway with antisense oligos as anticancer agents include those targeted to mutant p53, *bcl-2*, protein kinase C, protein kinase A, *c-raf* kinase, and Ha-*ras* *(4–10)*. Clinical trials of oligos with advanced antisense chemistry have also begun *(22)*. In this chapter, we are presenting the antisense anti-MDM2 oligos with advanced antisense chemistry as an example to illustrate the protocol for in vitro and in vivo evaluation of antisense oligo therapeutics in preclinical settings.

1.2. MDM2 as a Target for Cancer Therapy

Oncogene and tumor suppressor genes have been shown to play a major role in formation, growth and progression of human cancers. Activation of proto-oncogenes that promote cell growth, in combination with the inactivation of tumor suppressor genes that inhibit cell growth by means of growth arrest and induction of apoptosis, leads to tumor progression and malignancy. Perhaps the most important and studied tumor suppressor gene is p53 *(23)*. Abnormalities of the p53 tumor suppressor gene are among the most frequent molecular events in human and animal neoplasia. Studies have also shown that the tumor suppressor function of p53 can be inhibited without mutation. A major advancement in understanding the p53 pathway is the discovery of MDM2 and its role in controlling p53 levels *(24,25)*. There is an MDM2-p53 autoregulatory feedback loop that regulates intracellular p53 function: the MDM2 gene is a target for direct transcriptional activation by p53, and MDM2 protein is a negative regulator of p53 (reviewed in **ref. 26**). In addition, MDM2 protein interacts with other cellular proteins that are involved in cell cycle regulation, including pRb, E2F1/DP1, and p19ARF. Therefore, MDM2 plays a crucial role in cell cycle control and tumor transformation and growth. Like p53, MDM2 has become a target for rational drug design for cancer therapy *(25,26)*. Several recent excellent reviews provide a comprehensive discussion of the MDM2 oncogene and its functions as well as its interaction with various cellular proteins *(27–32)*.

MDM2 also has been shown to play a role in DNA damaging treatment. MDM2 is transcriptionally induced by p53 following DNA damage *(33,34)*. The MDM2 oncoprotein, in turn, binds to and directly blocks p53 function as a transcription factor and tumor suppressor and induces p53 degradation. This p53-MDM2 loop may play a role in p53-mediated response to DNA-damaging treatment in tumor cells and, therefore, can be modulated to improve the therapeutic effectiveness of DNA-damaging agents or radiation therapy.

The connection between MDM2 and cancer has been shown in many studies of human cancers. Overexpression of MDM2 is shown in a variety of human tumors and may be due to one or more of the following three mechanisms: 1) gene amplification *(35,36)*; 2) increased transcription *(37)*; or 3) enhanced translation *(38)*. Overexpression of MDM2 gene has been shown in many human tumors, including soft tissue tumors, osteosarcomas, esophageal carcinomas, brain tumor, breast cancer, ovarian carcinoma, cervical cancer, lung cancer, colon cancer, bronchogenic carcinoma, nasopharyngeal carcinoma, neuroblastomas, testicular germ-cell tumor, and urothelial cancers, as well as in pediatric solid tumors (reviewed in **refs. *26*** and ***35***). In general, human cancer cell lines or tumor tissues with MDM2 gene amplifications or overexpression often have wild-type p53 *(35)*, presumably inactivated by MDM2. Several studies have shown that overexpression of MDM2 is associated with poor prognosis in human cancers including osteosarcoma, soft tissue sarcoma, breast cancer, ovarian cancer, cervical cancer, oral squamous cell carcinoma, brain tumors, esophageal cancer, bladder cancer, leukemia, and large B cell lymphoma (reviewed in **ref. *26***).

It has been demonstrated that many cancer therapeutic agents exert their cytotoxic effects through activation of wild-type p53, and the restoration of wild-type p53 can increase the sensitivity of tumors to DNA-damaging agents *(39,40)*. However, the activation of p53 by DNA damage such as cancer chemotherapy and radiation treatment may be limited in cancers with MDM2 expression, especially those with MDM2 overexpression. Therefore, the inactivation of the MDM2 negative feedback loop may increase the magnitude of p53 activation following DNA damage, thus enhancing the therapeutic efficacy of DNA damaging drugs and radiation therapy. In the past, several strategies have been used to test the hypothesis that by disrupting p53-mdm2 interaction, the negative regulation of p53 by MDM2 is diminished and the cellular functional p53 level will increase, particularly following DNA damaging treatment, resulting in tumor growth arrest and/or apoptosis. These strategies included polypeptides that bind to MDM2 protein *(41)*, antibody against MDM2 protein *(42)*, as well as small molecular MDM2 inhibitors *(43)*. Recently, we have successfully identified anti-MDM2 antisense oligos that effectively inhibit MDM2 expression in tumor cells containing MDM2 gene amplifications *(44–46)*. We are now using the specific anti-MDM2 oligos designed with advanced chemistry as a research tool to investigate the role of MDM2 oncogene in the development and treatment of human cancers and, by using in vitro and in vivo approaches, to systematically evaluate these antisense oligos as therapeutic agents alone or in combination with other therapeutics. These studies will not only provide the proof of principle for anti-MDM2 oligonuleotides but also contribute to the evaluation of the usefulness of antisense therapy in general.

The selected antisense anti-MDM2 oligo has been shown to specifically inhibit the MDM2 expression in vitro *(44)*. Inhibition of MDM2 expression in cultured human cancer cell lines results in activation of p53 and induces apoptosis or cell cycle arrest. The p53 activation activity of the antisense oligo has been shown in all tested cell lines containing wild type p53 with various levels of MDM2 expression *(45)*. This oligo has no effect on levels of mutant p53, while MDM2 expression is inhibited in cells with mutant p53. In a recent study using advanced antisense chemistry (mixed-backbone oligos), we demonstrated that the new anti-MDM2 antisense oligo specifically inhibited MDM2 expression in cultured cells and in tumor tissues and had significant in vivo anti-tumor activity when administered alone, with synergistic effects being observed when used in combination with DNA damaging agents *(46)*.

2. Materials

All chemicals should be analytical grade or the highest grade available. All aqueous solutions should be prepared in sterile, distilled, deionized water or phosphate-buffered saline (PBS) buffer. All cell culture equipment and biological hood and culture media should be sterile or sterilized prior to use. Gloves should be worn for all operations. Toxic chemicals should be handled in a fume hood and disposed of safely. The test oligo, a 20-mer mixed-backbone oligo (5'-**UGA**CACCTGTTCTCAC**UCAC**-3') and its mismatched control (5'-**UG**T**CACCC**T**TTT**T**CA**T**UCAC**-3') were synthesized, purified, and analyzed as previously described *(17,19,44–46)*. Two nucleotides at the 5'-end and four nucleotides at the 3'-end are 2'-*O*- methylribonucleotides (represented by boldface letters); the remaining are deoxynucleotides. The underlined nucleotides of the control oligo are the sites of the mismatched controls compared with the antisense oligo. For both mixed-backbone oligos, all internucleotide linkages are phosphorothioate. The purity of the oligos was shown to be greater than 90% by capillary gel electrophoresis and polyacrylamide gel electrophoresis (PAGE), with the remainder being n-1 and n-2 products. The integrity of the internucleotide linkages was confirmed by ^{31}P NMR.

2.1. Materials for Cell Culture, Lipofectin®-Mediated Oligonucleotide Transfection, and Combination Treatment of Cultured Tumor Cells

1. Cell culture dishes (60-mm), 6-well or 24-well plates or flasks (25 mm^2 or 75 mm^2).
2. 1.5-mL microfuge tubes.
3. 15- or 50-mL centrifuge tubes.
4. Cell scrapers.
5. Microscope.
6. Hemacytometer.
7. Lipofectin (Cat. no. 18292-011 or 18292-037; Life Technologies, Gaithersburg, MD).
8. Human colon cancer cell line LS174T (American Type Culture Collection, Rockville, MD).

9. Cell culture medium MEM with 0.1 m*M* nonessential amino acids and 10% fetal bovine serum (FBS).
10. PBS (phosphate-buffered saline).
11. 0.25% trypsin/0.1% EDTA.
12. 0.4% trypan blue viability stain.
13. Penicillin-streptomycin.
14. Oligonucleotides (0.1 m*M* in PBS).
15. Chemotherapeutic agents adriamycin, CPT and HCPT *(47–50)*.

2.2. Western Blot Analysis

1. Power supply.
2. Electrophoresis apparatus (Bio-rad Protean II).
3. Casting stand.
4. Clamps.
5. Glass plates.
6. Spacers (0.75–1.5 mm).
7. Inner cooling core.
8. Buffer chamber.
9. Chamber lid with attached electrodes.
10. Teflon combs with 1–20 teeth (matched to spacer width).
11. Vacuum pump.
12. Erlenmeyer side-arm flask.
13. Hamilton pipet or pipetter with gel loading tips (narrow diameter).
14. Blotting apparatus.
15. Buffer tank.
16. Gel holder cassette.
17. Fiber pads (2 per gel).
18. Lid with electrodes.
19. Cooling unit.
20. Membrane appropriate for application, nitrocellulose, nylon, or polyvinylidine fluoride (PVDF).
22. Whatman 3MM filter paper (precut or cut to fit gel).
23. Shallow dish for assembling gel sandwich.
24. Plastic wrap.
25. X-ray film.
26. X-ray cassette.
27. Film developer.
28. RIPA cell lysis buffer: 150 m*M* NaCl, 50 m*M* Tris-HCl, pH 7.4, 1% sodium deoxycholate, 0.1% sodium dodecylsulfate (SDS), 1% Triton X-100, 1 m*M* protease inhibitor phenylmethylsulfonyl fluoride (PMSF) (Sigma Cat. no. p8340, 50 μL/mL; unstable in aqueous solutions; must be added fresh).
29. 4X Tris-HCl/SDS: 1.5 *M* Tris-HCl, pH 8.8, 0.4% SDS.
30. 4X Tris-HCl/SDS: 0.5 *M* Tris-HCl, pH 6.8, 0.4% SDS.

31. Acrylamide/bisacrylamide solution: 29. 2% acrylamide, 0.8% bisacrylamide, w/v.
32. 10% SDS solution.
33. 10% Ammonium persulfate in H_2O.
34. 2X SDS sample buffer: 0.1 M 4X Tris-HCl/SDS, pH 6.8, 20% (w/v) glycerol, 4% (w/v) SDS, 0.5 M dithothreitol (DTT), 0.001% (w/v) bromophenol blue.
35. 5X Running buffer stock solution: 0.125 M Tris base, 0.96 M glycine, 0.5% (w/v) SDS.
36. 1X Running buffer.
37. Protein molecular weight standards for PAGE.
38. H_2O-saturated isobutyl or isoamyl alcohol.
39. 1X Transfer buffer: 25 mM Tris base, 192 mM glycine, 20% v/v methanol, pH 8.3.
40. 25 mM sodium phosphate.
41. TBS (Tris buffered saline): 100 mM Tris-HCl, pH 7.5, 150 mM NaCl.
42. TBST (TBS-Tween 20): 100 mM Tris-HCl, pH 7.5, 150 mM NaCl, 0.1% Tween 20.
43. Blocking reagent: (5% non-fat milk in TBST).
44. Primary antibodies: MDM2 (SMP-14) monoclonal antibody (Santa Cruz Biotechnology, Inc.); p53, p21, and β-actin monoclonal antibodies (Oncogene Research Products, Boston, MA).
45. Secondary reagent: HRP-conjugated anti-Ig G (Cat. no. 170-6516; Bio-Rad laboratories).
46. Enhanced chemiluminescence (ECL) detection reagents (Amersham).

2.3. Additional Materials for Microculture Tetrazolium (MTT) Assay

1. 0.22-μm filter for reagent preparation.
2. 96-well plates.
3. 96-well microplate reader.
4. RPMI-1640 cell culture medium lacking phenol red.
5. Dimethyl sulfoxide (DMSO).
6. MTT (3-[4,5-dimethylthiazol-2-yl]-2,5-diphenyltetrazolium bromide; Sigma Cat. no. M5655).

2.4. Additional Materials for In Vivo Animal Models

1. 175-mm^2 cell culture flasks or 100-mm culture dishes.
2. Microisolator cages with sterile bedding, food and water and cage card with animal identification information.
3. 1-cc syringes with 26-G syringe needles.
4. Sterilized animal feeding needles, 18/50 mm, curved tube style.
5. Calipers for measuring tumor diameters.
6. Balance for body weight measurement.
7. Ear tags and ear puncher for identification of animals.
8. Chlorhexiderm disinfectant.

9. Sterile gauze.
10. Culture medium without FBS or antibiotics.
11. 70% ethanol.
12. 0.9% NaCl (physiological saline, sterile).
13. Drug preparations: Oligonucleotides (various concentrations in physiological saline); chemotherapeutic agents: adriamycin in physiological saline campto-thecin (CPT) and 10-hydroxycamtothecin (HCPT) in cotton seed oil.
14. Solution for sample preparation for pathology analysis: Add 735 mL of absolute alcohol (100%) into 315 mL of deionized H_2O, then add 117 mL of formalin (37% w/v formaldehyde solution).

2.5. Animals

Animal use protocols should be reviewed and approved by the Institutional Committee on Animal Use and Care. Pathogen-free 4 to 6-wk-old female nude mice or C.B.-17-*scid/scid* mice should be accommodated for 5 d for environmental adjustment prior to study. Animals should be housed in 12 h/12 h light/dark cycle and fed with sterile commercial diet and given sterile water *ad libitum*. Cages and bedding materials should be autoclaved. Laboratory coat, gloves, eye-glasses, and mouth mask should be worn during animal care and treatment.

3. Methods
3.1. Assay for In Vitro Effects of Oligos on Cultured Human Colon Cancer LS174T Cells
3.1.1. Transfection of Cells with Oligos for Western Blot Analysis

All procedures should be carried out under sterile conditions.

1. Trypsinize cells when ~80% confluent and resuspend in MEM medium containing 1% FBS with antibiotics. Plate $3–5 \times 10^5$ cells per 60-mm dish.
2. Incubate cells for 18 h at 37°C in 5% CO_2, then remove medium and refeed with 2.5 mL MEM/1% FBS without antibiotics.
3. Prepare 1 mM and 0.1 mM stock solution of oligonucleotides in sterile PBS. Keep in –20°C until use.
4. Mix 22 μL of lipofectin with 0.25 mL of serum-free minimum essential medium (MEM) and keep it at room temperature for 45 min prior to use.
5. To a separate tube, add 6 μL of 0.1 mM oligo stock solution to 0.25 mL serum-free medium (final concentration, 200 nM). For preparation of other concentrations of oligos, dilution from 0.1 mM oligo stock solution is needed.
6. Combine the lipofectin mixture (from **step 4**) and oligo solutions (from **step 5**) and incubate at room temperature for 10 min.

7. Add 0.5 mL of Lipofectin-oligo mixture to each 60-mm dish. The final oligo concentration is 200 nM. (For preparation of other concentrations of oligonucleotides, *see* **step 5**).

8. Incubate at 37°C for 20–24 h, then remove medium and wash cells with 1 mL ice-cold PBS for each dish.

9. Add 100–200 μL of lysis buffer (RIPA) with PMSF.

10. Scrape cells from the plate and transfer to a microfuge tube. Put the tube on ice for 10 min.

11. Centrifuge the cell suspension at 14,000g, 4°C, for 10 min.

12. Transfer the supernatant to a clean microfuge tube. The cell lysate is ready for protein determination and Western blot analysis. If necessary, store the lysate at –80°C until analysis.

3.1.2. Transfection of Cells with Oligos in 24-Well Plates and Determination of Viable Cell Number

1. Trypsinize cells when ~80% confluent and resuspend in medium containing 10% FBS with antibiotics. Plate 3–5 × 10^4 cells per well for a 24-well plate.

2. Incubate cells at 37°C, 5% CO$_2$ for 18 h. Remove medium and refeed with 0.2 mL MEM/1% FBS lacking antibiotics per well.

3. Mix 2.2 μL of Lipofectin with 0.05 mL serum-free medium. Incubate at room temperature for 45 min.

4. To a separate tube add 0.6 μL of 0.1 mM oligo stock solution to 0.05 mL serum-free medium (*see* **Subheading 3.1.1., step 5**).

5. Combine the lipofectin mixture (from **Subheading 3.1.1., step 4**) and oligo solutions (from **Subheading 3.1.1., step 5**) and incubate at room temperature for 10 min.

6. Add 0.1 mL of lipofectin-oligo mixture to each well. The final oligo concentration is 200 nM and the final Lipofectin concentration is 7 μg/mL. Treat control wells with Lipofectin mixture only.

7. Incubate at 37°C for 20–24 h. Remove the medium and wash the cells twice with 0.5 mL of PBS.

8. To count viable cells, add 0.5 mL of 0.25% trypsin to each well.

9. Incubate plates at 37°C for 5–10 min or until cells come off.

10. Pipet cells up and down to dissociate them.

11. Dilute 100 μL of the cell suspension with 100 μL of 0.4% trypan blue viability stain and mix well and then incubate the cells for 3 min at room temperature.

12. Examine the cells under a microscope and count viable cells using a hemacytometer. Count cells within 5 min of adding dye to prevent nonspecific staining.

13. Data analysis for growth inhibition study: Calculate the average cell counts for a minimum of 4 fields and multiply the average count by 2 × 10^4 to obtain the actual cell number in each well. Calculate the mean, standard deviation (SD) and standard error (SE) for counts from replicate wells. Calculate the percentage of

viable cells after drug treatment relative to the number of cells in control wells treated with Lipofectin® only. Plot the cell numbers or percentage of surviving cells versus drug concentration for a dose/response curve and determine IC_{50}. Compare cells treated with test oligo and its mismatched control to determine the sequence specificity.

3.1.3. Transfection of Cells with Oligos for MTT Assay

1. Trypsinize cells and count. Adjust cell density to 2×10^4 cells/mL in MEM supplemented with 10% FBS.
2. Plate 0.1 mL of cell suspension per 96-well plate (2000 cells/well). Incubate overnight at 37°C.
3. Prepare Lipofectin and oligo solutions in MEM without serum at four times the final concentration. Dilute Lipofectin 1:36 in MEM to prepare 28 μg/mL solution (4X). Incubate for 30–45 min at room temperature.
4. Prepare the oligo solutions in MEM to obtain 4X stock solutions.
5. Combine equal volumes of 4X Lipofectin and 4X oligo solutions and incubate at room temperature for 10 min.
6. Combine equal volumes of Lipofectin/oligo mixture and MEM/1.6% FBS. Final serum concentration is being 0.8%.
7. Add 0.1 mL of Lipofectin/oligo/MEM solution to each well.
8. Incubate cells at 37°C in 5% CO_2 for the desired transfection time (18–48 h). In studies with combination treatment, chemotherapeutic agents at various concentrations are added after 18–24 h transfection.
9. Incubate cells at 37°C, 5% CO_2 for an additional 3–5 d.
10. Perform MTT assay when control cells reach 90% confluence.

3.1.4. MTT Assay

1. Prepare a 5 mg/mL stock solution of MTT in PBS. Filter the solution using 0.2-μm filter to remove undissolved particles. Store solution at 4°C in the dark for up to 1 mo.
2. Remove the cell culture medium from cells in a 96-well plate and replace with prewarmed (37°C) 0.2 mL of MEM without serum.
4. Multiply 50 μL by the total number of wells to calculate the volume of MTT solution required.
5. Dilute 5 mg/mL MTT solution in MEM immediately before use to prepare a 2 mg/mL working solution.
6. Add 50 μL of the 2 mg/mL MTT solution to each well. Two to four control wells should be incubated with MEM without MTT to determine background absorbance values.
7. Incubate the plates for 2–4 h at 37°C.
8. Observe plates under the microscope during incubation to estimate optimum incubation time with the MTT reagent. The presence of blue granules inside

the cells indicates viable cells. Incubation time may vary with different cell lines, since the efficiency of MTT uptake by cell lines may differ. Once the optimum incubation time has been determined, use the same incubation period for all future studies.

9. Carefully remove the MTT solution from the wells at the end of the incubation.
10. Add 150 µL of DMSO to each well with a multichannel pipet to solubilize dye crystals. Pipet up and down to mix samples.
11. Read plates at 540 nm using a microplate reader. The purple color will remain stable for a few hours. Subtract background values obtained for control wells minus MTT reagent from sample OD values. Determine mean, standard deviation, and error for repeated samples.
12. Plot the relative OD values against drug concentrations to illustrate the dose-dependent effect of oligos on in vitro cell growth.

3.2. Western Blot Analysis to Determine the Effects of Oligos on Target Gene Expression

3.2.1. Preparation of Cell Lysates from Cultured Cells or Tumors

1. For cultured cells, remove culture medium and wash cells twice with cold PBS. Place the cell culture dishes on ice.
2. Add 0.5 mL of cold cell lysis (RIPA) buffer per 60-mm dish.
3. For tumor tissue, homogenize tumor tissue (500 mg) in 2.5 mL RIPA buffer containing freshly added PMSF (50 µL/mL). Keep the tissue homogenate on ice throughout the procedure.
4. Centrifuge the cell lysate at 14,000g for 5 min at 4°C.
5. Remove the supernatant and transfer to a clean tube.
6. Quantify total protein concentration of supernatant using a standard protein assay, e.g., modified Lowery assay (Pierce).

3.2.2. Protein Gel Electrophoresis (SDS-PAGE)

1. Fractionate proteins by 5–15% SDS-PAGE. Use unstained or prestained molecular weight markers to monitor protein migration in the gel.
2. Adjust the power supply to 200 V using a constant voltage setting. Set the timer for the desired running time, generally 35–45 min.

3.2.3. Transfer Proteins to Membrane

1. Prepare and refrigerate transfer buffer and fill the cooling chamber with water and freeze in advance.
2. Remove the gel from the apparatus and equilibrate the gel in transfer buffer for 15–30 min, depending upon gel thickness. This will remove buffer salts from the gel and prevent it from shrinking during transfer. Always wear gloves when handling membrane to prevent contamination.

3. Cut membrane to fit gel. Mark one corner of membrane with soft pencil or small cut to identify membrane orientation with respect to the gel. Wet membrane by slowly sliding it into transfer buffer. Allow it to soak for 15 min.
4. Obtain precut filter paper or cut Whatman 3MM paper to fit the membrane. Thoroughly wet the filter paper in transfer buffer.
5. Fill the buffer tank about half-full with transfer buffer and install a cooling unit with ice.
6. Assemble the gel sandwich.
7. Transfer protein to the membrane at 100 V for 1 h or 30 V overnight.

3.2.4. Immunoblotting

1. Block nonspecific sites on membranes in 5% blocking solution for 1–2 h at room temperature.
2. Transfer the membranes to a small container for antibody incubation. Minimize volume of antibody solution to conserve valuable reagents, but use enough solution to completely cover membrane without drying during incubation.
3. Dilute the primary antibody in TBST. Optimum antibody dilution may have to be determined empirically. For commercial antibodies, consult the product data sheet for suggested antibody concentration. In this study, antibodies are diluted as follows: Anti-MDM2: 1:1000; Anti-p53: 1:1000; Anti-p21; 1:1000; and Anti-β-actin: 1:5000.
4. Incubate membrane with primary antibody for 1–3 h at room temperature or overnight in the cold room.
5. Wash membranes three times for 15 min using a large volume of TBST (~200–400 mL per wash). For best results, do not reduce incubation time or wash volume to avoid high or uneven background.
6. Dilute HRP-conjugated secondary antibody in TBST (1:3000) or consult product data sheet for recommended dilution.
7. Incubate the membrane with secondary antibody for 1 h at room temperature.
8. Wash membranes three times for 15 min using a large volume of TBST (~200–400 mL per wash).
9. Pour off the final wash solution and lightly blot excess liquid from the membrane.
10. For chemiluminescence detection, combine equal volumes of ECL solutions 1 and 2.
11. Place the membrane on a piece of plastic wrap.
12. In the darkroom, add the detection reagent mix to membrane with protein side up. Incubate for exactly one minute.
13. Pour off excess detection reagent and wrap membrane with plastic wrap. Avoid wrinkles in the plastic wrap, which may cause artifacts on the film.
14. Expose the membrane to x-ray film for 1 min, and immediately develop film.
15. Adjust the exposure time to obtain satisfactory band intensities. Complete film exposures within a short interval, as the chemiluminescence reaction has a short half-life and the signal will begin to fade with long delays.

3.2.5. Data Analysis: Imaging and Densitometry

1. Orient the film according to position of lanes on gel and identify sample lanes. Observe band intensities and positions relative to protein standards. In the present study, the presence of MDM2 protein is at about 90 kDa molecular weight.
2. Examine the film for artifacts that may arise during washing, detection, or film exposure steps.
3. Note the presence of any unexpected bands which may derive from nonspecific or cross-reactive binding of primary or secondary antibody. Be aware that the possibility of nonspecific signal increases with the use of polyclonal antisera or unpurified antibody.
4. If desired, quantify protein levels using densitometry, a technique that measures optical density values for selected areas of the film. Quantitative analysis requires equivalent amounts of protein in each sample loaded on the gel.
5. It is important not to overexpose film to obtain accurate quantitative data. The film will become saturated at high band intensities and additional signal will not be resolved.

3.3. In Vivo Effects of Oligos on Human Colon Cancer LS174T Xenografts in Nude Mice

3.3.1. Establishment of Animal Model

1. Culture human colon LS174T cells in 175-mm^2 flasks or 100-mm dishes under the aforementioned conditions.
2. Harvest tumor cells in the exponential growth phase by trypsinization.
3. Combine cells and transfer to 50 mL centrifuge tubes. Centrifuge them at 800g for 5 min.
4. Remove the supernatant and wash the cells twice with medium lacking serum and antibiotics.
5. Remove a small volume of the cell suspension before the last centrifugation and count the cells using a hemacytometer. Calculate the total cell number by multiplying cell density (cells/mL) by the volume of cell suspension.
6. Centrifuge tubes again for 5 min at 800g to collect cells.
7. Add the necessary volume of culture medium lacking serum to the cells. Pipet up and down to obtain a homogeneous cell suspension (10^8 cells/mL).
8. Transfer the cell suspension to a 1-cc syringe with a 26-gauge needle.
9. Inject 0.2 mL of the cell suspension (10^7 cells) subcutaneously into the left inguinal area of the mouse. Use proper precaution and techniques to handle immunodeficient animals. Label each cage card with the date and type of cells injected.
10. Observe animals for tumor growth and clinical signs every day. When tumors are easily visible, begin to measure tumor diameter (cm) with calipers and record the tumor measurements.
11. The following formulae are used to calculate tumor mass and volume: mass (mg) = 0.5 (long diameter)(short diameter)^2 × 1000; volume (mm^3) = [0.25 × (short

diameter + long diameter)]^3 × 4.18879 × 1000. Note that the calculation [0.25 × (short diameter + long diameter)] corresponds to the average tumor radius.

3.3.2. Treatment of Animal Model

1. When tumors reach ~80–200 mg, treatment with oligos and chemotherapeutic agents begins.
2. Animals are randomly divided into treatment groups and controls (6–10 animals/ group). Calculate the mean, SD, and SE in mass and volume for each group. Label the cage card with the date, experiment and treatment group numbers, and the drug, dose and frequency. In the study, the following groups are included: untreated control (saline); control oligos (three doses); test oligos (three doses); chemotherapeutic agents (at minimum tolerated dose, MTD); test oligo plus chemotherapeutic agents; and control oligo plus chemotherapeutic agents. Oligos should be given ip or iv. HCPT or CPT should be given orally by gavage.
3. Tumors should be measured at least twice a week. For very fast growing tumors, it may be necessary to measure tumors every other day. Clinical observation and body weight monitoring are needed. In general, when tumor reaches 10% of the body weight or animals develop severe toxicity owing to tumor growth or treatment toxicity, the animals should then be sacrificed.
4. Final measurements and tumor size calculations should be performed prior to sacrificing animals and removing tumors.
5. At the end of the experiment, confirm that final measurements and calculations have been performed for each animal. Pathology examination of tumor and host tissues may be performed.

4. Notes

1. Although the design of antisense oligos is theoretically straightforward (to identify a complementary oligonucleotide on the basis of the nucleotide sequence of the mRNA), the selection of an effective and specific antisense oligo is largely based on experience and trial-based experiments. In the design of anti-MDM2 oligos, more than 12 oligos were initially tested and significant difference in activity was found. Since certain oligo sequences such as CpG and GGGG have been shown to have sequence-dependent non-antisense effects, these sequences should be avoided to demonstrate sequence-specific antisense effects. In addition, since PS-oligos have certain side effects and undergo extensive metabolism in vivo, advanced antisense chemistry may be needed in in vivo studies.
2. In this protocol, Lipofectin® is used to facilitate the in vitro cellular uptake of oligos and can be replaced by other lipids. Of note, the ratio of lipids/oligo will affect the results of uptake. The cytotoxicity of Lipofectin® without oligo may affect the results of in vitro cell killing study of oligos.
3. In general, decreased levels of protein can be evidence for antisense effects. However, this is not sufficient, especially if a dose-dependent relationship is not demonstrated. Proper controls, e.g., random, sense, or mismatched sequence, should be used. Decreased and/or degraded mRNA can be further evidence for

antisense effects. In addition, functional evidence is desired. In our studies, we have shown the antisense effect of anti-MDM2 oligos by demonstrating not only decreased MDM2 protein expression and decreased mRNA levels, but also increased p53 levels and function (p21 induction and induced apoptosis) *(44–46)*.

4. In vivo effects. The in vivo effects of antisense oligos can be complex. Proper controls should be used and a dose-dependent relationship should be demonstrated. In vivo decreased protein or mRNA levels of target gene should be demonstrated. In addition, host conditions (strains of animals, sex, and age), tumor size, route of administration, schedule and duration of treatment may affect the results of the study.

Acknowledgments

Experimental studies in our laboratory were supported by a grant from the National Institute of Health, National Cancer Institute to R. Zhang (R01 CA 80698).

References

1. Zamecnik, P.C. (1996) History of antisense oligonucleotides, in *Antisense Therapeutics* (Agrawal, S., ed.), Humana Press, Totowa, NJ, pp. 1–12.
2. Stein, C. A. and Cheng, Y. C. (1993) Antisense oligonucleotides as therapeutic agents. Is the bullet really magical? *Science* **261,** 1004–1012.
3. Diasio, R. B. and Zhang, R. (1997) Pharmacology of therapeutic oligonucleotides. *Antisense Nucl. Acid Drug Dev.* **7,** 239–243.
4. Agrawal, S. (1996) Antisense oligonucleotides: towards clinical trial. *Trends Biotech.* **14,** 376–387.
5. Crooke, S. T. (1998) *Antisense Research and Applications*, Springer-Verlag, Berlin.
6. Wickstrom, E. (1998) *Clinical Trials of Genetic Therapy with Antisense DNA and DNA Vectors*, Marcel Dekker, New York.
7. Kushner, D. M. and Silverman, R. H. (2000) Antisense cancer therapy: the state of the science. *Curr. Oncol. Rep.* **2,** 23–30.
8. Monia, B. P., HolmLund, J., and Dorr, F. A. (2000) Antisense approaches for the treatment of cancer. *Cancer Invest.* **18,** 635–650.
9. Gewirtz, A. M. (2000) Oligonucleotide therapeutics: a step forward. *J. Clin. Oncol.* **18,** 1809–1811.
10. Zhang, R. and Wang, H. (2000) Antisense oligonucleotides as anti-tumor therapeutics. *Recent Res. Dev. Cancer* **2,** 61–76.
11. Zhang, R., Yan, J., Shahinian, H., et al. (1995) Pharmacokinetics of an oligodeoxynucleotide phosphorothioate (GEM 91) in HIV-infected subjects. *Clin. Pharmacol. Ther.* **58,** 44–53.
12. Zhang, R., Diasio, R. B., Lu, Z., et al. (1995) Pharmacokinetics and tissue disposition in rats of an oligodeoxynucleotide phosphorothioate (GEM 91) developed as a therapeutic agent for human immunodeficiency virus type-1. *Biochem. Pharm.* **49,** 929–939.

13. Zhang, R., Lu, Z., Zhao, H., et al. (1995) In vivo stability, disposition, and metabolism of a "hybrid" oligonucleotide phosphorothioate in rats. *Biochem. Pharmacol.* **50**, 545–556.

14. Zhang, R., Iyer, P., Yu, D., et al. (1996) Pharmacokinetics and tissue disposition of a chimeric oligodeoxynucleotide phosphorothioate in rats following intravenous administration. *J. Pharm. Exp. Ther.* **278**, 971–979.

15. Agrawal, S. and Zhang, R. (1997) Pharmacokinetics of phosphorothioate oligonucleotide and its novel analogs, in *Antisense Oligodeoxynucleotides and Antisense RNA as Novel Pharmacological and Therapeutic Agents* (Weiss, B., ed.), CRC Press, Boca Raton, FL, pp. 58–78.

16. Agrawal, S. and Zhang, R. (1997) Pharmacokinetics of oligonucleotides, in *Oligonucleotides as Therapeutic Agents. CIBA Foundation Symposium 209*, Wiley, Chichester, pp. 60–78.

17. Agrawal, S. and Iyer, R. P. (1995) Modified oligonucleotides as therapeutic and diagnostic agents. *Curr. Opin. Biotechnol.* **6**, 112–119.

18. Agrawal, S., Zhang, X., Zhao, H., et al. (1995) Absorption, tissue distribution and in vivo stability in rats of a hybrid antisense oligonucleotide following oral administration. *Biochem. Pharm.* **50**, 571–576.

19. Agrawal, S., Jiang, Z., Zhao, Q., et al. (1997) Mixed-backbone oligonucleotides as second generation antisense oligonucleotides: In vitro and in vivo studies. *Proc. Natl. Acad. Sci. USA* **94**, 2620–2625.

20. Agrawal, S. and Zhang, R. (1998) Pharmacokinetics and bioavailability of oligonucleotides following oral and colorectal administrations in experimental animals, in *Antisense Research and Applications* (Crooke, S., ed.), Springer-Verlag, Heidelberg, pp. 525–543.

21. Wang, H., Cai, Q., Zeng, X., Yu, D., Agrawal, S., and Zhang, R. (1999) Anti-tumor activity and pharmacokinetics of a mixed-backbone antisense oligonucleotide targeted to RIα subunit of protein kinase A after oral administration. *Proc. Natl. Acad. Sci. USA* **96**, 13,989–13,994.

22. Chen, H. X., Marchall, J. L., Ness, E., et al. (2000) A safety and pharmackinetic study of a mixed-backbone oligonucleotide (GEM231) targeting the type I protein kinase A by two-hour infusion in patients with refractory solid tumors. *Clin. Cancer Res.* **6**, 1259–1266.

23. Prives, C. and Hall, P. A. (1999) The p53 pathway. *J. Pathol.* **187**, 112–126.

24. Piette, J., Neel, H., and Marechal, V. (1997) Mdm2: keeping p53 under control. *Oncogene* **15**, 1001–1010.

25. Cahilly-Snyder, L., Yang, F. T., Francke, U., and George, D. L. (1987) Molecular anlaysis and chromosomal mapping of amplified genes isolated from a transformed mouse 3T3 cell line. *Somat. Cell Mol. Genet.* **13**, 235–244.

26. Zhang, R. and Wang, H. (2000) MDM2 oncogene as a novel target for human cancer therapy. *Curr. Pharm. Design* **6**, 393–416.

27. Momand, J. and Zambetti, G. P. (1997) Mdm-2: "big brother" of p53. *J. Cell Biochem.* **64**, 343–352.

28. Prives, C. (1998) Signaling to p53: breaking the MDM2-p53 circuit. *Cell* **95,** 5–8.
29. Lozano, G. and Montes de Oca Luna, R. (1998) MDM2 function. *Biochim. Biophys. Acta* **1377,** M55–M59.
30. Juven-Gershon, T. and Oren, M. (1999) Mdm2: the ups and downs. *Mol. Med.* **5,** 71–83.
31. Freedman, D. A., Wu, L., and Levine, A. J. (1999) Functions of the MDM2 oncoprotein. *Cell. Mol. Life Sci.* **55,** 96–107.
32. Freedman, D. A. and Levine, A. J. (1999) Regulation of p53 protein by MDM2 oncoprotein-Thirty eighth G.H.A. Clowes memorial award lecture. *Cancer Res.* **59,** 1–7.
33. Barak, Y., Juven, T., Haffner, R., and Oren, M. (1993) MDM2 expression is induced by wild type p53 activity. *EMBO J.* **12,** 461–468.
34. Perry, M. E., Piette, J., Zawadzki, J. A., Harvey, D., and Levine, A. J. (1993) The mdm-2 gene is induced in response to UV light in a p53-dependent manner. *Proc. Natl. Acad. Sci. USA* **90,** 11,623–11,627.
35. Momand, J., Jung, D., Wilczynski, S., and Niland, J. (1998) The MDM2 gene amplification database. *Nuc. Acids Res.* **26,** 3453–3459.
36. Watanabe, T., Hotta, T., Ichikawa, A., Kinoshita, T., Nagai, H., and Uchida, T. (1994) The MDM2 oncogene overexpression in chronic lymphocytic leukemia and low-grade lymphoma of B-cell origin. *Blood* **84,** 3158–3165.
37. Landers, J. E., Haines, D. S., Strauss, J. F., and George, D. L. (1994) Enhanced translation: a novel mechanism of mdm2 oncogene overexpression identified in human tumor cells. *Oncogene* **9,** 2745–2750.
38. Landers, J. E., Cassel, S. L., and George, D. L. (1997) Translational enhancement of mdm2 oncogene expression in human tumor cells containing a stablized wild-type p53 protein. *Cancer Res.* **57,** 3562–3568.
39. Dorigo, O., Turla, S. T., Lebedeva, S., and Gjerset, R. A. (1998) Sensitization of rat glioblastoma multiforme to cisplatin *in vivo* following restoration of wild-type p53 function. *J. Neurosurg.* **88,** 535–540.
40. Nielsen, L. L. and Maneval, D. C. (1998) p53 tumor suppressor gene therapy for cancer. *Cancer Gene Ther.* **5,** 52–63.
41. Bottger, A., Bottger, V., Sparks, A., Liu, W. L., Howard, S. F., and Lane, D. P. (1997) Design of a synthetic Mdm2-binding mini protein that activates the p53 response in vivo. *Curr. Biol.* **7,** 860–869.
42. Midgley, C. A. and Lane, D. P. (1997) P53 protein stability in tumor cells is not determined by mutation but is dependent on Mdm2 binding. *Oncogene* **15,** 1179–1189.
43. Arriola, E. L., Lopez, A. R., and Chresta, C. M. (1999) Differential regulation of p21/waf-1/cip-1 and mdm2 by etoposide: etoposide inhibits the p53-mdm2 autoregulatory feedback loop. *Oncogene* **18,** 1081–1091.
44. Chen, L., Agrawal, S., Zhou, W., Zhang, R., and Chen, J. (1998) Synergistic activation of p53 by inhibition of MDM2 expression and DNA damage. *Proc. Natl. Acad. Sci. USA* **95,** 195–200.

45. Chen, L., Lu, W., Agrawal, S., Zhou, W. Zhang, R., and Chen, J. (1999) Ubiquitous induction of p53 in tumor cells by antisense inhibition of MDM2 expression. *Mol. Med.* **5,** 21–34.

46. Wang, H., Oliver, P., Zeng, X., et al. (1999) MDM2 oncogene as a target for cancer therapy: an antisense approach. *Intl. J. Oncol.* **15,** 653–660.

47. Cai, Q., Lindsey, J. R., and Zhang, R. (1997) Regression of human colon cancer xenografts in SCID mice following oral administration of water-insoluble camptothecins, natural product topoisomerase I inhibitors. *Int. J. Oncol.* **10,** 953–960.

48. Zhang, R., Li, Y., Cai, Q., Liu, T., Sun, H., and Chambless, B. (1998) Preclinical pharmacology of the natural product anticancer agent 10-hydroxycamptothecin, an inhibitor of topoisomerase I. *Cancer Chemother. Pharm.* **41,** 257–267.

49. Takimoto, C. H. and Arbuck, S. G. (1996) The camptothecins, in *Cancer Chemotherapy and Biotherapy* (Chabner, B. A. and Longo, D. L., eds.), Philadelphia: Lippincott Raven Publishers, pp. 463–484.

50. Liu, W. and Zhang, R. (1998) Upregulation of p21/[WAF1/CIP1] in human breast cancer cell lines MCF-7 and MDA-MB-468 undergoing apoptosis induced by natural product anticancer agents 10-hydroxycamptothecin and camptothecin through p53-dependent and independent pathways. *Int. J. Oncol.* **12,** 793–804.

VIII

GENOMICS

19

Pharmacogenetic Analysis of Clinically Relevant Genetic Polymorphisms

Christine M. Rose, Sharon Marsh, Margaret-Mary Ameyaw, and Howard L. McLeod

1. Introduction

1.1. Pharmacogenetics

With the recent publication of the human genome sequence, there has been an expanse of publicly available resources for pharmacogenomics research. Early estimates predicted that over 3 million single nucleotide polymorphisms (SNPs) are present in the human genome, with over 1.42 million already deposited in the public databases *(1)*. SNPs in coding and control regions of genes can cause significant inter-individual variation in the resulting protein function and activity, leading to important differences in disease susceptibility and drug metabolism. This expansion in valuable SNPs has stimulated the development of a number of detection methods *(2)*. We describe protocols for three distinct methods (allele-specific polymerase chain reaction (PCR), PCR-restriction fragment length polymorphism (PCR-RFLP), and Pyrosequencing) as examples of ways to assay clinically relevant polymorphisms.

Allele-specific PCR is the quickest of the three methods, involving two PCR reactions per sample and direct visualization of the resulting product using agarose gel electrophoresis. However, it relies heavily on achieving specificity of the primers for the variant alleles and a degree of optimization is necessary for each assay.

PCR-RFLP is a very robust technique utilizing the gain or loss of a restriction enzyme recognition sequence at the site of the SNP. However, not all SNPs are within recognition sequences and often, alternative analysis methods are

From: *Methods in Molecular Medicine, vol. 85: Novel Anticancer Drug Protocols*
Edited by: J. K. Buolamwini and A. A. Adjei © Humana Press Inc., Totowa, NJ

necessary. In addition, the enzymes required to cut the PCR products are expensive.

Pyrosequencing produces specific sequence data in the form of peaks on a pyrogram. This robust method does not require the presence of an enzyme site and PCR product and internal primer sites can vary in size and position. However, the Pyrosequencing reaction is costly and requires specialized equipment, and so is not always an available resource.

1.2. Allele-Specific PCR and PCR-RFLP Assays for Analysis of TPMT SNPs

A genetic polymorphism in thiopurine methyltransferase (TPMT) nicely illustrates both allele-specific and RFLP SNP analysis methods. TPMT catalyzes the S-methylation of thiopurine drugs to inactive metabolites *(3,4)*. Patients with low TPMT activity are at high risk for severe toxicity from standard doses of mercaptopurine or azathioprine *(5)*. There are currently 8 variant *TPMT* alleles known to be associated with low TPMT enzyme activity *(5)*. In all populations studied, mutant alleles have been present in individuals categorized as having low TPMT activity *(5–8)*. Identification of individuals with low-activity *TPMT* alleles will allow for prospective strategies to reduce patient risk of toxicity.

Three distinct alleles (*TPMT***2*, *TPMT***3A*, *TPMT***3C*) are responsible for >85% of TPMT deficiency. The *TPMT***2* allele is caused by a G238C single nucleotide polymorphism leading to an amino acid substitution (Ala80Pro) *(5)*. This SNP is easily assessed in individuals by allele-specific PCR. This technique involves carrying out two separate PCR reactions, both of which contain a common primer plus a primer specific for either the wild-type or the mutant allele. The results are visualized using electrophoresis on an agarose gel. Wild-type samples will only give a PCR product when the wild-type primer is used, mutant alleles only when the mutant primer is used. Heterozygous samples will produce a product in both PCR reactions.

The *TPMT***3A* allele is caused by 2 SNPs, G460A and A719G, leading to amino acid substitutions Ala154Thr and Tyr240Cys *(5)*. *TPMT***3C* contains only the A719G SNP *(5)*. Both of these alleles are assessed using a PCR-RFLP method. This technique takes advantage of restriction enzymes that cut only at specific nucleotide sequences. The PCR fragment is digested with the appropriate restriction enzyme, which will cut only in the presence of a specific sequence. If the wild-type sequence is the recognition sequence (e.g., G460A), electrophoresis on an agarose gel will yield smaller fragments than the uncut PCR fragment. If the mutant allele is present, the restriction recognition site is abolished and the fragment remains undigested. A patient heterozygous for both wild-type and mutant alleles will give a combination of uncut and cut fragments on an agarose gel. If the restriction enzyme recognition sequence is only present in the mutant allele (e.g., A719G) the reverse pattern will occur.

1.3. Analysis of SNPs Using Pyrosequencing

Pyrosequencing relies on the production of pyrophosphate during the incorporation of nucleotides into DNA for the analysis of SNPs. A PCR reaction is carried out and an internal primer is hybridized in the PCR product in the region of the SNP. Individual nucleotides are then added to extend the primer using the PCR product as the template. When a nucleotide is incorporated, the released pyrophosphate acts as a substrate for ATP-sulfurylase, releasing ATP. The ATP is used by luciferase resulting in the emission of light. A cooled charge-coupled detection (CCD) camera records the light and this is displayed as a peak on a pyrogram. The remaining nucleotides are then removed from the assay by degradation with apyrase. When a sample is homozygous wild-type, a peak will occur for the wild-type nucleotide and not for any other nucleotides and vice versa for homozygous mutant. When a sample is heterozygous, half-sized peaks will occur for both nucleotides on the pyrogram *(9)*.

2. Materials
2.1. Allele-Specific PCR and PCR-RFLP
2.1.1. PCR

1. Genomic DNA (50–100 ng/(L).
2. AmpliTaq Gold PCR Master Mix 2X (Applied Biosystems, California, USA). 250 U (0.05 U/µL) AmpliTaq Gold DNA polymerase, GeneAmp PCR Gold Buffer (30 mM Tris HCl, 100 mM KCl, pH 8.05), 400 µM deoxynucleotide triphosphates (dNTP), 5 mM MgCl$_2$.
3. High Purity water (MilliQ 18.2 M × cm or equivalent).
4. Reverse and forward oligonucleotide primers for specific TPMT SNPs (Sigma/Genosys, The Woodlands, TX, USA).
5. Polypropylene PCR tubes.
6. Thermal cycler for DNA amplification.

2.1.2. Agarose Gel Electrophoresis

1. Agarose, electrophoresis grade (Promega Corporation, Madison, WI).
2. 1X Tris-Acetate EDTA (TAE) diluted from stock (50X TAE: 242 g Tris base, 57.1 mL glacial acetic acid, 100 mL 0.5 M ethylene diamine tetraacetic acid (EDTA) in 1 L distilled water, pH 8.0).
3. Ethidium Bromide solution at 10 mg/mL (Promega Corporation, Madison, WI).
4. 100-bp DNA Ladder 250 µg (New England Biolabs, Beverly MA, USA).
5. 5X Sample Loading Dye: 30% v/v glycerol, 0.25% w/v bromophenol blue, 0.255 w/v xylene cyanol FF.
6. Horizontal Gel Electrophoresis Apparatus with combs.

7. Power Supply for Electrophoresis Apparatus.
8. Ultraviolet Transilluminator.

2.1.3. RFLP

1. Restriction Enzymes MwoI and AccI (New England Biolabs, Beverly MA, USA).
2. Water Bath.

2.2. Pyrosequencing

2.2.1. PCR

1. Genomic DNA (10–50 ng).
2. Forward and reverse oligonucleotide PCR primers, one will need to be biotinylated (Sigma-Genosys, The Woodlands, TX, USA).
3. AmpliTaq Gold PCR Master Mix 2X (Applied Biosystems, California, USA): 250 U (0.05 U/μL) AmpliTaq Gold DNA polymerase, GeneAmp PCR Gold Buffer (30 mM Tris HCl, 100 mM KCl, pH 8.05), 400 μM dNTP, 5 mM MgCl$_2$.
4. 96-well thin wall PCR tray (Labsource, Chicago, IL).
5. High Purity water (MilliQ 18.2 M × cm or equivalent).
6. Thermal Cycler for DNA Amplification.

2.2.2. Pyrosequencing

1. Internal primer (Sigma-Genosys, The Woodlands, TX, USA).
2. 2X Binding Wash Buffer II, pH 7.6: 10 mM Tris-HCl, 2 M NaCl, 1 mM EDTA, 0.1% Tween 20.
3. Dynabeads M280 Streptavidin (Dynal AS, Oslo, Norway).
4. Eppendorf Thermomixer R (Brinkmann, Westbury, NY).
5. PSQ96 Instrument and Software (Pyrosequencing AB, Uppsala, Sweden).
6. PSQ96 Plate Low (Pyrosequencing AB, Uppsala, Sweden).
7. PSQ96 Sample Prep Tool Cover (Pyrosequencing AB, Uppsala, Sweden).
8. PSQ96 Sample Prep Workstation (Pyrosequencing AB, Uppsala, Sweden).
9. PSQ96 SNP Reagent Kit (Pyrosequencing AB, Uppsala, Sweden).
10. Dry Bath Incubator (Fisher Scientific, Pittsburgh, PA).
11. 10X Annealing Buffer: 200 mM Tris-Acetate, 50 mM Mg(OA$_c$)$_2$, pH 7.6.
12. 0.50 M NaOH.
13. PSQ96 Sample Prep Thermoplate (Pyrosequencing AB, Uppsala, Sweden).

3. Methods

3.1. TPMT G238C Allele-Apecific PCR Assay

3.1.1. PCR Reaction

This assay uses two primer sets and therefore two reactions are to be performed per sample.

Table 1
Thermal Cycling Conditions for TPMT G238C

Step	Temperature	Time	Cycles
Hold	95°C	10 min	1
Denature	94°C	1 min	35
Anneal	55°C	2 min	35
Extend	72°C	1 min	35
Hold	72°C	5 min	1

1. Add 1 µL template DNA to each of two reaction tubes clearly marked wildtype or mutant.
2. Prepare a cocktail mix for PCR as follows (per reaction): Mix 1 (wildtype specific): 0.5 µL primer 1 (wildtype specific), 0.5 µL primer 3, 8 µL ddH$_2$O, 10 µL AmpliTaq Gold PCR Master Mix; Mix 2 (mutation specific): 0.5 µL primer 2 (mutant specific), 0.5 µL primer 3, 8 µL ddH$_2$O, 10 µL AmpliTaq Gold PCR Master Mix. Primer 1 (5′-GTA TGA TTT TAT GCA GGT TTG 3′); Primer 2 (5′-GTA TGA TTT TAT GCA GGT TTC 3′); Primer 3 (5′-TAA ATA GGA ACC ATC GGA CAC 3′) (*see* **Notes 1–6**).
3. Mix cocktail mixes well.
4. Aliquot 19 µL of cocktail mix into each reaction tube. The final reaction volume is 20 µL (*see* **Note 7**).
5. Place in a thermal cycler using the following conditions:

3.1.2. Agarose Gel Analysis

1. Prepare a 2% agarose gel as follows: 2 g agarose, 100 mL 1X TAE. Melt the agarose in a microwave oven until boiling to ensure proper mixing. After the agarose is properly mixed add 5 µL ethidium bromide. Pour into gel box with combs. Remove any bubbles that may form. After gel has polymerized, add 1X TAE to cover the gel, and remove the comb.
2. Run the two reactions side by side (wildtype/mutant) after adding 5 µL of loading dye to each sample.
3. Load 10 µL of 100 bp DNA ladder in the first well of each gel followed by the PCR products.
4. Run at 150 V for 30 min, then visualize on a UV transilluminator (*see* **Note 8**).

3.1.3. Results

A PCR product of approx 250 bp will be produced by this method (*see* **Fig. 1**).

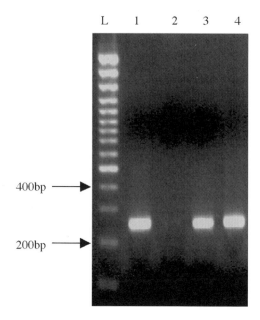

Fig. 1. Electrophoresis patterns for allele specific PCR analysis of nucleotide 238 using primer E and C (lanes 1 and 3) or D (lanes 2 and 4). L—100 bp DNA ladder; the patient analyzed in lanes 1 and 2 was homozygous wild type and in lanes 3 and 4 was heterozygous for the G238C mutation.

3.2. TPMT G460A PCR/RFLP Assay

3.2.1. PCR Reaction

1. Add 1 μL template DNA.
2. Cocktail mix (per reaction): 0.5 μL primer P460Fb (0.3 μM), 0.5 μL primer P460Rb (0.3 μM), 8 μL ddH$_2$O, 10 μL Amplitaq Gold PCR Master Mix. P460Fb (5'-AGG CAG CTA GGG AAA AAG AAA GGT G-3'); P460Rb (5'-CAA GCC TTA TAG CCT TAC ACC AG G-3') (*see* **Notes 1–6**).
3. Mix cocktail mixes well.
4. Aliquot 19 μL of cocktail mix into each reaction tube containing genomic DNA. The final reaction volume is 20 μL (*see* **Note 7**).
5. Place in a Thermal cycler using the conditions described in **Table 2**.
6. Check that the PCR reaction was successful by running a 5 μL aliquot on a 2% agarose gel (PCR product 694 bp). Mix 5 μL PCR product and 1 μL of dye.
7. Load into 2.5% agarose gel in TAE with ethidium bromide.
8. Load 10 μL of 100 bp DNA ladder in the first well of each gel followed by the PCR products.
9. Run at 150 V for 30 min, then visualize on a UV transilluminator.

Table 2
Thermal Cycling Conditions for TPMT G460A

Step	Temperature	Time	Cycles
Hold	95°C	10 min	1
Denature	94°C	1 min	35
Anneal	55°C	2 min	35
Extend	72°C	1 min	35
Hold	72°C	5 min	1

3.2.2. RFLP Analysis

1. Mix 5 µL PCR reaction, 3 µL 10X buffer (*see* **Note 9**), 1 µL MwoI enzyme, and 21 µL dH$_2$O (prepare master mix for high sample number).
2. Incubate at 60°C for 1 h.
3. Mix 20 µL reaction mixture with loading dye and run on 2.5% agarose gel as above (*see* **Note 8**).

3.2.3. Results

A 694 bp PCR product will be produced by this method (*see* **Fig. 2**, lane 1).

3.3. TPMT A719G PCR/RFLP Assay

3.3.1. PCR Reaction

1. Add 1 µL template DNA.
2. Cocktail mix (per reaction)
   0.5 µL primer P719Fb (0.3 µ*M*)
   0.5 µL primer P719Rb (0.3 µ*M*)
   8 µL ddH$_2$O
   10 µL Amplitaq Gold PCR Master Mix
   P719Fb (5′-GAG ACA GAG TTT CAC CAT CTT GG-3′); P719Rb (5′-CAG GCT TTAGCA TAA TTT TCA ATT CCT C-3′) (*see* **Notes 1–6**).
3. Mix cocktail mixes well
4. Aliquot 19 µL of cocktail mix into each reaction tube containing genomic DNA. The final reaction volume is 20 µL (*see* **Note 7**).
5. Place in a Thermal cycler using the conditions described in **Table 3**.
6. Check that the PCR reaction was successful by running a 5 µL aliquot on a 2.5% agarose gel (PCR product 373 bp). Mix 5 µL PCR product and 2 µL of dye.
7. Load into 2.5% agarose gel in TAE with ethidium bromide (5 g/200 mL TAE and 10 µL ethidium bromide).
8. Load 10 µL of 100 bp DNA ladder in the first well of each gel followed by the PCR products.
9. Run at 150 V for 30 min, then visualize on a UV transilluminator.

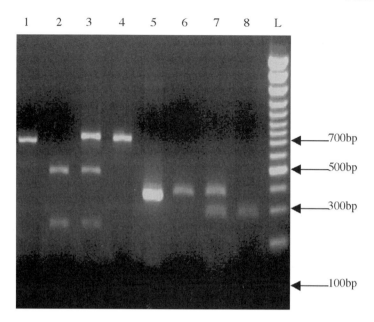

Fig. 2. Lanes 1–4: PCR-RFLP analysis of nucleotide 460: 1—Undigested (694 bp); 2—homozygous wild type (443 bp and 251 bp); 3—heterozygous (694 bp, 443 bp, and 251 bp); 4—homozygous mutant (694 bp). Lanes 5–8: PCR-RFLP analysis of nucleotide 719: 5—Undigested (373 bp); 6—homozygous wild-type (373 bp); 7—heterozygous (373 bp, 283 bp, and 90 bp); 8—homozygous mutant (283 bp and 90 bp).

3.3.2. RFLP Analysis

1. Add 5 µL of PCR product to fresh reaction tube.
2. Add 3 µL of 10X buffer (*see* **Note 9**), 1 µL AccI and 21 µL of ddH$_2$O to each tube (prepare master mix for high sample number).
3. Incubate at 37°C for 1 h.
4. Add loading dye and run digests on 2.5% agarose gel then visualize on a UV transilluminator (*see* **Note 9**).

3.3.3. Results

A 373 bp PCR product will be produced by this method (*see* **Fig. 2**, lane 5).

3.4. Pyrosequencing

3.4.1. Primer Design

Initially, three primers will need to be ordered: forward and reverse PCR primers (one of which is biotinylated) and an internal sequencing primer.

Table 3
Thermal Cycling Conditions for TPMT A719G

Step	Temperature	Time	Cycles
Hold	95°C	10 min	1
Denature	94°C	1 min	35
Anneal	58°C	2 min	35
Extend	72°C	1 min	35
Hold	72°C	5 min	1

1. The forward and reverse PCR primers can be designed using ABI Prism Primer Express software or a comparable primer design software. The primers should be 15–30 bases in length, the T_m should be between 50–60°C, they should have little predicted secondary structure, and the product size can be anywhere between 25–700 bp. Once the PCR primers have been chosen, an internal primer will be need to be designed.
2. Design internal primers using technical support at www.pyrosequencing.com. The internal primer can lie within 10 bases of the SNP, the T_m should be about 50°C, it should be 15–20 bases in length, and it should also have little predicted secondary structure.
3. After the internal primer has been chosen, then the PCR primer for the opposite strand will need to be biotinylated.

3.4.2. PCR Reaction

1. For a 20 µL reaction add the reaction components described in **Table 4** (*see* **Notes 1–6**).
2. Perform PCR at the optimal annealing temperature using the conditions described in **Table 5** (*see* **Notes 7** and **10**).
3. Check the PCR on a 2.5% agarose gel by adding 5 µL PCR product to 5 µL of 5X loading dye. Make sure there is no contamination and the PCR product is the predicted size (*see* **Note 11**).

3.4.3. Immobilization of PCR Product

1. Add 20 µL of 2X Binding Wash Buffer II and 60–175 µg Dynabeads to each reaction (amount of Dynabeads depends on the size of the PCR product, typically 15 µL for <300 bp PCR product, 30 µL for >300 bp PCR product) (*see* www.pyrosequencing.com for details).
2. Vortex on an Eppendorf thermomixer 1400 rpm at 65°C. (Vortex 15 min for PCR products <300 bp. Vortex 30 min for PCR products >300 bp) (*see* **Note 12**).
   Note: While the PCR is on the thermomixer the workstation can be set up as follows: Plate #1—empty, Plate #2—50 µL 0.5 *M* NaOH, Plate #3—100 µL 1X annealing buffer, Plate #4—40 µL 1X annealing buffer and 5 µL sequencing primer in three-fold excess of the PCR-primers (3–15 pmols).

Table 4
PCR Reaction Components

Component	Volume
Genomic DNA (10–50 ng/µL)	1 µL
Forward PCR primer (1–5 pmol/µL)	0.5 µL
Reverse PCR primer (1–5 pmol/µL)	0.5 µL
Amplitaq Gold PCR Master Mix (2X)	10 µL
High purity water	8 µL
Total reaction volume	20 µL

Table 5
Thermal Cycling Conditions for Pyrosequencing

Step	Temperature	Time	Cycles
Hold	95°C	10 min	1
Denature	94°C	30 sec	45–55
Anneal	55–65°C	30 sec	45–55
Extend	72°C	60 sec/kb	45–55
Hold	72°C	5 min	1

3.4.4. Strand Separation

1. After immobilization is complete, transfer the reactions from the PCR plate to PSQ96 plate #1.
2. Attach the PSQ96 Sample Prep Tool Cover onto the PSQ96 Sample Prep Tool. Place the Prep Tool into plate #1 and push the handle downwards. Wait 30–60 s to allow capture of the beads before transferring the beads to plate #2.
3. With the handle in the down position, transfer the beads from plate #1 to plate #2. Once the sample prep tool is in plate #2, pull the handle up and shake the tool gently to release the beads into the NaOH. Allow the beads to incubate in the NaOH for one minute.
4. Place the PSQ96 Sample Prep Tool back into plate #2, recapture the beads and release into plate #3. After release, recapture and then release the beads into plate #4.
5. Place plate #4 in the PSQ96 Sample Prep Thermoplate and place on the Dry Bath Incubator. Incubate for 2 min at 80°C.
6. After two minutes, take the PSQ96 Sample Prep Thermoplate off the dry bath incubator and place on the lab bench to cool for about five minutes before removing the PSQ96 plate from the thermoplate (*see* **Note 13**).

3.4.5. Sequencing

1. The SNP sequence will first need to be entered. Open the PSQ96 Instrument Control panel. Under modules choose SNP entry, then enter your SNP name and the sequence to analyze starting at the 3′ end of the sequencing primer up to or past the SNP. Choose check, an order of dispensation along with a bar graph will appear displaying the three theoretical results. Save the results and exit. After exiting from SNP entry, choose Application and enter your user name and password. Choose SNP analysis and the Instrument PSQ appears, then Enter run ID, kit ID, and plate ID. Move to Process parameter, choose method and select your SNP name. Left click and drag to choose the wells in which you are analyzing.
2. Allow the cartridge and solutions to equilibrate to room temperature and then dispense 200 µL of each enzyme into the appropriate location in the cartridge. Then add 620 µL of high purity water to the substrate and enzyme and pipet immediately into the cartridge (*see* **Note 14**).
3. Place the PSQ96 plate and the cartridge in the machine and choose run on the instrument control panel. First the enzyme and then substrate will be added, followed by the dNTPs in the correct dispension order. The pyrogram will display the results in real time.

3.4.6. Analysis

1. When the instrument has completed the run the results can be analyzed. Under Modules, choose SNP evaluation and the PSQ96 Evaluation AQ will appear. Under unanalyzed data, double click on the run that was completed and then select analyze.
2. Analyze all wells according to the theoretical results displayed and then save the results.

4. Notes

1. In order to prevent cross contamination when performing PCR, use sterile techniques and autoclaved equipment.
2. Oligonucleotide primers are diluted to 1 nmol/µL and stored at –80°C. A 1 in 100 dilution of this stock solution is used for PCR.
3. Remember to vortex all solutions before pipetting, briefly pulse in a microcentrifuge to bring reagents down from the sides and underneath the lid.
4. All PCR reagents are stored at –20°C. Thaw PCR reagents on ice before use.
5. Determine the quantity of cocktail mix required by allowing for about 3–5 extra samples to be set up.
6. Remember to include a negative control consisting of all the PCR reagents minus the template DNA for each set of PCR reactions.

A

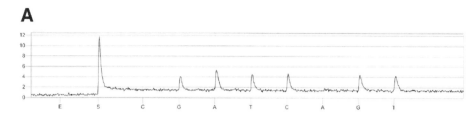

B

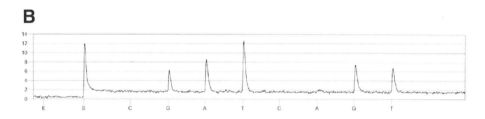

C

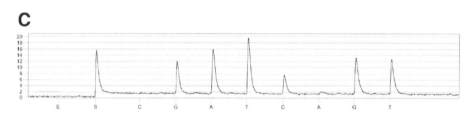

Fig. 3. Pyrogram of MDR1 c3435t SNP. The sequence to analyze is GATC /TGT:
(**A**) C/C homozygous wild-type; (**B**) T/T homozygous mutant; (**C**) C/T heterozygous.
Pyrogram courtesy of Christi Ralph.

7. For thermal cyclers without heated lids, the PCR reaction mixture needs to be overlaid with mineral oil to facilitate adequate and even heating of the tubes and prevent evaporation of the mixture.
8. It is useful to load base pair markers in the first and/or last lanes of the gel. This will help orientate the gel.
9. Restriction enzymes are supplied with a 10X reaction buffer.
10. Before performing PCR on precious samples, run a temperature gradient to find the optimal annealing temperature using a temperature scale between 55–70°C. T_m calculators are not always correct.
11. After PCR, if background is showing as a smear on the agarose gel, less cycles may need to be done to reduce background and get a higher concentration of PCR product.
12. PCR trays must be nonskirted to fit correctly in the Eppendorf Thermomixer.
13. After strand separation is complete the PSQ96 plate may be sealed and can sit at room temperature for 4–6 h, at 4°C for 48 h, or it can be frozen for 6 mo.

14. After adding water to the substrate and enzyme, they can be kept on ice for one day or can be frozen for one month.

Acknowledgments

This work is supported in part by the NIH Pharmacogenetics Research Network (U01 GM63340) and the Siteman Cancer Center.

References

1. The International SNP Map Working Group (2001) A map of human genome sequence variation containing 1.42 million single nucleotide polymorphisms. *Nature* **409,** 928–933.
2. Kwok, P. Y. (2001) Methods for genotyping single nucleotide polymorphisms. *Annu. Rev. Genomics Hum. Genet.* **2,** 235–258.
3. Krynetski, E.Y., Tai, H-L., Yates, C.R., et al. (1996) Genetic polymorphism of thiopurine methyltransferase: clinical importance and molecular mechanisms. *Pharmacogenetics* **6,** 279–290.
4. Weinshilboum, R. (2001) Thiopurine pharmacogenetics: clinical and molecular studies of thiopurine methyltransferase. *Drug Metab. Dispos.* **29,** 601–605.
5. McLeod, H. L., Krynetski, E. Y., Relling, M. V., and Evans, W. E. (2000) Genetic polymorphism of thiopurine methyltransferase and its clinical relevance for childhood acute lymphoblastic leukemia. *Leukemia* **14,** 567–572.
6. Ameyaw, M. M., Collie-Duguid, E. S., Powrie, R. H., Ofori-Adjei, D., and McLeod, H. L. (1999) Thiopurine methyltransferase alleles in British and Ghanaian populations. *Hum. Mol. Genet.* **8,** 367–370.
7. Hon, Y. Y., Fessing, M. Y., Pui, C. H., Relling, M. V., Krynetski, E. Y., and Evans, W. E. (1999) Polymorphism of the thiopurine S-methyltransferase (TPMT) gene in African Americans. *Hum. Mol. Genet.* **8,** 371–376.
8. McLeod, H. L., Coulthard, S., Thomas, A. E., et al. (1999) Analysis of thiopurine methyltransferase variant alleles in childhood acute lymphoblastic leukemia. *Br. J. Haematol.* **105,** 696–700.
9. Ronaghi, M. (2001) Pyrosequencing sheds light on DNA sequencing. *Genome Res.* **11,** 3–11.

20

Gene Expression Microarrays

Christopher P. Kolbert, William R. Taylor, Kelly L. Krajnik, and Dennis J. O'Kane

1. Introduction

New methods have been developed for determining and monitoring gene expression levels during pathologic or therapeutic processes. In particular, nucleic acid microarrays provide information about the expression levels of thousands of genes during a single experiment. Advances in nucleic acid sequencing technology and the subsequent burgeoning of public sequence databases have resulted in the availability of a vast amount of sequence information for both known genes and expressed sequence tags (ESTs). These data have been used in the design and creation of clone sets utilized as probes during microarray expression profiling analysis. Several different microarray platforms exist, which make use of either oligonucleotides or cDNA amplification products spotted onto solid or semisolid substrates. Perhaps the most well known use of oligonucleotides for microarray analysis is the GeneChip™ system (Affymetrix Inc., Emeryville, CA). A GeneChip™ consists of a silicon wafer containing hundreds of thousands of oligonucleotide probe sets designed to interrogate specific genes. To control for nonspecific hybridization, two different probe sets are created to interrogate each gene. One probe set matches the target sequence perfectly and is called the "perfect match" (PM). The other probe set, known as the "mismatch" (MM) is identical to the "perfect match" set, with the exception that there is a single nucleotide mismatch in the center position of each probe. A photolithographic process is used to synthesize the gene-specific oligonucleotide probes directly on the surface of the wafer, which is then encapsulated in a plastic cartridge for ease of use. RNA transcripts are reverse transcribed to cDNA, which then undergoes an in vitro transcription in the presence of biotin-labeled nucleotides to form labeled cRNA. The

From: *Methods in Molecular Medicine, vol. 85: Novel Anticancer Drug Protocols*
Edited by: J. K. Buolamwini and A. A. Adjei © Humana Press Inc., Totowa, NJ

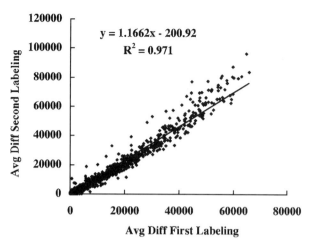

Fig. 1. Total RNA from a colon tumor was extracted, converted to cDNA, then to cRNA, and split into two portions. Each portion was separately labeled and hybridized to a high-density gene expression array (HU95A, Affymetrix). The resulting average difference values for the fluorescence signal for each gene was calculated for both arrays and graphed against each other. Approximately a 16% difference was found for the same RNA preparations. The general cut-on is 2- or 2.5-fold over- or under-expression for identifying genes of interest.

cRNA is fragmented, then hybridized to the microarray chips. A streptavidin phycoerythrin conjugate is added to induce fluorescence of the labeled fragments, the chips are washed, and then scanned for fluorescence with a confocal scanning microscope. Two separate microarray chips or chip sets are required for each gene expression analysis; one for the experimental or treated sample and one for the control sample. Images derived from the scanning process for the two microarrays are analyzed within the Affymetrix software platform and the hybridization-related intensities are assigned numerical values. The mean difference of the PM and MM probe intensity is used as the relative indicator of gene expression. A representative scatter plot of an RNA sample that was labeled and hybridized to two different microarrays is shown in **Figure 1**. Providing the Affymetrix protocols are followed exactly each time, reproducible results can be obtained. Approximately 62,000 genes and ESTs can be evaluated using the 5 microarrays in the high-density human gene set (U95). Candidate genes identified from high-density microarrays can then be examined on a larger number of RNA samples using lower cost custom spotted arrays. This is the focus of the following discussion.

Custom spotted microarrays can be prepared using oligonucleotide capture sequences, cDNA, or cDNA fragments. The overall protocol for utilizing custom spotted cDNA microarrays is shown in **Figure 2**. Oligonucleotide capture sets needed to spot custom arrays are commercially available, but are expensive. cDNA microarrays, while less specific, are relatively less expensive to produce. cDNA microarrays consist of PCR-amplified products that are spotted onto a glass or membrane substrate. Glass microscope slides are coated with polylysine, aminosilane, or aldehyde in order to facilitate nucleic acid binding. Nylon or nitrocellulose is used as a substrate for membrane arrays. During microarray experimentation with cDNA or EST products, total or polyA RNA is labeled with a fluorescent reporter or a radioisotope, such as Cy3 and Cy5, ^{33}P, or ^{32}P.

Unlike the Affymetrix GeneChip™ system, a single hybridization reaction is performed when using Cy3 and Cy5 as reporter molecules. Control and experimental RNA species, labeled with their respective fluorophore, are pooled and hybridized to an array spotted with cDNA or EST clone inserts. Following the hybridization, the slides are washed and centrifuged to minimize reagent-associated image distortions. Subsequently, they are scanned and the images analyzed to derive the hybridization-related intensities.

There are many array spotters and scanners that are available commercially. Some models are designed for high volume arraying and come with robotic plate stackers and environmental controls. Others are designed for moderate volume arraying. One such system is the Affymetrix 417 arrayer and 418 scanner (formerly built and marketed by Genetic MicroSystems). The Affymetrix 417 arrayer is a robotic system that employs proprietary Pin and Ring™ technology for spotting nucleic acids onto glass slides. Unlike some pin structures that hold minute sample volumes, the ring apparatus apparently reduces the effect of dehydration on spot volume and morphology by picking up and retaining approximately 1.5 µL of sample from a microwell. A solid pin is then forced down through the droplet, depositing 35–50 pL of sample at each spot location. With a center-to-center spot distance of 375 µm and 9 mm between each of the four pins, the system can place thousands of spots onto a 25 × 75-mm glass slide. The arrayer platen or workspace holds three 96 or 384-well plates and 42 microscope slides. A plexiglass enclosure protects the slides and microwell plates from contamination by dust particles. Environmental conditioning is not provided, however, individual laboratories may retrofit the system for humidity control.

The 417 arrayer is controlled by proprietary software, which allows the user to configure each spotting session with unique parameters. It is essential that clone identifications are tracked throughout the spotting process. We currently use Clonetracker™ (Biodiscovery Inc., Los Angeles, CA), which tracks clones by creating software-specific arrayer files that are linked to text files containing the identity and location of each clone in its respective microwell plate.

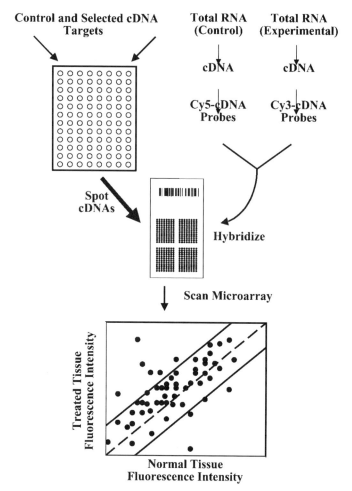

Fig. 2. The preparation of custom spotted arrays is presented. cDNAs of interest, including controls, are amplified in microwell plates and spotted on coated glass slides. Total RNA from control and treated tissues are separately converted to cDNA and labeled with cyanine dyes to permit two-color fluorescence analysis. The labeled cDNAs are mixed and hybridized overnight to the spotted slide. Following washing, the slide is scanned sequentially for Cy5 and Cy3 fluorescence and the images combined and analyzed for expression changes. The solid lines indicate the twofold over- and under-expression cut-offs. Candidate genes lying outside these cut-offs should be verified for expression levels by real-time PCR.

Table 1
Clones Used as Controls on Microarray Slides

ATCC cDNA clones	ATCC item number
Lys	87482
Phe	87483
Trp	87485
Dap	87486
human gamma-actin mRNA	365085
human deoxycytidylate deaminase	366960
human IMP dehydrogenase type 1 mRNA	364574
human hydroxymethylglutaryl-CoA lyase mRNA	364629
human phosphoglycerate mutase mRNA	363913
human serine dehydrase mRNA	363647
human ALAS1 mRNA for delta-aminolevulinate synthase	361298
human cytosolic aspartate aminotransferase mRNA	359365
human alpha-N-acetylgalactosaminidase mRNA	354938
human AMP deaminase	354744

The Affymetrix 418 scanner is a confocal, epifluorescence microscope for imaging of glass slides containing samples labeled with Cy3 or Cy5 fluorescent dyes. The instrument contains two fluorophore excitation lasers, with excitation spectra at 532 and 635 nm, respectively. The protocols below describe how to prepare customized spotted cDNA microarrays.

2. Materials

1. cDNA control clones (*see* **Table 1**).
2. PCR reagents (Applied Biosystems, Foster City, CA): 1X PCR buffer, 15 m*M* MgCl$_2$, vector-specific PCR primers, dNTPs, sterile deionized water, Taq Gold polymerase.
3. PCR supplies (Applied Biosystems): 96-well microplates, caps.
4. PCR purification system: Millipore Multiscreen PCR (Millipore Inc., Bedford, MA).
5. Plasmid DNA extraction, Qiagen Plasmid Miniprep, (Qiagen, Inc, Valencia, CA).
6. Dimethylsulfoxide (DMSO) (Sigma Chemical, St. Louis, MO).
7. 96-well microplates for clone spotting (Corning Costar, Corning, NY).
8. RNA purification kit: Qiagen RNeasy (Qiagen, Inc, Valencia, CA).
9. Cy3 and Cy5-labeled dUTP (Amersham Pharmacia Biotech, Inc., Piscataway, NJ).

10. RNA labeling and reverse transcription (RT) reagents: (Superscript II RT buffer, Superscript II RT, dNTPs, dithiothreitol (DTT); Invitrogen Life Technologies, Carlsbad, CA; ethylene diamine tetraacetic acid (EDTA), NaOH, HCl; Sigma Chemical, St. Louis, MO).
11. GFX PCR DNA and Gel Band Purification kit (Amersham Pharmacia Biotech, Inc., Piscataway, NJ).
12. Hybridization solution components: formamide, sodium citrate/sodium chloride (SSC), sodium dodecylsulfate (SDS), (Invitrogen Life Technologies, Carlsbad, CA), Poly(A)-DNA, COT1-DNA (Amersham Pharmacia Biotech, Inc., Piscataway, NJ).
13. CMT-GAPS slides (Corning Inc., Corning, NY).
14. Thermal cycler.
15. 42°C water bath.
16. 80°C dry oven.
17. UV box.
18. Speed vacuum.
19. Centrifuge with plate holder.
20. Spectrophotometer.
21. 95°C heating block.
22. Hybridization cartridges (Telechem International Inc., Sunnyvale, CA).
23. Array spotter (Affymetrix 417).
24. Array scanner (Affymetrix 418).
25. Glass microscope slides, 1×3 inches (25×75 mm).
26. Poly-L-lysine (Sigma Chemical, St. Louis, MO).

3. Methods

3.1. Introduction

A number of protocols are available for preparing spotted expression microarrays *(1–3)*. Although published protocols are good starting points, they may require optimization by individual laboratories in order to develop routine procedures that produce acceptable limits of variation from one experiment to another. The protocols used to fabricate and analyze spotted cDNA gene expression microarrays produced in this laboratory were performed according to protocols described by Hegde et al. *(2)* with some modifications. An excellent internet site where these protocols are updated regularly is supported by The Institute for Genomic Research *(3)*.

3.2. Controls

A number of sources of variation are introduced into each microarray experiment that is performed. Control cDNA products must be printed onto each microarray slide to allow compensation for variations, such as variation in the fluorescent probe labeling and hybridization efficiencies.

3.2.1. Clones for Normalizing Signals

In our laboratory, I.M.A.G.E. control clones are chosen from a set determined to have similar gene expression levels in most tissue types *(2)* and are listed in **Table 1**. Since these genes are assumed to exhibit no differential expression in various tissues, they should have equal intensities in both the Cy5 and Cy3 fluorophor emission channels. The intensities of these controls should fall on a line of equality with slope equal to 1.0.

3.2.2. Spiked Hybridization Controls

Prokaryotic clones used with Affymetrix GeneChips™ (Affymetrix, Emeryville, CA) are spiked into the RNA hybridization mixture as additional controls. These include genes encoding phenylalanine, tryptophan, lysine, and Dap (*see* **Table 1**). These sequences are absent from the human genome and verify proper RNA labeling.

3.2.3. Amplification of Control Clones and Experimental cDNA Targets

Control clone inserts are prepared from the host bacteria that contain a plasmid insert encoding the control or experimental target genes. The host bacterial strains are grown overnight in liquid culture and the plasmid DNA is then extracted by heat denaturation at 95°C or by plasmid preparation (Qiagen Plasmid Miniprep, Qiagen Inc., Valencia, CA). The isolated DNA is subsequently amplified by standard PCR methods. The same approach is used to amplify the DNA segments of genes or ESTs to be incorporated on the microarray. Target genes can either be obtained from custom libraries prepared in the laboratory or purchased from commercial sources (I.M.A.G.E. clones, Unigene clusters, or ESTs).

3.2.3.1. PCR Amplification Mix

Target amplification is performed using vector-specific primers. 2 µL of DNA sample extract are added to 98 µL of PCR master mix that contains: 1X PCR buffer II, 2.5 mM MgCl$_2$, 200 µM each dNTP, 100 pmol each primer, and 2.5 U Taq Gold DNA polymerase (Applied Biosystems, Foster City, CA). PCR primers are designed using the sequences of the common restriction nuclease sites originally included in the plasmids. The restriction sites are described by the vendors. The advantages of designing primers that contain common sequences are that few unique primers are needed to amplify a large number of different control genes and the same thermal cycling conditions can be used for many of the clones.

3.2.3.2. THERMAL CYCLING CONDITIONS

Sample nucleic acids are denatured at 95°C for 10 min to form single strand DNA templates. The subsequent thermal cycling conditions are: anneal primers to the target DNA at 52°C for 30 s; extend the primers at 72°C for 2 min; denature the double strand DNA amplicons at 95°C for 30 s in order to prepare for the next cycle. The control genes and cDNA targets are amplified for 35 cycles using these conditions and then allowed to extend at 72°C for 10 min in order to ensure completion of full-length products.

3.2.3.3. PURIFICATION AND QUANTIFICATION OF AMPLICONS

Amplified gene products are purified by removing unincorporated primers and dNTPs using a 96-well microplate according to the manufacturer's instructions (Millipore Multiscreen PCR, Millipore Inc., Bedford, MA). The purified amplicons are eluted with 70 μL sterile deionized H_2O. Five microliter aliquots are analyzed using a 2% agarose gel (Seakem GTG, FMC Bioproducts, Rockland, ME) to determine amplification integrity based upon discrete bands for each amplicon of the correct molecular size. The amplified products are then quantified by spectrophotometry.

3.2.3.4. PREPARATION OF CONTROL SAMPLES AND cDNA TARGETS FOR SPOTTING

Amplified DNA products are dried to completion using a speed vacuum centrifuge. The DNA amplicons are resuspended in 20 μL of 50% DMSO in preparation for spotting on the coated glass slides. Other protocols require resuspending the amplicons in spotting solutions containing 3X SSC alone or 3X SSC containing 0.1% Sarkosyl. Control and target cDNA sequence amplicons can be stored for several months at –20°C. It is most convenient to store the amplicons in 96-well microwell plates for ease of handling for spotting applications and in order to enter the identifying information for all samples into a computer program that permits tracking the samples. Clone identifications and well locations are recorded in a tab-delimited text file, which is then imported into the software application Clonetracker™ (Biodiscovery Inc., Los Angeles, CA) and used to link amplicon identity to spot position on the glass arrays.

3.3. Preparation of Glass Slides for Spotting

Glass substrates must be modified in order to retain nucleic acids. Coated slides are available commercially in a variety of formats, and are convenient for preparing spotted microarrays, but are rather expensive. We routinely use aminosilane-coated glass slides (CMT-GAP slides, Corning Inc., Corning, NY). These slides retain large amplified DNA fragments very tightly (≥500 bases) and demonstrate very low background, but are unsuitable for smaller fragments. An inexpensive alternative is to prepare polylysine-coated glass slides as described below.

3.3.1. Coating Slides with Poly-L-Lysine

Several protocols are available for coating microscope slides with polylysine. We currently use a protocol created by Brown and co-workers, details of which are available on their laboratory's internet site *(4)*. Following is a summary of this protocol.

3.3.1.1. CLEANING THE SLIDES

Glass slides are cleaned by soaking in 2.5 M NaOH solution (70 g NaOH, 280 mL sterile deionized H_2O, 420 mL 95% ethanol) for 2 h with agitation. Immediately after cleaning, the slides are rinsed 4x in fresh deionized H_2O to remove NaOH and ethanol.

3.3.1.2. COATING THE SLIDES

Polylysine solution is prepared by adding 70 mL of poly-L-lysine (Sigma Corp., St. Louis, MO) to 70 mL tissue culture phosphate-buffered saline (PBS) in 560 mL water. Slides are placed into polylysine solution and agitated for 1 h, then rinsed 5× with fresh deionized H_2O. The polylysine coated slides are then centrifuged for 5 min at 28*g* and dried in a 45°C oven for 10 min. Exposure to open air should be minimized to avoid dust particles.

3.3.1.3. QUALITY CONTROL

Before using the coated slides, test the slide surface of each batch by placing drop of water onto a slide. The droplet should form discrete drops due to the hydrophobic properties of properly prepared slides. In addition, perform a test printing on at least one slide per batch to assess the overall spot quality and morphology.

3.4. Spotting the Slides with Target DNA

Protocols for spotting cDNA expression arrays will vary for different robotic arrayers. The arrayer protocol described below is used with the Affymetrix Model 417 arrayer. This arrayer is convenient for spotting small custom expression arrays of several hundred to a few thousand cDNAs and controls. In some laboratories, this arrayer has been utilized to construct larger expression arrays, but one might argue it would be easier and more cost-effective to purchase commercial arrays for large-scale gene expression analyses involving more than a few thousand cDNAs.

3.4.1. cDNA Target Samples and Controls

Thaw the amplified cDNA targets and controls (*see* **Subheading 3.2.3.4.**). Resuspend the materials and mix for 10–15 min.

3.4.2. Preparing the Arraying Robot for Spotting Slides

1. Turn on the vacuum (either house or pump). Ensure that a vacuum of at least 700 mbar (950 mbar if using a vacuum pump) can be obtained. The vacuum aids in drying the pins following washing.
2. Move the gantry to the right corner of the plate.
3. Make sure that the water container is full (ultrapure water) and the waste container is empty.
4. Place a few pieces of paper towel over the wash stations and prime them until the flow is continuous.

3.4.3. Calibrating the Arrayer

Calibration should be performed once a month, when new plate or slide types are used, and when new plate or slide lots are used.

1. Mix a 1 : 1000 dilution of blue food coloring in the appropriate spotting solution. Pipet 10–30 μL aliquots in wells A1, A2, B1, B2 of a 96-well plate (Nunc, cat. no. 442587). Place the plate into the leftmost plate location on the arrayer. Place a slide in locations 1 and 19 of the arrayer.
2. Pin Calibration: Select **Calibrate: Pin/Ring calibration, New Pin** from the software menu. The gantry will move the spotting pins over the slide at position 19. Press the down arrow on the dialogue box until the pins lightly touch the slide. Then click down two more times. Push the **Set** button, then the **Apply** button. This adjusts and sets the pin contact with the glass slide.
3. Ring Calibration: Select **Ring Calibration** and **New Ring** from the menu. The gantry will move the spotting pins over the A1, A2, B1, B2 wells, respectively. Press the down arrow until the rings are immersed in the food coloring. Be sure not to force the ring into the bottom of the plate. Then click **Set** and **Apply**.
4. Pin Test: Select **Pin Test** from the **Calibrate: Calibration Test and Adjustment** pull down menu. When finished, scan the slide using the red laser. The lines of the pin test grids should be within two lines of each other. An array test can also be performed to see how many spots can be created from a single ring full of solution. The array test creates four (one per pin) grids of 400 spots each.

3.4.4. Databases and Software Settings

In order to track the gene identities and locations of each spot, sample designations and microwell plate locations are typed into a spreadsheet using the column headings Plate ID, Row, Column, Ref. The file is then saved as tab-delimited text and imported into the plate database of Clonetracker™.

1. Choose **New** from the **File** menu. Type in the requested information and save the new set.
2. Choose **Plates** from the **Database** pulldown menu. Browse to find the appropriate text file and select it.
3. Choose **Select** from the **Plates** pulldown menu. A dialog box will appear. Find the appropriate plate file and drag it into the left half of the box. This will specify the appropriate data set.
4. Save the Clonetracker™ file.

3.4.5. The Arrayer File

"The arrayer file" that is created by Clonetracker™ allows the user to configure appropriately the location of spots on the glass slides and specifies to the arraying robot the sample wells to be utilized on specific microplates.

1. Turn on the arrayer and boot up the arrayer software on the desktop.
2. Select the arrayer software pull down menu and select **File** and **Open**. Then select the appropriate arrayer file that was created in Clonetracker™ and configure the run to your specifications.

3.4.6. Final Setup and Adjustments

The final set-up procedure positions the microwell plates on the platen and prepares the arraying robot to spot the coated slides.

1. Place a 96-well microplate into the leftmost plate station. Orient the plate so that the A1 well is in the lower left corner of the station. Subsequent plates should be placed from left to right.
2. Select the **Calibration Pull Down Menu** and highlight the **Pin/Ring Calibration** selection. The gantry will move the pins over the plate.
3. Align the plate so that the rings traverse down into the center of the wells. This will allow proper alignment of the pins over the microwells.
4. Cancel the calibration.
5. Place the correct number of coated slides into the slide positions. It may be necessary to tape the corners of the slides closest to the wash stations to ensure that the slides are placed appropriately.
6. Double-check to ensure that all settings are correct, then click **Start**. The arraying robot will now start spotting the samples from the microwell plates onto the coated slides.

3.5. RNA Preparation, cDNA Synthesis, and Probe Labeling

3.5.1. Basic Considerations

All reagents used for RNA preparation must be treated with diethylpyrocarbonate (DEPC) and RNase free. Either total RNA or purified mRNA can be used in these protocols, however isolation of total RNA is faster and minimizes losses of mRNA during subsequent isolation steps.

1. RNA Isolation: A number of RNA isolation procedures may be used to prepare total RNA. Good quality RNA is essential to the gene expression experiment. In some cases where a cell line or tissue over-expresses RNAses, two different sequential RNA isolation procedures may be required (Trizol followed by RNeasy, for example). In most cases, total RNA is readily and reliably extracted from tissue or cells using a Qiagen RNeasy Kit according to the manufacturer's instructions (Qiagen Inc., Valencia, CA).

2. Assessing RNA Quality: RNA quality is assessed by assaying each sample by microcapillary electrophoresis (Agilent Lab on a Chip, Model 2100 Bioanalyzer, Agilent Inc., Palo Alto, CA). Total RNA samples (1 µL) are pipetted into the wells of the microcapillary chip, the chip is placed into the Bioanalyzer, and an electric current is applied, causing the RNA to be separated by size. The ratios of the ribosomal RNA peaks and the absence of peaks between the 18S rRNA and 5S RNA/mRNA region are used as indicators of whether the sample is intact (*see* **Fig. 3A**) or substantially degraded (*see* **Fig. 3B**). Degraded samples do not provide reliable results and should not be utilized in experiments for measuring gene expression.

3. RNA Quantification: RNA is quantified by spectrophotometry at 260 nm and 280 nm (Spectrafluor Plus, Tecan, Durham, NC). This instrument utilizes UV-transmitting microwell plates, and allows a large number of samples to be quantified rapidly. Typically, 10 µg of total RNA is used for each hybridization. Total RNA samples can be prepared in advance and stored at −80°C until needed.

3.5.2. cDNA Probe Synthesis and Probe Labeling

RNA is readily degraded by ubiquitous ribonucleases in the cellular and surrounding environments. For this reason, precautions must be taken in order to maintain sample quality. Lab workers should wear gloves when handling samples and reagent containers and all reagents should be RNase free. During the labeling procedure, RNA samples are converted to stable cDNA by reverse transcription. Fluorescent cyanine dyes are incorporated into the cDNA: red excited Cy5 for labeling experimental samples; green excited Cy3 for normal or control samples.

1. Oligo-dT hybridization: Four microliters of oligo dT primer (0.5 µg/µL dT_{12}–dT_{18}) is added to 10 µg total RNA (or 2.0 µg mRNA) in a total volume of 10 µL. The prokaryotic Affymetrix control clones Lys, Phe, Dap, and Trp are spiked into each reaction at concentrations of 1.52 p*M*, 3.04 p*M*, 15.2 p*M* and 152 p*M*, respectively. RNA samples are mixed and vortexed briefly, then incubated at 70°C for 10 min and chilled on ice. Overhead room lights are turned

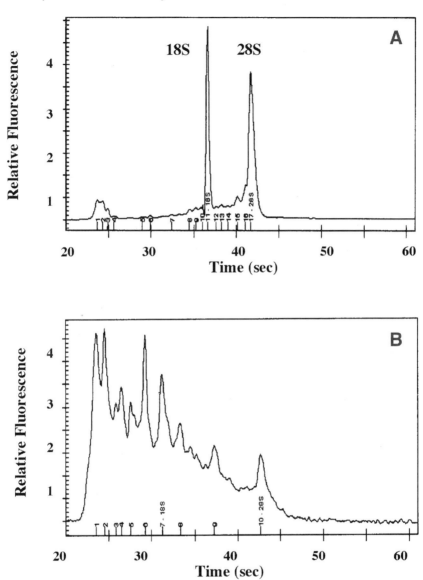

Fig. 3. Analysis of total RNA. (**A**) Migration profile of acceptable, intact total RNA. The 28S and 18S RNA is intact suggesting little sample degradation. Components representing small RNAs (mRNA, tRNA, and 5S RNA) are indicated. The run time is approx 90 s per sample. (**B**) An RNA sample submitted for labeling, but rejected due to the substantial sample degradation.

off to minimize photo-bleaching of the fluorescent dyes used in the labeling protocol.

2. Prepare the Reverse Transcription-Labeling Master Mix. Included in each labeling reaction are 6 μL of 5X first strand Superscript II buffer (250 m*M* Tris-HCl, pH 8.3, 375 m*M* KCl, 15 m*M* MgCl$_2$), 3 μL of 0.1 *M* DTT, 0.6 μL of low dTTP mix (25 m*M* each dATP, dGTP, dCTP; 5 m*M* dTTP) and 5.4 μL of DEPC-treated double distilled water. To the RNA samples prepared in **Subheading 3.5.1.1.**, add 15 μL of the master mix, 3 μL of 1 m*M* Cy3 dUTP for control samples or Cy5 dUTP for experimental samples (vortex briefly), and 2 μL of Superscript II RT (200U/μL). Mix thoroughly and incubate at 42°C for 2 h. Centrifuge the tubes very briefly and place on ice. Add 1.5 μL of 20 m*M* EDTA, pH 8.0 and vortex. Add 1.5 μL of 0.5 *M* NaOH and vortex to mix. Incubate at 70°C for 10 min. Cool to room temperature and add 1.5 μL of 0.5 *M* HCl. At this stage, fluorescent dUTPs have been incorporated into the synthesized cDNAs.

3. cDNA Probe Purification: Each labeled probe is purified according to manufacturer's instructions for the GFX™ PCR DNA and Gel Band Purification kit (Amersham Pharmacia Biotech Inc., Piscataway, NJ). Briefly, place a GFX column into a collection tube and add 500 μL of capture buffer. Transfer the probe to the column and mix thoroughly by pipetting up and down several times. Centrifuge columns at full speed for 30 s. Add 500 μL of wash buffer and centrifuge at full speed for 30 s. Transfer the column to a new 1.5 mL microcentrifuge tube and elute by adding 50 μL of 10 m*M* Tris, pH 8.0. Dry the probe to completion in a speed vacuum (20–30 min; 42°C). Resuspend the probe in 10 μL of DEPC ddH$_2$O. Combine the probes for a total of 20 μL. Store at –20°C until ready to use.

3.6. Hybridizing cDNA Probes to Spotted DNA Targets

Successful hybridization requires several steps including blocking sites on the coated microarray slide to prevent non-specific hybridization, the hybridization itself, and washing the slides to remove unhybridized materials. Each of these steps needs to be optimized.

3.6.1. Prehybridization to Block Non-Specific Binding Sites

1. Prepare pre-hybridization solution (5X SSC, 0.1% SDS, 1.0% bovine serum albumin). Place slides into pre-hybridization solution and incubate for 45 min at 42°C.

2. Wash the slides in double distilled water 5×. Immerse slides in room temperature isopropanol and centrifuge for 5 min at 28*g*. Slides should be hybridized soon after pre-hybridization.

3.6.2. Hybridization

1. Combine the labeled control and experimental cDNA probes in equal proportions in a 1.5 mL microcentrifuge tube. Add 1 μL of COT1-DNA (20 μg/μL) and

Poly(A)-DNA (20 μg/μL), mix well. The COT1-DNA is a common repeat sequence and is used to decrease non-specific hybridization.

2. Denature the cDNA by heating at 95°C for 3 min. Centrifuge the probe at high speed for 1 min. Add an equal volume of 2X hybridization solution (50% formamide, 10X SSC, and 0.2% SDS) heated to 42°C.
3. Place a glass coverslip over the grid area of the slide. Pipet the hybridization solution containing the Cy3/Cy5-labeled RNA mixture onto the slide adjacent to the coverslip. The solution will move by capillary action under the coverslip.
4. Place the slide into a hybridization cartridge (Telechem International Inc., Sunnyvale, CA) and pipet 20 μL of 3X SSC into each end.
5. Place the cover on top of the cartridge and tighten the screws.
6. Place the cartridge into a 42°C water bath and hybridize overnight.

3.6.3. Washing the Microarray Slide

1. After 16–18 h of incubation, remove the cartridge from the water bath and loosen the screws.
2. Place the slide into a wash solution containing 1X SSC/0.1% SDS (preheated to 42°C) and rotate for 5 min. The coverslip should fall off during the wash.
3. Next, place the slide into a wash solution containing 0.1X SSC/0.1% SDS (room temperature) and rotate for 5 min.
4. Finally, place the slide into a solution of 0.1X SSC (room temperature) and rotate for 5 min.
5. Spin slide in rack at approx 28*g* for 5 min. Scan immediately.

3.7. Scanning and Data Analysis

Images are created with the Affymetrix (GMS) 418 scanner. Slides are scanned by using both red and green excitation lasers operating at 635 and 532 nm, respectively. Laser power and PMT signal output are calibrated to generate the optimal visual image. Red and green images are analyzed by using Imagene (Biodiscovery Inc., Los Angeles, CA). Normalization is performed to account for experiment-related variation and background subtraction is conducted locally for each spot. Images are superimposed and the mean numerical values associated with each probe are extracted. A combination of software applications including Spotfire DecisionSite™ (Spotfire Inc., Cambridge, MA) and Microsoft Excel (Microsoft Corp., Redmond, WA) are used for final data reduction.

3.7.1. Procedure for Scanning the Microarray

1. Turn on the Affymetrix 418 scanner.
2. Start up the appropriate software on the desktop of the scanner computer.
3. Place the slide into scanner and gently push forward until it stops.

4. Turn the laser dial to the appropriate fluorescence emission color. From the Run Menu, select **Start**. Specify the size of the scan, the red laser, and the photomultiplier tube (PMT) gain that should be used. Then click **Start**.

5. Also, under the **Start** pulldown menu, select **Calibrate**. This will allow the user to change the PMT as the scan is proceeding. Repeat the scan using the green excitation laser.

3.8. Data Extraction

There are several good software applications for the initial data extraction procedure. Our laboratory currently uses Imagene (Biodiscovery, Los Angeles, CA) for this process. Software versions can vary considerably, thus a description of the process will not be included in this summary. In general, the respective images for the Cy3 and Cy5 scans are superimposed so that the arrayed spots are aligned properly. The range of spot diameters is measured and a grid is then created to define the spot locations. Normalization parameters are configured to account for the experimental design and the mean pixel intensity for each spot is then calculated. Many algorithms exist for normalization of data and a description of each is beyond the scope of this discussion. Generally, our laboratory normalizes spotted array data in multiple ways in order to assess the overall quality of the data. Separation data normalizations against the I.M.A.G.E. clones, spiked prokaryotic clones, and all of the arrayed spots may reveal the most appropriate analysis technique for specific data sets. The normalized dataset can then be imported into other software applications for final data reduction.

4. Notes

1. Although the protocols presented have been reliable in our hands, it is important to optimize protocols to ensure that they work optimally in each laboratory environment.

2. If different spotting robots are used, temperature and humidity control must be considered in order that sample concentration does not occur (minimized with 50% DMSO spotting solutions), and that the pins do not dry out during the spotting process. Quill type pins are more susceptible to drying than the pin and ring system utilized on the Affymetrix 417 arrayer. However, this pin configuration results in using more sample volume because of the ring.

3. When first performing labeling for custom spotted arrays, it is imperative to determine if there is a label-dependent bias introduced by the dyes. Cy3 and Cy5 are incorporated at different rates into nucleic acids. It is advisable to reverse the labeling dyes in an experiment to ascertain if this bias is significant. For example, instead of using Cy5 to label the normal sample, use it to label the treated sample material.

4. Cyanine dyes are photolabile. Cy5 is more labile than Cy3. Accordingly, the Cy5 channel should be scanned first to minimize photobleaching.

5. Data analysis programs vary from facility to facility. Data that can be saved in a comma- or tab-delimited formats, compatible with Microsoft Excel, permits easy exchange of raw data with colleagues and facilitates data analysis by other programs.

References

1. DeRisi, J., Penland, L., and Brown, P. O. (1996) Use of a cDNA microarray to analyze gene expression patterns. *Nat. Genet.* **14,** 457–461.
2. Hegde, P., Qi, R., Abernathy, K., et al. (2000) A concise guide to cDNA microarray analysis. *Biotechniques* **29,** 548–562.
3. http://www.tigr.org/tdb/microarray/protocolsTIGR.shtml
4. http://brownlab.stanford.edu/protocols.html

21

Methods for Isolation and Genetic Analysis of Circulating Tumor DNA in Patient Plasma

Tomoya Kawaguchi, Will S. Holland, and Paul H. Gumerlock

1. Introduction

Nanogram quantities of DNA circulating in blood are present in healthy subjects *(1,2)*. A number of recent studies have shown that tumor DNA is shed in either plasma or serum of cancer patients *(3–11)*. Further, the plasma of cancer patients is enriched in DNA, up to four times the amount of free DNA compared to plasma from normal controls *(4)*. Specific mutations found in genes in the primary tumors, but not present in the patient's genomic DNA, can also be identified in the DNA from plasma, demonstrating that the source of the DNA in plasma is the tumor *(5,6)*. Abnormalities detected include microsatellite alterations, immunoglobulin rearrangements, and hypermethylation of several genes *(7–10)*. Anker, et al. reported that 7 of 14 colorectal cancer patients (50%) had a codon 12 *K-Ras* mutation within their primary tumor, and identical mutations were found in the plasma DNA of 6 of those 7 patients (86%). Mutant DNA was not found in the plasma specimens of 7 patients whose tumors tested negative for *K-Ras* alterations or in healthy controls *(5)*. Lauschke, et al. also reported that *K-Ras* mutations were detected in 22 of 30 colorectal tumor tissues, and the same mutation was identified in the serum samples of 6 of the patients *(6)*. Also in that study, mutations of the *APC* gene were identified in 25 of 65 tumors, and 20 of these 25 patients showed the identical mutation in their serum samples. Genetic abnormalities mirroring those of the primary tumor have also been found in the blood of patients with many other types of cancer, including cancers of the lung, head and neck, breast, liver, and pancreas.

From: *Methods in Molecular Medicine, vol. 85: Novel Anticancer Drug Protocols*
Edited by: J. K. Buolamwini and A. A. Adjei © Humana Press Inc., Totowa, NJ

These studies have opened a new research area, indicating that plasma DNA might eventually be a suitable target for the development of noninvasive diagnostic, prognostic, and follow-up tests for many type of cancers. In this chapter, our laboratory's approach for the extraction of DNA shed in plasma is detailed. Furthermore, we have demonstrated the use of cancer patient plasma DNA in studies of both *K-Ras* codon 12 mutations and -tubulin (*TUBB*) mutations, which may be important genes for predicting chemotherapy response *(12,13)*.

2. Materials
2.1. Extraction of DNA

1. Patient peripheral blood: 5–10 mL.
2. QIAamp DNA mini kit (QIAGEN Inc., Valencia, CA).
3. ddH$_2$O.
4. 1.5-mL microcentrifuge tubes.

2.2. PCR Reactions

1. 10X PCR buffer: 100 mM Tris-HCl, 500 mM KCl, including 25 mM MgCl$_2$ (Roche Molecular Biochemicals, Indianapolis, IN).
2. dNTP mix (10 mM stock solution of each deoxynucleotide triphosphate, final concentrations 0.2 mM).
3. 5 U/µL of *Taq* DNA polymerase (Roche Molecular Biochemicals).
4. 20 µM stock solution of each PCR primer (final concentrations for *K-Ras* and *TUBB* are 2.5 µM and 0.5 µM, respectively) (*see* **Table 1**).
5. ddH$_2$O.
6. Thermal cycler.
7. 2.0% agarose gel.
8. Buffer H (Roche Molecular Biochemicals).
9. Restriction enzyme, 10 U/µL of *Mva I* (Roche Molecular Biochemicals).
10. 100 bp DNA Ladder (Promega, Madison, WI).
11. Electrophoresis gel box.
12. Power supply.

3. Methods
3.1. Extraction of DNA from Human Plasma

1. Blood (5–10 mL) is obtained in a purple-top tube (containing ethylene diamine tetraacetic acid (EDTA) to prevent clotting).
2. Centrifuge the blood sample at 800g for 15 min at 4°C soon after taking the blood from the patient to separate plasma from red blood cells and the white blood cell buffy coat.
3. Remove plasma and buffy coat separately from the samples, and freeze and store at –80°C until further use.

Table 1
Sequence for PCR primer (5′ → 3′)

KRas (1), forward: ACTGAATATAAACTTGTGGAGTTGGACCT
KRas (2), reverse: TCAAAGAATGGTCCTGGACC
KRas (3), reverse inside: TAATATGTCGACTAAAACAAGATTTACCTC
TUBB (1), forward: AAGGAGATACATCCGAGGGAATTAT
TUBB (2), reverse: AATGACCAGACGGAGTAATCGG
TUBB (3), forward inside: CTTTTCTCCTGACTGGCATTCC

---

4. Using 200 μL of plasma, perform the DNA extraction according to standard procedures with the commercial kit (QIAamp DNA mini kit, QIAGEN). Finally, elute the DNA in a volume of 50 μL ddH$_2$O using a single elution step. The DNA can be stored at −20°C until further use.
5. The sequences of oligonucleotides used as primers for *K-Ras* exon1 and *TUBB* exon 4 amplification are listed in **Table 1**.

3.2. K-Ras *Codon 12 Point Mutation Detection*

For detecting *K-Ras* codon 12 point mutations, plasma DNA is examined using a two-stage RFLP-PCR assay *(13)*. Human non-small cell lung cancer (NSCLC) A549 cells are used as a mutation control, and human prostate cancer LNCaP cells are used as a wild-type control.

1. For the 1st PCR, mix 10X PCR buffer (2.0 μL), dNTPs (0.4 μL), *K-Ras* primer 1 (2.5 μL), *K-Ras* primer 2 (2.5 μL), ddH$_2$O (12.4 μL), *Taq* DNA polymerase (0.2 μL), and template DNA (5.0 μL).
2. Perform PCR in a thermal cycler under the following conditions: 1 min at 94°C, followed by 35 cycles of 1 min at 94°C, 1 min at 55°C, and 30 s at 72°C, and a final extension of 10 min at 72°C.
3. Mix the PCR product (10 μL), buffer H (2 μL), restriction enzyme *MvaI* (1 μL), and ddH$_2$O (7 μL) for enzyme digestion. Incubate at 37°C for at least 2 h.
4. For hemi-nested 2nd PCR, mix 10X PCR buffer (2.0 μL), dNTPs (0.4 μL), *K-Ras* primer 2 (2.5 μL), *K-Ras* primer 3 (2.5 μL), ddH$_2$O (12.4 μL), *Taq* DNA polymerase (0.2 μL), and the digested 1st PCR product (5.0 μL).
5. Perform the 2nd PCR in a thermal cycler using the same cycling conditions as above. Mix the 2nd PCR product (10 μL), buffer H (2 μL), restriction enzyme *MvaI* (1 μL), and ddH$_2$O (7 μL) for 2nd enzyme digestion. Incubate at 37°C for at least 2 h.
6. Electrophorese the PCR product in a 2% agarose gel and visualize with ethidium bromide staining under UV light, and photograph it or digitally image it. All oncogenic activating mutations at codon 12 can be detected using this assay (*see* **Fig. 1**).

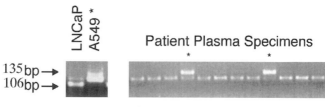

Fig. 1. *K-Ras* Mutation Detection in Cancer Patient Plasma by the RFLP-PCR Assay. Detection of codon 12 *K-Ras* point mutation after amplification with RFLP-PCR technique and digestion with *Mva I*. The 106 bp wild-type band and the 135 bp mutant band can be discriminated easily with this assay on a 2% agarose gel. Note that in the two cell line controls, LNCaP shows the 106 bp wild-type band while A549 shows the 135 bp mutant band. Also patient specimens in lanes 4 and 9 show the presence mutant *K-Ras* DNA in their plasma.

3.3. β-Tubulin (TUBB) Mutation Analysis

For detecting β-tubulin mutations, plasma DNA is examined using a hemi-nested PCR assay followed by direct sequencing.

1. For 1st PCR, mix 10X PCR buffer (2.0 µL), dNTPs (0.4 µL), β-tubulin primer 1 (0.5 µL), β-tubulin primer 2 (0.5 µL), ddH$_2$O (16.4 µL), *Taq* DNA polymerase (0.2 µL), and template DNA (2.0 µL).
2. Perform PCR in a thermal cycler under following conditions: 1 min at 94°C, 35 cycles of 30 s at 94°C, 1 min at 55°C, and 90 s at 72°C, and a final extension of 10 min at 72°C.
3. For hemi-nested 2nd PCR, mix 10X PCR buffer (2.0 µL), dNTPs (0.4 µL), β-tubulin primer 1 (0.5 µL), β-tubulin primer 3 (0.5 µL), ddH$_2$O (16.4 µL), *Taq* DNA polymerase (0.2 µL), and the PCR products from the first reaction (2.0 µL).
4. Perform PCR in a thermal cycler under the same cycling conditions as in the 1st PCR reaction.
5. Electrophorese the PCR product on a 2% agarose gel and visualize with ethidium bromide staining under UV light, and photograph it or digitally image it to confirm amplification of the exon 4 (*see* **Fig. 2**).
6. The PCR products should then be purified before being used for sequencing. A commercial kit is available which will accomplish this (QIAquick PCR Purification Kit, QIAGEN Inc.).
7. Single strand sequencing is done according to our previously published protocol *(14)*.

4. Notes

1. There may be no difference between plasma and serum when extracting DNA, but it is preferable to use and stock plasma, which also includes proteins, for future studies.

Patient Plasma Specimens

1239 bp ⟶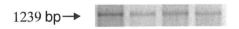

Fig. 2. Amplification of β-tubulin (*TUBB*) Exon 4 from Cancer Patient Plasma. Amplification products are often not seen after the 1st PCR due to the small amount of DNA (data is not shown). However, the 2nd hemi-nested PCR results in easy detection of the 1239 bp product on a 2% agarose gel. Following this amplification, the products can be directly sequenced as previously described *(14)*.

2. The amount of DNA we collected from plasma was too small (less than 5 ng/μL) to obtain an accurate concentration reading from a spectophotometer. As such, the volume of template DNA we used was not dependent upon the concentration.

3. In our experience, to obtain the highest concentration of DNA possible, a single elution step of 50 μL ddH$_2$O is recommended as mentioned above. To obtain a larger yield of DNA, we have found that two elution steps of 200 μL ddH$_2$O each give a better yield, although the DNA is at a lower concentration. This may necessitate precipitating the DNA in order to increase the concentration for the PCR reactions.

4. A hot block start, where the thermal cycler is already at the initial denaturation temperature, should be performed to prevent non-selective primer template hybridization when doing PCR.

5. Contamination can be a serious problem in carrying out PCR. A set of micropipettors should be devoted exclusively to preparation of the reaction mixtures at a designated PCR clean workstation set apart from the rest of the laboratory. PCR products should be handled with a separate set of micropipettors at a different area in the laboratory, and added after the reaction mixtures have been set up at the clean workstation.

6. In terms of *KRas* PCR, even after the first digestion, there is still undigested wild-type DNA that will be amplified in the second PCR reaction. The second digestion is necessary to discriminate between the mutant and undigested wild-type DNA.

7. At least one β-tubulin exon 4 PCR primer should be designed in an intronic region to prevent the potential amplification of spliced pseudogenes.

8. *Taq* DNA polymerase can make errors during PCR amplification. When PCR products are to be sequenced, a higher fidelity enzyme such as *Pfu* should be used instead of *Taq*.

References

1. Steinman, C. R. (1975) Free DNA in serum and plasma from normal adults. *J. Clin. Invest.* **56,** 512–515.
2. Raptis, L. and Menard, H. A. (1980) Quantiation and characterization of plasma DNA in normals and patients with systemic lupus erythematosus. *J. Clin. Invest.* **66,** 1391–1399.

3. Stroun, M., Anker, P., Maurice, P., Lyautey, J., Lederrey, C., and Beljanski, M. (1989) Neoplastic characteristics of the DNA found in the plasma of cancer patients. *Oncology* **46**, 318–322.

4. Shapiro B., Chakrabaty M., Cohn, E., and Leon, S. A. (1983) Determination of circulating DNA levels in patients with benign or malignant gastrointestinal diseases. *Cancer* **51**, 2116–2120.

5. Anker, P., Lefort, F., Vasioukhin, V., et al. (1997) K-ras mutations are found in DNA extracted from the plasma of patients with colorectal cancer. *Gastroenterology* **112**, 1114–1120.

6. Lauschke, H., Caspari, R., Friedl, W., et al. (2001) Detection of APC and K-ras mutations in the serum of patients with colorectal cancer. *Cancer Detect. Prev.* **25**, 55–61.

7. Sozzi, G., Musso, K., Ratcliffe, C., Goldstraw, P., Pierotti, M. A., and Pastorino, U. (1999) Detection of microsatellite alterations in plasma DNA of non-small cell lung cancer patients: a prospect for early diagnosis. *Clin. Cancer Res.* **5**, 2689–2692.

8. Kornacker, M., Jox, A., Vockerodt, M., et al. (1999) Detection of a Hodgkin/Reed-Sternberg cell specific immunoglobulin gene rearrangement in the serum DNA of a patient with Hodgkin's disease. *B. J. Haematol.* **106**, 528–531.

9. Esteller, M., Sanchez-Cespedes, M., Rosell, R., Sidransky, D., Baylin, S. B., and Herman, J. G. (1999) Detection of aberrant promoter hypermethylation of tumor suppressor genes in serum DNA from non-small cell lung cancer. *Cancer Res.* **59**, 67–70.

10. Ivy H. N., Wong, Y. M., Lo, D., et al. (1999) Detection of aberrant *p16* methylation in the plasma and serum of liver cancer patients. *Cancer Res.* **59**, 71–73.

11. Levi, S., Urbano-Ispizua, A., Gill, R., et al. (1991) Multiple K-ras codon 12 mutations in cholangiocarcinomas demonstrated with a sensitive polymerase chain reaction technique. *Cancer Res.* **51**, 3497–3502.

12. Monzó M., Rosell, R., Sánchez, J. J., et al. (1999) Paclitaxel resistance in non-small-cell lung cancer associated with β-tubulin gene mutations. *J. Clin. Oncol.* **17**, 1786–1793.

13. Rodenhuis, S., Boerrigter, L., Top, B., et al. (1997) Mutational activation of the K-ras oncogene and the effect of chemotherapy in advanced adenocarcinoma of the lung: a prospective study. *J. Clin. Oncol.* **15**, 285–291.

14. Shi, X. B., Gumerlock, P. H., Wellman, A. A., et al. (1993) Rapid PCR construction of a gene containing Lym-1 antibody variable regions. *PCR Methods Applications* **3**, 46–53.

IX

Cell Lifespan/Longevity

22

The Use of Early Sea Urchin Embryos in Anticancer Drug Testing

David Nishioka, Vanessa Marcell, Meghan Cunningham, Merium Khan, Daniel D. Von Hoff, and Elzbieta Izbicka

1. Introduction

In vitro anticancer drug testing is routinely performed on cell lines established from various types of malignant tumors. The use of these cell models has proved effective in determining the worthiness of potential drugs for further testing at the clinical level. They provide a system in which a potential drug may be added to a living culture of tumor cells and the drug's effects on cell proliferation and/or more specific mitotic events may be determined. However, in order for the effectiveness of a drug to be determined, it must be tested in some instances over many cell generations. It is particularly important for telomerase- and telomere-interactive drugs whose effects on telomere shortening may become apparent only after many cell cycles. This need for accurate testing carries with it certain operational problems, all related to the fact that cell generation times may be prolonged up to 24 h in some tumor cell lines: (1) the cell culture medium becomes depleted of nutrients over several cell cycles and must be replaced regularly; (2) the drug must also be replaced when the culture medium is replaced; (3) the drug may degrade over prolonged periods in culture and may need to be replaced more often than medium changes; (4) the elevated temperature (37°C) may accelerate drug breakdown; (5) the time and expense of maintaining the cells and drugs over a sufficient number of cell cycles for reliable drug testing is considerable; and (6) there are no convenient internal markers for cell viability separate from the cell proliferation and chromosomal effects that are already being determined. In this

From: *Methods in Molecular Medicine, vol. 85: Novel Anticancer Drug Protocols*
Edited by: J. K. Buolamwini and A. A. Adjei © Humana Press Inc., Totowa, NJ

chapter, we describe the use of fertilized sea urchin eggs as a novel cell system for anticancer drug testing in which the above problems are addressed.

Sea urchins have long provided a model system for studying fertilization and early embryonic development (reviewed in **refs. *1–5***). Mature specimens are induced to shed eggs and sperm readily and abundantly upon injection of isosmotic KCl into their coelomic cavities, and fertilization is easily achieved by suspending the two gametes together in sea water. Within a minute after insemination, the extracellular vitelline layer of the fertilized egg elevates and hardens to form the fertilization envelope within which the embryo undergoes cell division every 60 min to the blastula stage. In *Lytechinus pictus*, at a refrigerated temperature of 18°C, the blastula stage is reached within 15 h, at which time the embryo secretes a proteolytic hatching enzyme that dissolves the fertilization envelope and allows the embryo to emerge as a spherical, ciliated, free-swimming blastula. Composed of a single layer of cells that surrounds a spherical inner blastocoelic cavity, this relatively undifferentiated embryo soon enters the first stage of gastrulation in which cells at the vegetal pole undergo side-by-side columnar elongations to form the vegetal plate. Specific cells within the vegetal plate, the primary mesenchyme cells (PMCs), soon become pulsatile and lose contact with adjacent cells before invading the blastocoelic cavity at the vegetal pole. After PMC ingression, the remaining vegetal plate invaginates to form the early archenteron (primitive gut). Cellular proliferation and rearrangements within the archenteron result in the extension and elongation of this narrowing tube, the tip of which eventually fuses with cells lining the animal hemisphere of the blastocoelic cavity to form the mouth. Meanwhile, the PMCs localize at the base of the elongating archenteron before undergoing fusions into long, cable-like syncitia that synthesize and secrete the larval skeleton, the main spicules of which support the oral arms of the pluteus larva. Development through the blastula and gastrula stages to the pluteus larva stage is easily achieved under laboratory conditions in less than 72 h. Thus, early sea urchin embryogeny consists of very rapid cell divisions to the blastula stage, followed by a slowing of the cell cycle and differentiation into a swimming larval form with well developed digestive and skeletal systems.

In this chapter, we show that anticancer drugs may be tested over 10 cell cycles in less than 24 h in early developing sea urchin embryos. Therefore, their antiproliferative effects can be observed without replacement of the medium or drug, and the drug is tested at the reduced temperature of 18°C. Additionally, the many developmental markers described above, such as the production of a hatching enzyme and hatching, the production of cilia and swimming, the invagination of vegetal plate cells and gastrulation, and the migration of PMCs and larval spicule formation can all be used as easily observable, collateral viability markers.

Living sea urchin embryos, owing to their large size, are easily observed under the light microscope. Fixed embryos too, at both the light and electron microscopic levels, have long been used to correlate embryonic stages with particular cellular and/or molecular changes. Although the qualitative changes in morphology are easily recognized in living and fixed embryos, the quantitative changes in cell number have been more difficult to determine because the embryos are three dimensional and may consist of several layers of cells, especially in the post-blastula stages of development. Reported here is a procedure that facilitates this quantification by placing all of the nuclei and chromosomes of the embryo in the same focal plane. After specifically staining the nuclei and chromosomes with the DNA-specific Feulgen reaction, the embryos are mounted on a microscope slide and squashed under a cover glass. The slides are then thoroughly frozen on a bed of dry ice before the cover glasses are popped off and the slides with adherent embryos are dipped into ethanol. After air-drying, the dehydrated embryos are mounted permanently under a cover glass with one drop of Permount mountant. At ×400 magnification, all of the nuclei and chromosomes, stained a deep magenta color, are observed in one focal plane and are easily counted through the gastrula stage of development. Focus in one plane is compromised at higher magnifications and is lost at the pluteus larva stage, when thick oral arms supported by a well-developed skeletal system have developed. Nevertheless, prior to the pluteus larva stage and at low to middle magnifications, the nuclei in each embryo are quantifiable. Additionally, the nuclei and chromosomes are readily observable through a fluorescence microscope equipped for green excitation and red fluorescence, and the slides may be stored indefinitely at room temperature. Therefore, the nuclei may be quantified and the chromosomes may be observed at any time after preparation of the slides.

2. Materials

1. *Lytechinus pictus* sea urchins purchased from Marinus, Inc. (Long Beach, CA).
2. Refrigerated aquaria containing Instant Ocean synthetic sea water at 15°C.
3. 0.55 M KCl solution.
4. Syracuse dishes.
5. 10-mL beakers.
6. Artificial sea water: 423.0 mM NaCl, 9.0 mM KCl, 9.27 mM CaCl$_2$, 22.94 mM MgCl$_2$, 25.5 mM MgSO$_4$, 0.18 mM NaHCO$_3$ *(4)*.
7. Ethanol: acetic acid, 3:1 (Carnoy's fixative, made fresh).
8. Ethanol:acetic acid, 1:1 (made fresh).
9. 45% acetic acid solution.
10. 1.0 M HCl solution.
11. Schiff's reagent: Dissolve 1 g basic fuchsin (Difco) in 180 mL boiling water, cooling to 50°C, and add successively, 20 mL 1 M HCl and 2 g potassium metabisulfite. After swirling for 2 min, the solution is allowed to sit at room

temperature in the dark for 24 h. The resulting straw-colored solution is decolorized by adding 1 g activated charcoal and shaking for 1–2 min. After filtering through paper, the colorless solution is stored in a dark bottle at 4°C.

12. Microscope slides.
13. Cover glasses, 22 × 22 mm.
14. Dry ice.
15. Razor blade.
16. Forceps.
17. Coplin microscope slide jars.
18. 95% ethanol.
19. Absolute ethanol.
20. Permount histological mounting medium (Fisher).

3. Methods

3.1. Embryo Cultures

Lytechinus pictus sea urchins were purchased from Marinus, Inc. (Long Beach, CA) and maintained at 15°C in refrigerated aquaria containing Instant Ocean synthetic sea water. Spawning was induced by intracoelomic injection of 0.55 M KCl. Semen was shed directly into Syracuse dishes and maintained undiluted at 4°C until use. Eggs were shed into beakers containing artificial sea water (ASW) prepared according to the Woods Hole formula of Harvey *(4)*, dejellied by agitation, and allowed to settle through three changes of ASW. For monospermic fertilization, 0.01 vol freshly prepared stock sperm suspension (1 drop undiluted semen in 5 mL ASW) was added to a 1% egg suspension stirred at 60 rpm with motor-driven Teflon paddles. Ten minutes after insemination, the fertilized eggs were allowed to settle, and the supernatant ASW containing sperm was aspirated and replaced with fresh ASW. The embryos were cultured at 18°C with agitation.

3.2. Feulgen Staining of Nuclei and Chromosomes

At measured times after insemination, 5 mL aliquots of the 1% embryo cultures were centrifuged and the supernatants were aspirated. The pelleted embryos were resuspended in 5 mL Carnoy's fixative (ethanol:acetic acid, 3:1) for at least 1 h. After fixation, the embryos were pelleted and resuspended successively in (1) 5 mL ethanol:acetic acid, 1:1, for 5–15 min, (2) 5 mL 45% acetic acid for 5–15 min, (3) 5 mL room temperature 1 N HCl for 1–2 min, (4) 5 mL 60°C 1 N HCl for 7–8 min, (5) 5 mL room temperature 1 N HCl for 1–2 min, (6) 0.5 mL Schiff's reagent for 90–120 min, and (7) 5 mL 45% acetic acid for at least 5 min. Samples of these embryos were placed on microscope slides, covered with cover glasses, and frozen on a bed of dry ice. After at least 30 min, the cover glasses were popped off using a razor blade, and the slides were immediately plunged into Coplin jars containing 95% ethanol for 5 min. The slides were then transferred to Coplin jars containing 100% ethanol for 5 min. After removing the slides and allowing them to air dry, the embryos were mounted with one drop of Permount (Fisher) under a cover glass.

3.3. Photomicrography

The embryos were observed and photographed with an Olympus BH-2 photomicroscope. For bright field black-and-white photos, a dark green filter was used to increase the contrast of negatives produced on Kodak Plus-X film.

3.4. Quantification of Nuclei

At each time point, 10–12 photomicrographs of randomly chosen embryos were sufficiently enlarged to facilitate nuclear counting. Each photomicrograph was scored under a transparent plastic sheet on which counted nuclei were marked. Nuclear counts were recorded with a hand-held counter.

4. Notes

1. The Feulgen reaction involves a mild acid hydrolysis of DNA that selectively removes purine bases and renders the exposed deoxyribose sugars (Schiff's bases) reactive with Schiff's reagent. Therefore, the most crucial step in the staining procedure is the timing of the hydrolysis in 1 N HCl at 60°C. In our experience, eight minutes produces the most vivid and nuclear-specific staining. The degree of squashing can be monitored microscopically and controlled by increasing or decreasing the volume of stained embryos placed on the slide before adding a coverslip and freezing on dry ice. Increased squashing can also be achieved by blotting excess 45% acetic acid from under the coverslip before freezing. To minimize fading, the final dehydrations should not exceed 5 min each in 95% and 100% ethanol.

2. **Figure 1** provides representative photomicrographs of Feulgen-stained sea urchin embryos through the pluteus stage (72 h) of development. As seen in these embryos, with the exception of the pluteus stage embryo, the nuclei remain separate from one another and within the same optical plane. This focus on all nuclei in one plane is dependent on the degree of squashing and the total magnification. In our experience, it is easily achieved up to ×400 but is compromised at ×1000. **Figure 1C** shows that Feulgen nuclear staining may also be viewed through a fluorescence microscope equipped with green excitation and red emission (rhodamine) filters; however, unlike nuclei stained with other fluorescent dyes, Feulgen-stained nuclei do not photobleach even after prolonged

exposures to incident light. Additionally, since the slides bearing these embryos are permanently mounted, they may be stored indefinitely at room temperature. At 4 h after fertilization (*see* **Figs. 1a–1c**) most of the embryos are at the 8- to 16-cell stage. Since cleavages are synchronous at this early stage, condensed mitotic chromosomes lined up on the metaphase plate are often observed (*see* **Fig. 1a**). Interphase nuclei at these early stages are larger and more diffuse than later stage nuclei, rendering them more difficult to observe with bright field light optics (*see* **Fig. 1b**). In this situation, the nuclei may be observed more easily with a fluorescence microscope equipped for rhodamine detection (*see* **Fig. 1c**). By 8 h post-fertilization (*see* **Fig. 1d**), the embryos consist of approx 200 cells. At 12 h (*see* **Fig. 1e**) and 16 h (*see* **Fig. 1f**), cleavages are no longer synchronous, so mitotic chromosomes may be observed among interphase nuclei. At 20 h (*see* **Fig. 1g**), the living blastula embryo consists of a single layer of cells surrounding a large spherical cavity, the blastocoel. Our squash preparations of these embryos are observed as circular arrays of quite evenly distributed nuclei and mitotic chromosomes with the three-dimensional depth imposed by the blastocoel effectively eliminated. By 24 h (*see* **Fig. 1h**), the primary mesenchyme cells have invaded the blastocoel at the vegetal pole and their nuclei are locally concentrated in an evenly distributed circular array of other nuclei. The archenteron (A), which has begun its invagination by 32 h (*see* **Fig. 1i**) and has lengthened by 40 h (*see* **Fig. 1j**), is seen as an elongating concentration of nuclei in squashed embryos. At 48 h (*see* **Fig. 1k**), when the archenteron has invaginated fully and its tip has fused with the cells at the opposite wall of the blastocoel to form the larval mouth, it is observed as a band of concentrated nuclei that crosses the circular array of nuclei. By 72 h (*see* **Fig. 1l**) the pluteus larva has developed prominent oral arms (OAs) supported by larval spicules. With the increased cell number and three-dimensional structure imposed by the development of the oral apparatus, squash preparations reveal highly localized concentrations of nuclei in this region of the embryo.

3. Since, within magnification limits (×400), all of the nuclei in our preparations are in the same focal plane, and since the spatial distributions of nuclei are sufficient to resolve individual nuclei (*see* **Fig. 1**), obtaining reliable nuclear counts was possible. Although resolution of individual nuclei lessens as the archenteron invaginates to produce several layers of cells in our squash preparations, the nuclei are still quantifiable in 48-h embryos with fully invaginated archenterons. Resolution of individual nuclei is compromised only after the oral arms have developed (*see* **Fig. 1l**). Nuclear counts in embryos up to the 48-h gastrula stage are shown on a logarithmic scale in **Figure 2**. The results are consistent with nuclear replications and cell divisions that occur approximately every hour for the first 8–10 h after fertilization. The number of nuclei increases exponentially to 592 ±110 in 12-h embryos, after which the rate of nuclear doublings decreases significantly, so that by 24 h after fertilization the number of embryonic nuclei is 1080 ± 57.7. By 48 h after fertilization, the number of nuclei increases to 1512 ± 82.5.

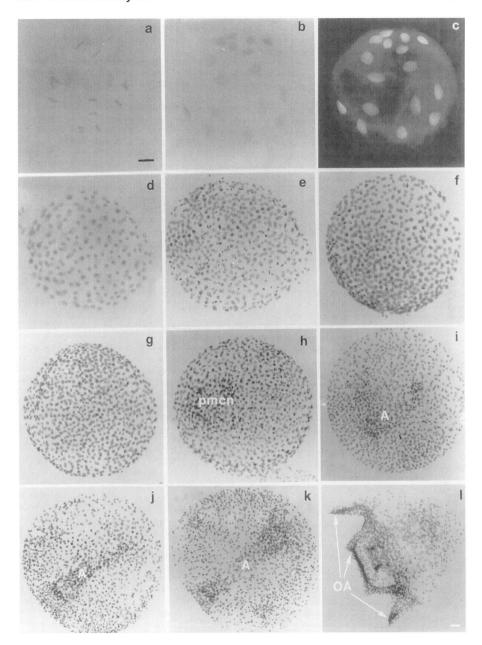

Fig. 1. Whole mount squash preparations of Feulgen-stained sea urchin embryos at varying times after fertilization: (a) 4 h; (b) 4 h; (c) same 4-h embryo as in "b" viewed with fluorescence optics; (d) 8 h; (e) 12 h; (f) 16 h; (g) 20 h; (h) 24 h; (i) 32 h; (j) 40 h; (k) 48 h; (l) 72 h. pmcn = primary mesenchyme cell nuclei; A = Archenteron; OA = Oral Apparatus. Black Bar = 20 μm, Plates a–k; White Bar = 20 μm, Plate 1.

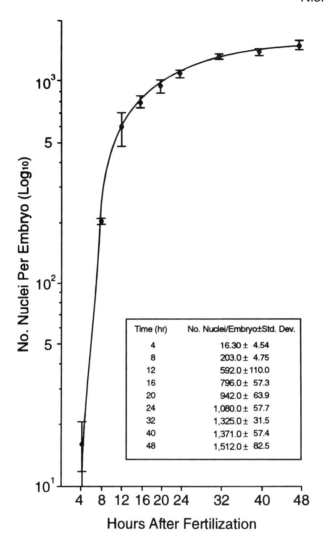

Fig. 2. Number of nuclei in *Lytechinus pictus* embryos cultured at 18°C through the late gastrula stage of development (48 h). Note that the number of nuclei are plotted on a logarithmic scale. The means ± Std. Dev. are also provided in tabular form (inset).

4. Rapid development to the blastula stage in sea urchin embryos is a capability that appears to be pre-programmed in the sea urchin egg during oogenesis. For example, it is known that to accommodate the rapid assembly of microtubules needed for the many mitotic spindles that form during early cleavage, large pools of unassembled tubulin are accumulated and stored in the egg during oogenesis. It is also known that development to the blastula stage can proceed normally

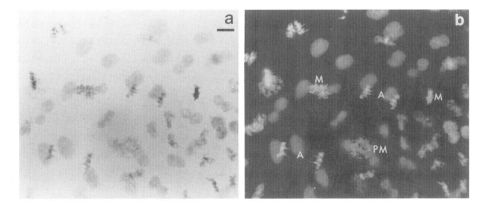

Fig. 3. High-magnification (x1000) photomicrographs of a Feulgen-stained 8-h sea urchin embryo. The same view of a whole mount squash preparation was photographed with (a) light and (b) fluorescence optics. PM = prometaphase chromosomes; M = metaphase chromosomes; A = anaphase chromosomes. Bar = 10 μm.

in the absence of RNA synthesis *(6,7)* confirming that a maternally-supplied pool of messenger RNA directs the increased protein synthesis that begins 5–10 min after fertilization *(8)*.

5. Photomicrographs of 8-h embryos taken at x1000 magnification are shown in **Figure 3**. At this magnification, the depth of field is exceeded so that only selected nuclei and mitotic chromosomes are in focus. Nevertheless, as observed with both light (*see* **Fig. 3a**) and fluorescence (*see* **Fig. 3b**) optics, mitotic chromosomes in all stages of mitosis are resolvable at this higher magnification. DNA-specific fluorescent dyes, such as DAPI and Hoechst, are also quite effective in selectively staining nuclei and chromosomes. However, these dyes photobleach quite rapidly and are usually applied to wet mounted embryos, in which far fewer chromosomes and nuclei appear in the same focal plane. Additionally, the slides may be viewed only once with an oil immersion objective lens. Although not all of the nuclei and chromosomes are in the same focal plane in our Feulgen-stained embryos, a high percentage are, and, since the embryos are permanently stained and mounted, the slides may be reviewed multiple times with an oil immersion lens, and without photobleaching.

6. As a first use of these techniques we determined the effects of 3′-azido-3′-deoxythymidine (AZT) on early sea urchin embryos. **Figure 4** compares representative control embryos with AZT-treated embryos at 10 h after fertilization. The video pictures of living embryos show a control embryo that has reached the blastula stage but has not yet hatched (*see* **Fig. 4a**). At this stage, the embryo composed of approximately 300 cells is ciliated and begins to rotate (swim) within the enveloping fertilization coat. In comparison, the AZT-treated embryo is composed of approximately 50 cells and lacks a definitive blastocoel (*see* **Fig. 4b**), but becomes ciliated and weakly motile within a fertilization

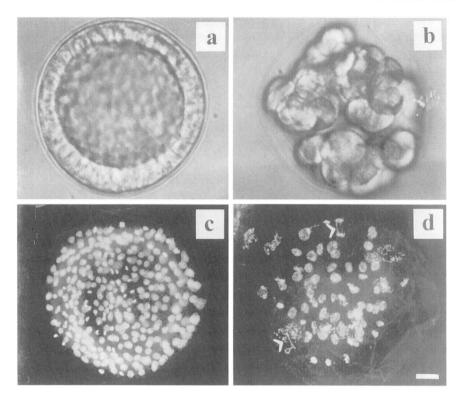

Fig. 4. Sea urchin embryos 10 h after fertilization. Video photomicrographs of (a) control embryos and (b) embryos cultured in the presence of 10 μM AZT. Fluorescence photomicrographs of (c) control embryos and (d) embryos cultured in the presence of 10 μM AZT. Arrowheads point to end-to-end chromosome fusions. Bar = 20 μm.

coat. Both control and AZT-treated embryos soon produce hatching enzyme and emerge as free swimming embryos, albeit with reduced motility in the AZT-treated embryos. Thus, although cell proliferation is apparently inhibited by AZT, the developmental markers of ciliogenesis and the production of hatching enzyme proceed on schedule, indicating that the inhibitory effects of AZT are more specific than those of a general toxin.

7. Corresponding Feulgen-stained embryos viewed with fluorescence optics are shown in **Figures 4c** and **4d**. The control embryo shows the normal number of nuclei for this stage of development (*see* **Fig. 4c**). The AZT-treated embryo on the other hand shows a reduced number of nuclei (*see* **Fig. 4d**) concomitant with the reduced number of cells observed in living embryos (*see* **Fig. 4b**). Additionally, the nuclei are more diffuse in AZT-treated embryos and the chromosomes show various abnormalities in comparison to control embryos. Most notably and

most consistently are end-to-end chromosome adhesions that persist well into anaphase and telophase of mitosis.

8. Recently, the techniques reported in this paper were used to determine the effects of telomere- and telomerase-interactive agents on early sea urchin embryos *(9)*. In addition to AZT, a telomerase inhibitor that can stack within the telomeric G-quadruplex and an antisense oligonucleotide to the telomerase RNA template were also shown to exert antiproliferative effects. On the other hand, an isomer of the G-quadruplex interactive agent, which cannot achieve planarity and which does not inhibit telomerase, as well as a control scrambled oligonucleotide showed no effects on cellular proliferation in sea urchin embryos. By viewing the treated embryos at high magnification, we have demonstrated that only the antiproliferative agents cause the abnormal end-to-end adherence of chromosomes during mitosis. Similar abnormalities have been observed in cells of a *Tetrahymena* strain containing a mutated telomerase RNA template *(10)* and in human cells containing a dominant negative allele of the human telomeric protein, TRF2 *(11)*.

9. Our results demonstrate several advantages of the sea urchin embryo system over cultured tumor cells for preclinical drug testing with a particular focus on telomerase- and telomere-interactive drugs. In standard tests, low concentrations of potential drugs must be administered to tumor cells over many cell cycles, oftentimes taking over a month to complete *(12)*. Sea urchin embryos, as shown here dividing every hour through the first 8–10 cleavages, allow tests over comparable numbers of cell cycles to be completed in hours. Additionally, well characterized developmental markers may be used to check for toxic effects of potential drugs on vital biological processes collateral to their antiproliferative effects. The results reported here further establish the developing sea urchin embryo as an additional and convenient non-mammalian model that may be used to evaluate the antiproliferative and chromosomal effects of potential therapeutic anticancer drugs.

Acknowledgments

This work was supported by a National Drug Discovery Grant (No. CA67760) from the National Cancer Institute, National Institutes of Health.

References

1. Czihak, C. (1975) *The Sea Urchin Embryo Biochemistry and Morphogenesis.* Springer, Berlin, Heidelberg, New York.
2. Giudice, G. (1973) *Developmental Biology of the Sea Urchin Embryo.* Academic Press, New York, London.
3. Giudice, G. (1986) *The Sea Urchin Embryo.* Springer, Berlin, Heidelberg, New York.
4. Harvey, E. B. (1956) *The American Arbacia and Other Sea Urchins.* Princeton University Press, Princeton, NJ.

5. Horstadius, S. (1973) *Experimental Embryology of Echinoderms.* Clarendon Press, Oxford, UK.
6. Gross, P. R. and Cousineau, G. H. (1964) Macromolecular synthesis and the influence of actinomycin D on early development. *Exp. Cell Res.* **33,** 368–395.
7. Vafa, O. and Nishioka, D. (1995) Developmentally regulated protease expression during sea urchin embryogenesis. *Mol. Reprod. Dev.* **40,** 36–47.
8. Epel, D. (1967) Protein synthesis in sea urchin eggs: A "late" response to fertilization. *Proc. Natl. Acad. Sci. USA* **57,** 899–906.
9. Izbicka, E., Nishioka, D., Marcell, V., et al. (1999) Telomere-interactive agents affect proliferation rates and induce chromosomal destabilization in the sea urchin embryo. *Anti-Cancer Drug Design* **14,** 355–365.
10. Kirk, K., Harmon, B., Reichardt, I., Sedat, J., and Blackburn, E. (1997) Block in anaphase chromosome separation caused by telomerase template mutation. *Science* **275,** 1478–1481.
11. van Steensel, B., Smorgorzewska, A., and de Lange, T. (1998) TRF2 protects human telomeres from end-to-end fusions. *Cell* **92,** 401–413.
12. Sharma, S., Raymond, E., Soda, H., et al. (1997) Preclinical and clinical strategies for development of telomerase and telomere inhibitors. *Ann. Oncol.* **8,** 1063–1074.

X

IN VIVO IMAGING

23

PET Screening of Anticancer Drugs

A Faster Route to Drug/Target Evaluations In Vivo

Anna Fredriksson and Sharon Stone-Elander

1. Introduction

Drug development engages many disciplines in the complex processes of designing, synthesizing, isolating, and subsequently testing the bioactivity of large new chemical libraries. The few candidates identified in the initial screening as the most promising potential drugs are selected and subjected to further testing in appropriate model systems. In vitro testing, as well as ex vivo and in vivo studies in animals are usually required before the best can proceed to clinical trials in humans. Only a small fraction of the compounds arising from lead compound optimizations are ever introduced as drugs.

Information about a compound's uptake, distribution and regional residence time is important, since these parameters are crucial for a drug's ability to exert its intended action in the designated target for the desired duration. One way to obtain such information is via ex vivo studies, i.e., to administer the (^{3}H- or ^{14}C-labeled) compound to animals, sacrifice them at different times, and thereafter analyze the regional distribution of the substance. Aside from cost and time considerations, a major drawback for this approach is the necessity of using a large number of animals at each time and at many different times for an accurate assessment of the dynamics of the compound's distribution. The fact that transport, receptor, excretion, and metabolic systems in humans do not necessarily function in the same way as those in animals can further confound the utilization of these results in the decision chain. Since even drug candidates that have shown promise in animal screening may be ineffectual in humans, information about the in vivo behavior of candidate drugs should preferably

From: *Methods in Molecular Medicine, vol. 85: Novel Anticancer Drug Protocols*
Edited by: J. K. Buolamwini and A. A. Adjei © Humana Press Inc., Totowa, NJ

also be acquired in humans early in the developmental process. Large, time-consuming, and expensive investments in broader preclinical and clinical studies with such false hits might thereby be prevented.

Positron emission tomography (PET) and single photon emission computed tomography (SPECT) are in vivo imaging techniques that track the distribution of radiolabeled substances known as tracers. A single PET study in one animal can provide dynamic information about the regional concentration of the tracer over the whole observation period, information that would otherwise require the sacrifice of a large number of animals and assumptions about the standardization of disease models between individual animals. This chapter will focus on the potential of the PET technique for drug screening, with a description of the method illustrated by work from our group (*1*) on one epidermal growth factor (EGF) receptor tyrosine kinase inhibitor, PD153035, as an example of rapid evaluation in animals. A brief discussion on the benefits and the limitations of the technique is included, as well as references for further reading.

1.1. The PET Technique

PET (*see* **Fig. 1**) is a "molecular" nuclear medicine technique which provides functional rather than morphological information (*see* **refs.** *2,3* for further information). Positron-emitting radionuclides are built into compounds of interest, here the drug candidates to be screened.

The positron emitted in each decay travels a few millimeters before colliding with its antiparticle, the electron. The two particles are annihilated and their combined mass is transformed into energy. The energy is in the form of two gamma photons, each of 511 keV, emitted at an angle of 180° (± 0.25°) from one another. The gamma photons are energetic enough to penetrate tissues and can therefore be externally detected by the PET camera. The simultaneous registration of two photons makes it possible to localize the decaying radionuclide somewhere along a straight line between the two registering detectors. The accumulated data are reconstructed and presented as color-coded maps of the concentration of radioactivity in different body regions. In addition to describing the biodistribution in given organs or regions, information about the kinetics of the uptake is also obtained.

The positron-emitters commonly used in PET are carbon-11, nitrogen-13, oxygen-15, and fluorine-18. Relevant physical data and typical production routes using dedicated medical cyclotrons are briefly presented in **Table 1** (for more cyclotron information *see* for example **ref.** *4*). Particularly, ^{11}C and ^{18}F are used for drug distribution studies, since they have favorable imaging

A **Dedicated medical cyclotrons**

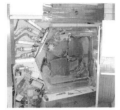

produce $^{11}CO_2$, $^{15}O_2$, $^{13}NO_3^-$, and $^{18}F^-$ on demand (as the MC17 pictured here). The radionuclides are subsequently transported to the hot lab.

B **Hot lab: conversion to radiotracers**
Radiotracers are produced as quickly as possible, with remote control and lead shielding for radiation protection.

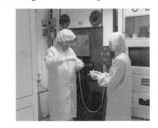

C **The radiotracer is delivered to the animal/patient lying in the scanner.** Different types of scanners may be required to match the particular demands of a given PET application.

(1) Dedicated Animal PET   (2) Human PET   (3) Hybrid PET (Clinical)

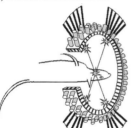

Coincidence Detection

See Note 4 for the different camera's prestanda.

D **PET studies of different processes are performed and analyzed**

The emission data collected are converted into images of tracer distribution, e.g.:

(1, 2) screenings in rat and monkey
(3, 4) cerebral and cardiac metabolism
(5) amino acid uptake
(6) receptor distributions
(7) maps of cerebral functions
(8) whole body studies

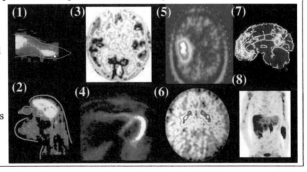

Fig. 1. The PET process step by step from radioisotope production (**A**) to PET images (**D**).

Table 1
**The Commonly Used PET Isotopes With Some Physical Data
and Nuclear Reactions for Their Formation**

Nuclide	Half-life	β^+ Energy	Production methods	Obtained as
^{15}O	2.07 min	1.72 MeV	$^{14}N(d,n)^{15}O$	$^{15}O_2$
^{13}N	9.96 min	1.19 MeV	$^{16}O(p,\alpha)^{13}N$	$^{13}NO_3^-$
^{11}C	20.4 min	0.96 MeV	$^{14}N(p,\alpha)^{11}C$	$^{11}CO_2$, $^{11}CH_4$
^{18}F	109.7 min	0.635 MeV	$^{18}O(p,n)^{18}F$, $^{20}Ne(d,\alpha)^{18}F$	$^{18}F^-$, $^{18}F_2$

Table 2
**Frequently Used ^{11}C and ^{18}F Labeling Precursors and the Different Kinds
of Functional Groups (Products) They, Respectively, Can Be Transformed
Into by Organic Synthesis**

^{11}C-labeling precursor → products	^{18}F-labeling precursors → products
$[^{11}C]R$-I (-OTf) → alkyl amines, alcohols, thiols	$[^{18}F]R$-I (-OTf) → alkyl amines, alcohols, thiols
^{11}CN → amines, amides, aldehydes, acids, esters	$[^{18}F]$Aryl nitriles, aldehydes → amides, amines, esters, acids
$^{11}CO_2$ → acids, aldehydes, alcohols	
^{11}C-acid chlorides → acids, amides, esters	$^{18}F_2$ (double/triple bond additions) → alkyl fluorides
^{11}C-organometallics, -ylides → C-C couplings	$CH_3COO^{18}F$ → aryl and alkyl fluorides

characteristics, longer half-lives, and they can be produced in high specific
radioactivity, which implies that the mass of the administered tracer will be
very small, even for large amounts of radioactivity. The radionuclide chosen for
labeling should be long-lived enough to permit observation of the biochemical
process, but not so long that radioactivity will be residing in the body long after
the investigation has ceased. Suitable labeling strategies determined by the
available arsenal of radiolabeling precursors (*see* **Table 2**) must be designed
and optimized. The short half-lives of the radionuclides are a determining
factor for the labeling strategies that can be used. Since the entire production
sequence should be performed in less than three half-lives of the nuclide, a
good deal of effort is made to specially design labeling precursors and the
unlabeled substrate so that the radiosyntheses can be achieved in as few steps as
possible. Methods for rapidly isolating, analyzing, and verifying the identity of
the radiotracer must also be developed and validated before it can be used in in

vivo experiments in animals or in humans. A specially equipped radiochemistry laboratory with ventilated lead-shielded hoods and remote control systems is required to minimize exposure of laboratory personnel to radiation.

Many different types of PET cameras with varying characteristics are available today (*see* **Fig 1C**). Ideally, the equipment should be chosen so that its prestanda is sufficient for the size of the systems studied and the amounts of radiotracer to be used (resolution and sensitivity, respectively). Appropriately timed protocols for the accumulation of data from the region(s) of interest must be chosen. Careful analyses of the PET images and the dynamic data, is of course crucial for successful evaluations. Compartmental modeling may sometimes be necessary for adequately describing the pharmacokinetics. Challenges of tracer behavior by loading with non-labeled drugs may also be performed in order to more accurately assess the specificity of the uptake and retention mechanisms.

1.2. The Tyrosine Kinase Inhibitor PD 153035

Observations indicating that the numbers of EGF receptors (EGFRs) are increased in many different cancers have provided an impetus for extensive research into developing drugs that target different components of this receptor/signaling system. One particularly persistent approach has focused on finding compounds that inhibit intracellular tyrosine kinase (TK) activity. Inhibition of TK prevents the receptor from phosphorylating and activating different downstream target proteins in the growth signal pathway, and thus interrupts the proliferative process.

The potent TK inhibitor PD 153035 (*see* **Table 3**, **1**), developed by Parke-Davis and first presented in Fry et al. in 1994 *(5)*, inhibits the EGFR TK to 50% (IC_{50}) at a concentration of about 29 pM. Both the selectivity of PD 153035 towards the EGFR TK compared to other TKs and its affinity are very high (inhibition constant $K_i \approx 5.2$ pM). These properties not only make PD 153035 an interesting candidate for this particular chemotherapeutic strategy, but are also excellent characteristics for potential ligands for in vivo imaging studies. By labeling the drug with appropriate radionuclides, studies with trace amounts of the compound could be performed to investigate its distribution in vivo without perturbing the system and, in diseased states, to determine whether the drug actually reaches its target.

2. Materials and Methods
2.1. Radiolabeling PD 153035 and/or Analogs

A number of approaches for radiolabeling PD 153035 or its analogs for tumor imaging have been presented (structures **2–12**, **Table 3**) *(6–15)*. The

Table 3
Molecular Structures of Different Analogs of PD 153035 Labeled
With Positron or Gamma Emitting Radionuclides

Structure no	R'	R''	n	W (2')	X (3')	Y (4')	Z (5')	References
PD 153035, **1**	Me	Me	0	H	Br	H	H	(5)
2	Me	Me	0	H	^{123}I	H	H	(6)
3	Me	Me	0	H	^{125}I	H	H	(6, 15)
[^{11}C]PD 153035, **4**	Me	^{11}C-Me	0	H	Br	H	H	(7)
5	Me	^{18}F-Et	0	H	Br	H	H	(7)
[^{11}C]PD 153035, **6**	R' or R'' = ^{11}C-Me, the other = Me		0	H	Br	H	H	(8, 9)
7	Me	Me	1	H	H	^{18}F	H	(10)
8	Me	Me	0	H	^{18}F	H	CF$_3$	(11)
9	Me	Me	0	^{18}F	H	Cl	Cl	(11)
10	Et	Et	1	H	H	^{18}F	H	(12)
11	Me	Me	0	H	Cl	^{18}F	H	(13, 14)
12	Et	Et	0	H	^{125}I	H	H	(15)

hypothesis has been that the reported increases in EGFRs would result in a higher uptake of radioactivity in tumors than in non-tumor tissue, i.e., a relatively high tumor to non-tumor (T/NT) ratio. If that is the case, radiolabeled PD 153035 and analogs could be clinically useful for detecting tumors and for quantifying EGFRs as a means of either predicting prognosis for therapy response or to follow tumor response to therapy, e.g., regression or progression.

The majority of labeling strategies presented so far have been directed toward the N-aryl group in PD 153035. Fluorine-18 has been introduced in different positions in either a substituted or unsubstituted phenyl ring (**7–11**). In some analogs, the bromine in PD 153035 was replaced by iodine-123 or -125 for planned in vivo (**2**) or in vitro applications (**3** and **12**), respectively. All the other labelings have been directed toward the alkoxy positions (**4–6**). The ^{18}F-labeled **5** is a fluoroethoxy analog whereas the ^{11}C-labeled **4** and **6** are structurally identical to the original PD 153035.

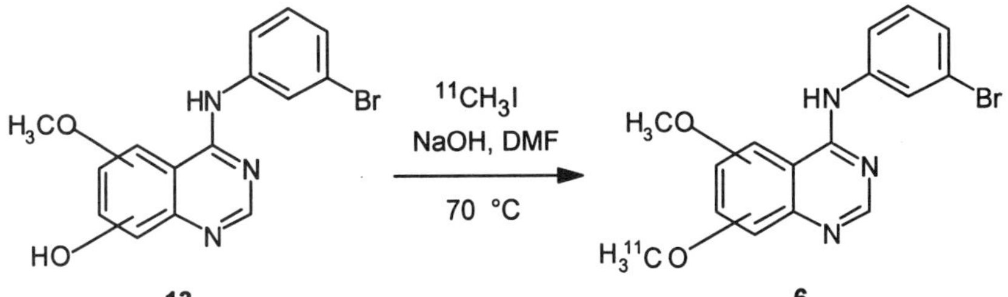

Fig. 2. Production of [^{11}C]PD 153035, **6**, by reaction of desmethyl PD 153035, **13**, with [^{11}C]CH$_3$I under alkaline conditions in dimethyl formamide (DMF).

The aryl ^{18}F-labeling strategies circumvented the problem of performing difficult new precursor syntheses that are multi-step radiosyntheses requiring the optimization of several consecutive transformations and isolations. Fluorine-18 has been introduced by aromatic nucleophilic substitution (fluorine for NO$_2$– or (CH$_3$)$_3$N$^+$– substitution in the case of **8**, **9** and of **7**, **10**, **11** respectively) on an activated benzaldehyde (for **7**), nitrobenzene (for subsequent reduction to the aniline) (for **8**, **9**, **11**), or benzonitrile (for reduction to the benzylamine) (for **10**). The corresponding ^{18}F-labeled aromatics were isolated and coupled to the 4-amino- (for **7**) or 4-chloro- (for **8–11**) 6,7-dialkoxyquinazoline to give the products (**7–11**). Incorporations of radioiodine on the phenyl rings were performed in a single radiochemical step by iododestannylation of the appropriate 4-(3′-trialkylstannylanilino)-6,7-dialkoxyquinazoline, giving compounds **2**, **3**, and **12**.

The other labeling strategies involving *O*-alkylation under basic conditions should, in principle, be simpler. However, our experience is that the monomethoxy precursor (**13**) is difficult to synthesize *(9)* and this has so far been a limiting factor. With carbon-11, the reaction steps must be as few and as fast as possible owing to the nuclide's 20 min half-life. In our strategy *(9)*, we first synthesized PD 153035, then cleaved one of the methoxy groups to obtain **13**. Via this route, the precursor obtained could be realkylated with one of the most commonly used labeling precursors, [^{11}C]iodomethane ([^{11}C]CH$_3$I). The radiosynthesis could thus be performed using standard, semi- or totally automated systems and, apart from its radioactive decay, the product, [^{11}C]PD 153035 (**6**), is identical to the authentic drug.

Briefly, **6** was synthesized by reacting [^{11}C]CH$_3$I with a large excess of **13** (0.9 mg, 2.6 μmol) for 7 min at 70°C *(see* **Fig. 2**). The product was separated from unreacted **13** and other reagents by semi-preparative reversed-phase high-performance liquid chromatography (HPLC), and the collected fraction containing **6** was evaporated to dryness. The residue was reconstituted in phosphate-buffered saline (PBS) and the solution sterile-filtered. The identity and the radiochemical purity of **6** were confirmed by analytical HPLC with UV- and radiodetection.

2.2. Imaging Procedure

In vivo studies of [^{11}C]PD 153035 were performed in rats using PET *(16)*. The biodistribution was assessed in one healthy rat, and the uptake of radioactivity in proliferating tissue was followed in three rats with tumor implants. A human neuroblastoma cell line (SH-SY5Y) was implanted subcutaneously on the lateral side of each hind leg, and the xenografts formed were used as tumor models. For the PET studies, the rats were anesthetized and placed (one at a time) on their backs in the PET camera so that the tip of their tail was out of the camera's field-of-view. Following the injection of **6** (15-23 MBq/kg rat, in 0.2 mL PBS), the photons produced in the decay process were registered by the PET camera for 65–80 min for each rat. Data collection intervals after iv radiotracer injection were initially very short (0.5–1 min during the first 5 min), but were progressively extended to longer samplings and were up to 10 min by the end of the study. Blood was also sampled at different times from the healthy rat so that plasma radioactivity could be measured.

2.3. Data Treatment

At the end of the experiment, the accumulated data were reconstructed using software provided with the PET camera. Color-coded images were generated which depict the regional distribution and concentration of radioactivity (left part of **Figs. 3** and **4**). All or part of the body studied can be displayed as tomographic slices through sagittal, coronal and/or transaxial planes. The uptake can be viewed from several perspectives, thereby making it easier to distinguish particular organs or region(s) of interest (ROI) from the surrounding tissue(s).

After a visual inspection to identify the different organs, ROIs of appropriate size were outlined directly on the transaxial images portrayed on the computer screen, and the concentration of radioactivity in these regions was calculated for each sampling period throughout the entire investigation. Examples of the kinetic (decay-corrected) data obtained for some of the defined ROIs, over organs and xenografts, are shown in the time-activity curves in **Figure 3** and **4** (right part), respectively.

Since the kinetic behavior of a compound can be described by the number of phases the time-activity curve contains, we used a curve-fitting program to find the smallest number of parameters needed to describe the curves appropriately. The number of phases corresponds to the number of exponential terms in the function describing the curve.

Coronal   Sagittal

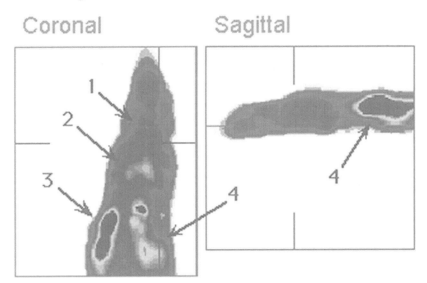

Fig. 3. Distribution of radioactivity after i.v. administration of [^{11}C]PD 153035 in a healthy rat (*see* **Acknowledgment**). **(Left)** Images are sums of data collected from 0–60 min and show the relative concentrations of radioactivity. Rat is on its back with head to the top of the coronal view and to the left in the sagittal view. The markers indicate the orientation of the planes with respect to each other. The lower body was out of the field-of-view. Arrows point out the uptake in (1) brain, (2) heart, (3) liver and (4) gastrointestinal tract. **(Right)** Time-activity curves calculated for organ ROIs delineated in different transaxial tomographic planes of the images from the healthy rat.

The pattern of radioactivity over time for the heart and the brain were similar in the healthy rat. The amounts of radioactivity were highest in the first sampling period. After the initial ca. 5 min, the time-activity curves are biphasic and in the second phase they have the same half-life (χ 13 min). In the liver, the peak radioactivity was reached after around 5 min and thereafter decreased in a monophasic manner (also with $t_{1/2}$ χ 13 min). The curve for the intestines is not as smooth as for the other organs. This is probably owing to difficulties in excluding other tissues and blood vessels when delineating ROIs for the intestines (in small animals). Distribution of radioactivity to (peak value later than 15 min) and extraction from (after peak $t_{1/2}$ $\approx$ 20 min) that region was slower than for the other regions examined.

The right part of **Figure 4** shows time-activity curves for ROIs placed over the left and right side tumors in one rat. On each side, two ROIs were placed in successive tomographic planes. The radioactivity uptake was higher in the right side tumor that also was larger (>2 mL) than the left side tumor (<0.5 mL).

Coronal   Transaxial

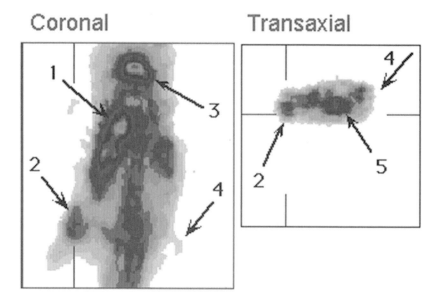

Fig. 4. Distribution of radioactivity after i.v. administration of $[^{11}C]PD$ 153035 in tumor-bearing rats (*see* **Acknowledgment**). (**Left**) Images are sums of data collected from 0–13 min. Rat is on its back with its head out of the field-of-view to the top of the coronal view. In the transaxial view, in which the rat's back is downwards, the green markers indicate the level of the coronal plane, i.e., the coronal view is a rather dorsal plane. The arrows point out the uptake in (1) liver, (2) tumor (left side), (3) heart, (4) tumor (right side) and (5) urinary bladder. Implant (4) was smaller, consisted of several small tumors, and the uptake was consequently barely discernable. (**Right**) Time-radioactivity curves calculated for tumor implant ROIs delineated in two successive transaxial tomographic planes on the right (Δ and ●) and on the left (× and +) sides. These data were obtained from another of the tumor bearing rats with implants that, on each side, had resulted in single tumors.

The washout of radioactivity from the left side was monophasic while it was biphasic from the right side. The half-life for the left side and the right side's second phase were of the same order of magnitude (χ 40–45 min).

3. Discussion

A major goal of the drug development process is to identify substances that exert their actions best at the site of disease and least with other, non-diseased tissues. After first finding out which drug(s) can induce the desired effect in the identified targets, optimizing therapy requires determining the most favorable balance between the amounts that must be administered and the amounts that are delivered to the site of disease. This is particularly important for anti-cancer drugs since low therapeutic indices may have serious consequences for the possibility of succeeding with treatment and minimizing toxic side-effects *(17)*. PET is one of the most sensitive methods available for directly assessing the pharmacokinetic characteristics of experimental compounds, if they can be properly labeled with a positron-emitting radionuclide *(18–20)*. Comparisons of the in vivo behavior of families of compounds arising from lead optimizations may shorten the preclinical validation period and help identify the most optimal drug more rapidly.

The example presented above illustrates the first steps in the series of experiments that can be performed with PET to evaluate the in vivo behavior of an experimental drug. In a single experiment in a control rat, information about the time dependencies for the concentrations of radioactivity in all tissues within the field-of-view was revealed. Radioactivity was taken up in organs known to contain EGF receptors, which is the first prerequisite if a desired interaction with the biological target is to be achieved in vivo. Dividing the tissue concentrations by the plasma radioactivity at each time interval can give a relative estimate of the plasma-tissue exchange rates. Peak concentrations and the times to reach them in each organ are easily seen in the time-activity curves.

Extrapolation of the measurements of radiotracer uptake to that of the drug requires additional information about the drug's metabolic stability in vivo. The photons registered by the PET camera do not provide information about whether labeled metabolites are formed and/or co-distributed with the intact drug. Such information is, however, often obtained in the course of the initial screening. The candidate can be labeled with the more long-lived radionuclides carbon-14 or tritium, administered to rodents, and metabolite analyses performed ex vivo after extracting the radioactivity from the tissue. If such information is available for the compound labeled in the same position, metabolite corrections may be made. If not, the usual next step of an in vivo evaluation of the positron-labeled tracers is to perform similar analyses. Information about the identity of tissue radioactivity is usually only obtainable from rodents, while plasma radioactivity from larger animals and humans is often analyzed to determine the percentage of intact drug as a correction factor for kinetic modeling of the tracer behavior *(21)*. The blood and tissue samples obtained from rodents are usually quite small, which can be a serious limiting factor for reliable counting statistics, particularly after long work-up procedures. While difficult to perform metabolite analyses rapidly enough with such a short-lived nuclide as carbon-11, it is not impossible if properly optimized methodology is used *(22)*.

If the tracer is unmetabolized during the period of observation or the metabolism can be accounted for, the radiotracer uptake data can be divided by the specific activity of the administered compound to estimate the drug's concentration in tissue with time. The ability to determine in vivo the area under the concentration-time curve for each target tissue is potentially beneficial for all drug evaluations. Furthermore, this type of approach is predicted to provide crucial information for chemotherapeutic strategies targeting specific tissues (e.g., antibody-based therapies), for which the more conventional monitoring of drug concentrations in plasma may be completely insufficient for predicting efficacy.

The binding and enzyme inhibition characteristics of PD 153035 in model systems have been carefully determined elsewhere, part of which was briefly related above in **Subheading 1.2.** Typically the next step in a preclinical screening is to test the compound in animal models of disease, if available. Most anti-cancer drugs are tested in rodents with xenografts from implanted specific cell lines. Here, with PET, the dynamics of the uptake of radioactivity in two tumor implants in each of three rats was observed for a total observation time up to 80 min. The implants differed in morphology, as determined post-mortem, and these differences affected the ease with which they were detected and the certainties in the resulting calculations. The uptake of radioactivity in all the implants was, however, higher than that in the immediate surrounding tissues. The ROIs could be drawn based on this target/non-target contrast and calculations of the concentrations with time were subsequently made. However, the tumors that were comparable to, or significantly larger than the spatial resolution of the PET camera, were more easily discernible, as shown in the example in **Figure 4** (left part). Using dedicated scanners with system resolution more attuned to small animal studies would further improve the capability of detecting very small, functionally aberrant lesions *(23,24)*.

The advantages of acquiring dynamic information from a single animal or several animals, particularly those with disease models, are obvious. Temporal information must otherwise be obtained by administering the drug to a much larger number of animals. Several are then sacrificed at each desired time interval and the amount of compound in the different organs is assayed. However, such ex vivo methods are particularly affected by inter-animal variations. The rate of administration, individual differences in organ functions, differences in anesthesia, and the like will all influence the timing of regional uptake and subsequent elimination. Although the same physiological variations occur in animals scanned with PET, continuous observations of the distribution in target as well as non-target tissues can facilitate the detection of such systemic variations.

Despite the power of the kinetic analyses achievable, PET in vivo screening cannot avoid many of the conventional problems of using animal models of disease. For example, xenograft heterogeneity and the differential vasculariza-tion can markedly affect the radiotracer's and the drug's distribution *(25)* and consequently, the conclusions drawn about its ability to trace or treat the diseased condition, respectively. In fact, a good deal of emphasis in drug development is currently being placed on improving animal models of disease. For that to be relevant, it must be possible to validate that the findings in sick animals can be extended to targeting and treating disease in humans. Since tracer doses of the compounds are used in PET screening, a subsequent step to performing in vivo evaluations in humans could be much more quickly performed and evaluated and could provide essential information about species similarities/differences in the pharmacokinetics of the drug.

The PET evaluation of radiolabeled drugs does not stop at simple calculations of its distribution to the targeted tissues as a function of time. Since drugs usually produce their therapeutic effects by interacting with specific receptors or by binding to molecules, it is common to follow up distribution studies with attempts to challenge or perturb the uptake of the radiotracer in order to demonstrate selectivity and specificity of these interactions in vivo. Direct observations of these pharmacological challenges can also help couple drug efficacy to the mechanisms of actions proposed from the initial in vitro screening in isolated systems. Once validated in animal studies, similar drug-receptor interaction studies in humans may also help assess the degree of receptor occupancy or enzyme inhibition during therapy.

PET can provide valuable pharmacokinetic and pharmacodynamic information for all phases of the drug discovery process, from early animal screening to pilot studies in humans and finally to evaluation of efficacy in different diseased states in humans. Integration of PET tracer research programs with those of industrial medicinal chemistry units has always been the most rapid method of finding the most selective and specific probes. More and more of the major pharmaceutical companies are realizing the benefits to be gained and are collaborating with established PET facilities or, in some cases, are even opening their own programs. Integration of pharmaceutical research with molecular imaging techniques is predicted to become even more important for the future focus on individualized therapeutic strategies.

4. Notes

1. A number of factors affect the capability of PET to resolve different structures. The PET isotopes all decay by emitting positrons with nuclide-specific energies (*see* β+-energies in **Table 1**). The positron's energy determines how fast and far (the positron range) it will travel in the tissue before it slows down enough to collide with an electron and the two gamma photons are emitted. Since the location of the actual decay is different than the site at which the detectable photons are emitted, the spatial resolution in the PET images is decreased. The higher the energy, the larger the positron range and the lower the resolution (i.e.,

resolution $^{18}F > ^{11}C > ^{13}N > ^{15}O$). The not-quite co-linear emission of the two photons leads to incorrect assignment of the location for the photon formation and thereby degrades resolution. Image resolution is also affected by scattered and random photons, by the camera's crystal geometry, and by uncertainty in "off-center" photon registrations. For a more in-depth discussion see, for example, Budinger et al. *(26)*. A resolution better than 1.5–2 mm is not probable.

2. PET cameras have a rather small axial field-of-view. The Siemens-CTI Ecat Exact HR used here has a field-of-view of 15 cm. Therefore, most, but not quite all, of the rat could be monitored at the same time. For larger animals and humans, dynamic studies of the whole body are, of course, even less feasible. The possibility of performing several dynamic studies covering a new segment each time is almost exclusively limited to inter-individual comparisons, since the radiation doses for intra-individual repeated studies are usually too high. When whole body scans are needed, SPECT or "hybrid"-PET may be used since they have larger field-of-views. However, the spatial and time (dynamic capacity) resolution in these cameras is poorer.

3. High-energy radioactivity is used in every step of the PET process, except in the data analysis. Personnel working in this field are trained in special handling techniques to keep their own exposure at a minimum. Administration of the radiotracers to human subjects also requires a careful estimation and minimization of their radiation dose exposure during the investigation. The studies in animals (rats or preferably monkeys) are used to identify the organ(s) with the highest absorbed dose. This information is then used to regulate the maximum amount of the tracer, which can be administered to humans. The radiation dose in "a typical" PET clinical study using $(2-^{18}F)$-2-fluoro-2-deoxy-D-glucose (FDG) is comparable to the amount normally received from background radiation during one year.

4. As presented in **Figure 1C**, different types of scanners may be required to match the particular demands of a given PET application: (1) Animal PET: resolution ≥ 1.8 mm, medium to high sensitivity, 2–8 cm axial length; (2) Human PET: resolution 3–10 mm, high sensitivity, 10–20 cm axial length; (3) Hybrid PET: resolution χ 4–6 mm, low to medium sensitivity, 40 cm axial length.

Acknowledgment

Parts of **Figures 3** and **4** are reprinted from Life Sciences, vol. 65, Fredriksson A., Johnström P., Thorell J. O., von Heijne G., Hassan M., Eksborg S., Kogner P., Borgström P., Ingvar M., Stone-Elander S.: In vivo evaluation of the biodistribution of ^{11}C-labeled PD153035 in rats without and with neuroblastoma implants, pp. 165–174, Copyright (1999), with permission from Elsevier Science.

References

1. Fredriksson, A., Johnström, P., Thorell, J.-O., et al. (1999) In vivo evaluation of the biodistribution of ^{11}C-labeled PD153035 in rats without and with neuroblastoma implants. *Life Sci.* **65,** 165–174.

2. Murray, I. P. C. and Ell, P. J. (ed.) (1994) *Nuclear medicine in clinical diagnosis and treatment.* Churchill Livingstone, London, UK.

3. Phelps, M. E., Mazziotta, J. C., and Schelbert, H. R. (ed.) (1986) *Positron emission tomography and autoradiography: Principles and applications for the brain and heart.* Raven Press, New York, NY.

4. McCarthy, T. J. and Welch, M. J. (1998) The state of positron emitting radionuclide production in 1997. *Sem. Nucl. Med.* **28,** 235–246.

5. Fry, D. W., Kraker, A. J., McMichael, A., et al. (1994) A specific inhibitor of the epidermal growth factor receptor tyrosine kinase. *Science* **265,** 1093–1095.

6. Mulholland, G. K., Winkle, W., Mock, B. H., and Sledge, G. (1995) Radioiodinated epidermal growth factor receptor ligands as tumor probes. Dramatic potentiation of binding to MDA-468 cancer cells in presence of EGF. *J. Nucl. Med.* **36,** P71.

7. Mulholland, G. K., Zheng, Q.-H., Winkle, W. L., and Carlson, K. A. (1997) Synthesis and biodistribution of new C-11 and F-18 labeled epidermal growth factor receptor ligands. *J. Nucl. Med.* **38,** P141.

8. Johnström, P., Fredriksson, A., Thorell, J.-O., et al. (1997) Synthesis and in vivo biodistribution of tyrosine kinase inhibitor, [methoxy-^{11}C]PD 153035. *J. Labelled Cpd. Radiopharm.* **40,** S377–S379.

9. Johnström, P., Fredriksson, A., Thorell, J.-O., and Stone-Elander, S. (1998) Synthesis of [methoxy-^{11}C]PD153035, a selective EGF receptor tyrosine kinase inhibitor. *J. Labelled Cpd. Radiopharm.* **41,** 623–629.

10. Lim, J. K., Riese II, D. J., Negash, K., Hawkins, R. A., and VanBrocklin, H. F. (1998) Synthesis and in vitro evaluation of epidermal growth factor receptor tyrosine kinase inhibitors. *J. Nucl. Med.* **39,** P20.

11. Mishani, E., Bonasera, T. A., Rozen, Y., Ortu, G., Gazit, A., and Levitski, A. (1999) Fluorinated EGFR-TK inhibitor-based tracers for PET. *J. Labelled Cpd. Radiopharm.* **42,** S27–S29.

12. Lim, J. K., Riese II, D. J., and VanBrocklin, H. F. (1999) Synthesis of 4-(4′-[^{18}F]fluorobenzylamino)-6,7-diethoxyquinazoline: a positron emitting radioprobe for the epidermal growth factor receptor. *J. Labelled Cpd. Radiopharm.* **42,** S693–S695.

13. Snyder, S. E., Whitmer, K. M., and Brown-Proctor, C. (1999) Synthesis of 3-chloro-4-[^{18}F]fluoroaniline as a synthon for epidermal growth factor receptor inhibitors for tumor imaging with PET. *J. Labelled Cpd. Radiopharm.* **42,** S522–S524.

14. Snyder, S. E., Sherman, P. S. and Blair, J. B. (2000) 4-(3-Chloro-4-[^{18}F]fluoro-phenylamino)-6,7-dimethoxyquinazoline: a radiolabeled EGF receptor inhibitor for imaging tumor biochemistry with PET. *J. Nucl. Med.* **41,** 233P.

15. Lim, J. K., Negash, K., Hanrahan, S. M., and VanBrocklin, H. F. (2000) Synthesis of 4-(3′-[^{125}I]iodoanilino)-6,7-dialkoxyquinazolines: radiolabeled epidermal growth factor receptor tyrosine kinase inhibitors. *J. Labelled Cpd. Radiopharm.* **43,** 1183–1191.

16. Ingvar, M., Eriksson, L., Rogers, G. A., Stone-Elander, S., and Widén, L. (1991) Rapid feasibility studies of tracers for positron emission tomography: High-

resolution PET in small animals with kinetic analysis. *J. Cereb. Blood Flow Metab.* **11,** 926–931.

17. Hustinx, R., Eck, S. L., and Alavi, A. (1999) Potential application of PET imaging in developing novel cancer therapies. *J. Nucl. Med.* **40,** 995–1002.
18. Saleem, A., Aboagye, E. O., and Price, P. M. (2000) In vivo monitoring of drugs using radiotracer techniques. *Adv. Drug Delivery Rev.* **41,** 21–39.
19. Fowler, J. S., Volkow, N. D., Wang, G.-J., Ding, Y.-S., and Dewey, S. L. (1999) PET and drug research and development. *J. Nucl. Med.* **40,** 1154–1163.
20. Bhatnagar, A., Hustinx, R., and Alavi, A. (2000) Nuclear imaging methods for non-invasive drug monitoring. *Adv. Drug Delivery Rev.* **41,** 41–54.
21. Osman, S., Lundkvist, C., Pike, V. W., et al. (1996) Characterization of the radioactive metabolites of the 5-HT$_{1A}$ receptor radioligand, [O-*methyl*-^{11}C]WAY-100635, in monkey and human plasma by HPLC: Comparison of the behaviour of an identified radioactive metabolite with parent radioligand in monkey using PET. *Nucl. Med. Biol.* **23,** 627–634.
22. Davenport, R. J., Law, M. P., Pike, V. W., Osman, S., and Poole, K. G. (1995) Propionyl-L-carnitine: Labelling in the *N*-methyl position with carbon-11 and pharmacokinetic studies in rats. *Nucl. Med. Biol.* **22,** 699–709.
23. Phelps, M. E. (2000) PET: The merging of biology and imaging into molecular imaging. *J. Nucl. Med.* **41,** 661–681.
24. Myers, R., Hume, S., Bloomfield, P., and Jones, T. (1999) Radio-imaging in small animals. *J. Psychopharm.* **13,** 352–357.
25. Pauwels, E. K. J., McCready, V. R., Stoot, J. H. M. B., and von Deurzen, D. F. P. (1998) The mechanism of accumulation of tumour-localising radiopharmaceuticals. *Eur. J. Nucl. Med.* **25,** 277–305.
26. Budinger, T. F., Brennan, K. M., Moses, W. W., and Derenzo, S. E. (1996) Advances in positron tomography for oncology. *Nucl. Med. Biol.* **23,** 659–667.

XI

MISCELLANEOUS PROTOCOLS

24

Assays for In Vitro and In Vivo Synergy

Beverly A. Teicher

1. Introduction

In the study of multi-modality therapy or combined chemotherapy, it is of interest to determine whether the combined effects of two agents are additive or whether their combination is substantially different from the sum of their parts *(1,2)*. While controversy and discussion continue and new methodologies continue in development, two methods for the determination of synergy/ additivity have emerged over the past 10 years as the main functional systems for the experimentalist and investigator in cancer. These are the median effect/combination index method and the isobologram method *(3–14)*. This chapter will discuss these methods and provide examples, but will not delve into the mathematical derivations associated with each. Both methods have been applied widely. One or the other method may be more applicable to the drug interaction being studied, often this cannot be determined until after the experiment is done. Unfortunately, the method for determination of synergy/additivity must be selected before the experiment is performed since each method requires attention to experimental design. Some investigators have applied both the median effect/combination index and the isobologram analyses to their work.

2. The Median-Effect Method

The median-effect and combination index method for the determination of additivity/synergy in experiments involving two agent combinations in cancer research has been popularized by the work of Chou and Talalay *(3–7)*, who not only described this approach to the assessment of additivity to the cancer research community but also provided a user friendly computer program for

From: *Methods in Molecular Medicine, vol. 85: Novel Anticancer Drug Protocols*
Edited by: J. K. Buolamwini and A. A. Adjei © Humana Press Inc., Totowa, NJ

analyzing data by this method *(8–12)*. The median-effect principle was obtained from the derivation of enzyme reaction rate equations and concentration or dose-effect relationship equations. The median-effect equation *(11,12)* states that:

$$f_a/f_u = (D/D_m)^m$$

where D is the dose or concentration of the agent; f_a and f_u are the fractions of the system affected and unaffected, respectively, by the dose D; D_m is the dose or concentration of the agent required to produce the median effect; and m is a coefficient signifying the sigmoidicity of the concentration or dose-effect curve. The median-effect equation can be used to describe many biological systems such as Michaelis-Menton and Hill enzyme kinetic relationships, the Langmuir physical adsorption isotherm, the Henderson-Hasselbach pH ionization relationship, the Scatchard equilibrium binding equation, and the many compound-receptor interactions *(3)*.

Chou and Talalay *(4,6)* went on to derive equations to describe two compound situations. For two compounds having similar modes of action where the effects of both compounds are mutually exclusive (i.e., parallel median effect plots for parent compounds and their mixtures) and for two compounds in which the effects are mutually nonexclusive (i.e., two compounds having different modes of action or acting independently), the general equation is:

$$[(f_a)_{1,2}/(f_u)_{1,2}]^{1/m} = [(f_a)_1/(f_u)_1]^{1/m} + [(f_a)_2/(f_u)_2]^{1/m} + [(f_a)_1(f_a)_2/(f_u)_1(f_u)_2]^{1/m}$$
$$= (D)_1/(D_m)_1 + (D)_2/(D_m)_2 + (D)_1(D)_2/(D_m)_1(D_m)_2$$

From this analysis, the combination index (CI) for quantifying synergism (greater-than-additive), summation (additive), and antagonism (less-than-additive) effects can be derived *(5,6)*:

$$CI = (D)_1/(D_x)_1 + (D)_2/(D_x)_2$$

for mutually exclusive compounds and

$$CI = (D)_1/(D_x)_1 + (D)_2/(D_x)_2 + (D)_1(D)_2/(D_x)_1(D_x)_2$$

for mutually nonexclusive compounds. Combination index (CI) values that are smaller than one indicate synergism (greater-than-additive) effect of the two agents, a combination index equal to one indicates summation (additivity) of the two agents, and a combination index value greater than one indicates antagonism (less-than-additive) effect of the two agents.

While the median effect analysis has been the subject of some controversy, as have other methods for assessment of additivity/synergy such as the isobologram method, it has gained wide spread use since it can readily be applied to many laboratory systems. Application of the median effect/combination index method requires specification in the experimental design such that the two agents being tested be combined in a constant ratio of doses or concentrations, in most cases *(11)*. The level of synergy/antagonism at various concentration or dose ratios for the two agents can be determined from the combination index calculation. The same can be done for different effect levels.

Gemcitabine (LY18801; 2',2'-difluorodeoxycytidine) is an analog of the natural pyrimidine nucleoside cytidine. The mechanism of action and metabolism of gemcitabine has been well characterized *(15,16)*. Deoxycytidine kinase activates gemcitabine to gemcitabine monophosphate, which is converted to the diphosphate and eventually the triphosphate. The triphosphate competes with deoxycytidine triphosphate for incorporation into DNA and results in chain termination one base pair beyond the point of insertion *(16,17)*. The addition of a base pair after gemcitabine triphosphate protects this lesion from excision by exonucleases. Gemcitabine cytotoxicity is proportional to the intracellular concentration of gemcitabine triphosphate and its incorporation into DNA. The diphosphate of gemcitabine exerts a time- and concentration-dependent inhibition of the enzyme ribonucleotide reductase, thereby diminishing intracellular deoxycytidine triphosphate and enhancing the incorporation of gemcitabine triphosphate into DNA *(15)*. In cell culture, gemcitabine causes accumulation of cells in the S phase of the cell cycle *(15,18,19)*. Gemcitabine is active against a number of solid tumors in vitro and has demonstrated activity against many solid tumor models including the CX-1 human colon cancer xenograft and the LX-1 human lung carcinoma xenograft in nude mice *(17–20)*. In Phase I human trials, gemcitabine was evaluated in a variety of schedules. The greatest efficacy with the least toxicity was demonstrated with a weekly schedule *(15)*. In Phase II human trials, gemcitabine demonstrated activity against small cell lung, non-small cell lung, breast, ovarian, pancreatic, myeloma, prostatic, renal, and bladder cancer *(21,22)*. Gemcitabine demonstrated a 22% objective tumor response rate in 331 patients diagnosed with non-small cell lung cancer receiving drug on a weekly schedule in a dose range of 800 mg/m^2 to 1250 mg/m^2.

Mitomycin C is the prototype bioreductive alkylating agent *(23–29)*. The cytotoxicity of mitomycin C is not cell cycle selective. Mitomycin C is metabolized, most efficiently by hypoxic cells, to an active alkylating species, which crosslinks the strands of DNA preferentially at guanine and thereby prevents DNA synthesis *(23–29)*. HT29 cell survival was assessed after exposure to gemcitabine or mitomycin C using a standard clonogenic assay. In one set of experiments, a non-cytotoxic concentration of gemcitabine and a concentration range of mitomycin C were combined. In a second set of experiments, combinations of gemcitabine and mitomycin C in various concentration ratios representing various levels of cytotoxicity were analyzed according to the median effect method *(6)*. The interaction of the two chemotherapeutic agents was quantified assuming a mutually nonexclusive interaction in calculating the combination index (CI). Aung et al. *(30)* found that a marked synergism (CI = 0.5–0.7) was produced by concurrent exposure to gemcitabine and mitomycin C. In contrast, sequential exposure led to additivity. These findings suggest that gemcitabine and mitomycin C may be a beneficial chemotherapeutic combination for the treatment of human malignancies.

Gemcitabine and cisplatin have different and potentially complementary mechanisms of action and thus are attractive candidates for drug combinations. Cisplatin is among the most widely used anticancer drugs with a broad spectrum of activity *(31)*. Intracellularly, cisplatin is hydrolyzed to an active species that forms primarily intrastrand crosslinks in DNA between adjacent guanines *(32–34)*. Studies have shown a schedule-dependent interaction between gemcitabine and cisplatin ranging from antagonism to synergy *(35–39)*. In anaplastic thyroid carcinoma cell lines, Voigt et al. *(40)* found that the combination of gemcitabine and cisplatin produced additive cytotoxicity when gemcitabine exposure preceded cisplatin exposure (CI = 1.0) and antagonism when cisplatin exposure preceded gemcitabine exposure (CI > 1.0). Van Moorsel et al. *(41)* examined interactions between gemcitabine and cisplatin in human ovarian and non-small cell lung cancer cell lines. Cells were exposed to the drug for 4, 24, and 72 h and synergy/additivity was assessed using median effect analysis and calculating a combination index. With cisplatin at an IC_{25}, the average CI's calculated for the combination at the IC_{50}, IC_{75}, IC_{90}, and IC_{95} after 4, 24, and 72 h of exposure were <1.0, indicating synergism. With gemcitabine at an IC_{25}, the CI's for the combinations with cisplatin after 24 h were <1.0 in each cell line, except for the H322 non-small cell lung cancer cell line that showed an additive effect. At 72 h exposure, all of the CI's were <1.0.

Irinotecan (7-ethyl-10-[4-(1-piperidino)-1-piperidino]carbonyloxycamptothecin; CPT-11) is a water soluble camptothecin analog which has a broad spectrum of antitumor activity including activity against multidrug resistant tumors *(42–46)*. The active metabolite of irinotecan, SN-38, inhibits the nuclear enzyme topoisomerase I by stabilizing the topoisomerase I-DNA cleavable complex resulting in the arrest of the DNA replication fork, thus causing DNA single strand breaks and ultimately cell death *(42,45)*. Bahadori et al. *(47)* applied both isobologram analysis and median effect analysis to growth inhibitory combinations of gemcitabine and irinotecan in human MCF-7 breast carcinoma cells and human SCOG small cell lung carcinoma cells. By isobologram analysis, the growth inhibition of the combination of gemcitabine and irinotecan exhibited synergy over a wide concentration range (gemcitabine:

0.1–3.0 μM; irinotecan: 5–60 μM). By median effect/combination index analysis (concentration ratio 1:1), the growth inhibition produced by gemcitabine and irinotecan was synergistic at lower concentrations (<0.1 μM) of the compounds in MCF-7 cells, but in SCOG cells synergy was achieved at concentrations greater than 1 μM (1–10 μM). Etoposide (VP-16), a widely used anticancer drug, inhibits the nuclear enzyme topoisomerase II forming a cleavage complex with the protein and DNA and resulting in double strand breaks in the DNA *(48–50)*. Etoposide has been reported to act synergistically with many DNA-interacting anticancer agents such as cisplatin and bifunctional alkylating agents although the mechanism of these interactions has not been fully elucidated. The interaction between gemcitabine and etoposide was examined by van Moorsel et al. *(51)* using median effect analysis with either a fixed molar ratio of the compounds or with a variable compound ratio. In the Lewis lung murine carcinoma cell line, the combination of gemcitabine and etoposide at a constant molar ratio (gemcitabine:etoposide = 1:4 or 1:0.125 after 4 or 24 h exposure, respectively) was synergistic (CI calculated at 50% cell growth inhibition = 0.7 and 0.8, respectively). After 24 and 72 h exposure to both compounds at a constant ratio, additivity was found in human A2780 ovarian cancer cells and ADDP, a cisplatin and etoposide resistant subline of A2780 cells, and human H322 non-small cell lung cancer cells (gemcitabine:etoposide = 1:500 for both exposure times). When cells were exposed to a combination of gemcitabine and etoposide for 24 or 72 h, with etoposide at its IC_{25} and gemcitabine over a concentration range, additivity was found in both the Lewis lung cells and the H322 cells; synergism was observed in the A2780 cells and the ADDP cells. Schedule dependency was found in the Lewis lung cancer cells such that when cells were exposed to gemcitabine 4 h prior to etoposide (constant molar ratio, total exposure time 24 h) synergism was found (CI = 0.5); however, additivity was seen when cells were exposed to etoposide prior to gemcitabine (CI = 1.6).

Paclitaxel, one of the most widely used anticancer agents, is an antimicrotubule agent isolated from the western Pacific yew tree *Taxus brevifolia (52–54)*. In cells, paclitaxel promotes microtubule assembly and stabilizes tubulin polymer formation, blocking cells in the late G2/M phase of the cell cycle *(55–57)*. Working in the human T24 bladder cancer cell line, Cos et al. *(58)* found that for the drug combination of paclitaxel and methotrexate, if cells were exposed to paclitaxel for 24 h and then to methotrexate for 24 h, or if cells were exposed to methotrexate for 24 h and then to paclitaxel for 24 h, the cytotoxicity was found to be synergistic by the combination index method. However, if the T24 cells were exposed to methotrexate and paclitaxel simultaneously then cytotoxic antagonism occurred between the drugs. A study from McDaid and Johnston *(59)* explored the interaction between 8-Cl-cAMP

(8-chloro-adenosine-3',5'-monophosphate), a cAMP analog, and paclitaxel. Two ovarian cancer cell lines, A2780 and OAW42, with differing sensitivity to both compounds, were tested using the fixed-ratio design and various scheduling regimens. The fixed ratio selected was the ratio equivalent to the ratio of the IC_{50}s for the compounds as single agents in each cell line. The 8-Cl-cAMP:paclitaxel fixed molar ratios were 6.25:1 for A2780 cells and 3448:1 for OAW42 cells. Simultaneous exposure of either cell line to 8-Cl-cAMP and paclitaxel resulted in a high level of synergism with CIs between 0.18 and 0.62 for A2780 cells and between 0.001 and 0.18 for OAW42 cells. Sequencing with paclitaxel exposure for 24 h prior to 8-Cl-cAMP was a very effective regimen; while sequencing with 8-Cl-cAMP prior to paclitaxel was the least effective regimen. The combination of paclitaxel and etoposide was examined in three human tumor cell lines, A549 non-small cell lung carcinoma, and MDA-231 and MCF-7 breast carcinoma (60). The single agent IC_{50} values for each compound in each cell line were used to design the ratios for the combination treatment regimens. Exposure schedules were 24 h simultaneous, 24 h sequential, and sequential 24 h with a 24-h intervening compound-free period. The data were analyzed using the median effect/combination index method. The simultaneous exposure results were less-than-additive cytotoxicity in two of the three cell lines. The sequential regimens and the sequential regimen with the intervening 24-h period resulted in synergistic cytotoxicity when either paclitaxel or etoposide exposure occurred first.

Vinblastine, an anticancer Vinca alkaloid compound, like paclitaxel is described as an antitubulin agent but unlike paclitaxel, vinblastine inhibits tubulin polymerization (61,62). Thus, the two compounds, paclitaxel and vinblastine, have the same protein target in cells but have distinctly different effects on that protein. Giannakakou et al. (63) maintained a constant concentration ratio of 1:1 for a study of the combination of paclitaxel and vinblastine in human KB epidermoid carcinoma cells and human MCF-7 breast carcinoma cells. Cytotoxicity studies carried out using the median effect method and the combination index analysis showed synergism when vinblastine and paclitaxel exposure occurred sequentially and antagonism for simultaneous exposure.

Methionine dependence, that is the increased requirement for methionine of tumor cells due to their proliferative thrust (64–72), is a common property of many tumor types and several potential therapeutic strategies have been developed to target methionine dependence. Methioninase from *Pseudomonas putida*, which degrades extracellular methionine to α-ketobutyrate, ammonia, and methanethiol (72), has been demonstrated to have antitumor efficacy in vitro and in vivo (71,73,74). Methioninase was shown to be synergistic in combination with 5-fluorouracil (74) and cisplatin (73,75). Miki et al. (72) used a gene therapy approach to methionine dependency. A recombinant adenovirus was prepared containing a MET gene (rAd-MET) as well as a control adenovirus (rAd). The combination therapy studies examined the cytotoxicity of the rAd-MET or rAd along with exposure to exogenous methioninase. The cytotoxicity of rAd-MET was tested using human OVCAR-8 ovarian cancer cells and human HT1080 fibrosarcoma cells. rAd-MET transduction of OVCAR-8 cells and HT1080 cells resulted in high levels of methioninase expression. The IC_{50} of rAd-MET in the OVCAR-8 cells was 2×10^6 plaque-forming units/well in a 96-well format while the IC_{50} for the rAd control virus was 20x higher. In the presence of the IC_{50} level of virus infection, the addition of 0.025 units/mL of methioninase inhibited the growth of 90% of the cells, while the same level of infection with the control virus along with methioninase inhibited the growth of 10% of OVCAR-8 cells. The synergistic effect of the combination of methioninase and rAd-MET was quantified by calculating the combination index (CI). The CIs for each combination of rAd-MET and methioninase tested in the OVCAR-8 cell line was <0.7 indicating synergy; while the same treatments with the rAd control virus resulted in CIs of 1.0 indicating additivity of the two agents.

3. Isobologram Methodology

The isobologram method is a generally valid procedure for analyzing interactions between agents, irrespective of their mechanisms of action or the nature of their mechanisms of action or the nature of their concentration- or dose-response relations (13). As with the median effect method, three possible conclusions can be drawn from the isobologram analyses, they are that the agents have zero interaction (additivity), that the agents exhibit synergy (greater-than-additivity), or that the agents exhibit antagonism (less-than-additivity). The isobologram method requires that if a combination is represented by a point and if the axes on the graph represent the two agents in the combination then the point lies on a straight line connecting the points where each of the two agents is present in zero concentration if the agents are non-interactive (13). In many situations in cancer research, either the response to an agent or its logarithm is linear with the logarithm of the concentration or dose of the agent (76–83). The equations would be:

$$E \text{ (dose or concentration)} = a + b \text{ (log dose or concentration)}$$

and $\quad$ log E (dose or concentration) = a + b (log dose or concentration),

then $\quad$ $$f_b^{-1}f_a (D_a) = 10^{(a_a - a_b)/b_b} \cdot D_a^{b_a/b_b},$$

and $\quad$ $$D_a[1 - D_a^{-b_a/b_b} \cdot 10^{(a_a - a_b)/b_b} \cdot d_b] - d_a = 0.$$

Several attempts have been made to simplify or modify the isobologram approach to provide for efficient experimental designs and observation over a wide range of effects. Tallarida et al. *(84)* presented a method employing a design in which the dose- or concentration-effect relation for each agent was used to generate theoretical composite additive total dose combinations in fixed agent proportions. This composite additive dose-effect relation is then compared with the data from the actual agent combination in the same proportion. Another simplified conceptual foundation for this form of analysis was developed and popularized by Steel and Peckman *(85)*, based on the construction of an envelope of additivity in an isoeffect plot (isobologram). This approach provides a rigorous basis for defining regions of additivity, supra-additivity, and sub-additivity and protection. This method of analysis is based on a clear conceptual formulation of the way that drugs or agents can be expected to show additivity. The first form of additivity is more conceptually simple and is defined as Mode 1 by Steel and Peckham *(85)*. For a selected level of effect (survival in this case) on a log scale, the dose of Agent A to produce this effect for the survival curve is determined. A lower dose of Agent A is then selected, the difference in effect from the isoeffect level is determined, and the dose of Agent B needed to make up this difference is derived from the survival curve for Agent B. For example, 3 mg of Agent A may be needed to produce 0.1% survival (3 logs of kill), the selected isoeffect. A dose of 2.5 mg of Agent A produces 1.0% survival (2 logs of kill). The Mode I isoeffect point for Agent B would thus be the level of Agent B needed to produce 1 log of kill, to result in the same overall effect of 3 logs of kill. In this instance, we might find that 4 mg of Agent B are needed to produce 1 log of kill.

Mode II additivity is conceptually more complex, but corresponds to the notions of additivity and synergy discussed in detail by Berenbaum *(13,14)*. For any given level of effect, the dose or concentration of Agent A needed to produce this effect is determined from the survival relationship. The isoeffect dose or concentration of Agent B is calculated as the amount of Agent B needed to produce this effect is determined from the survival relationship. The iso-effect dose or concentration of Agent B is calculated as the amount of Agent B needed to produce the given effect starting at the level of effect produced by Agent A. For example, 3 mg of Agent A may be needed to produce 0.1% survival (3 logs of kill). A dose of 2.5 mg of Agent A produces 1.0% (2 logs of kill). A dose of 6 mg of Agent B is needed to produce 3 logs of kill, and 2 logs of kill are obtained with Agent B at 5 mg. Thus, the Mode II isoeffect point with Agent A at 2.5 mg is equal to the amount of Agent B needed to take Agent B from 2 logs of kill to 3 logs of kill (6 mg – 5 mg = 1 mg). This can be conceptualized by noting that Agent A should produce 2 logs of kill and is, in this case, equal to 5 mg of Agent B. If Agent A + Agent B are identical in their mode of action, then 1 mg more of Agent B should then be equivalent in effect to 6 mg of Agent B. Graphically, on a linear dose scale, Mode II additivity is defined as the straight line connecting the effective dose or concentration of Agent A alone and the effective dose or concentration of Agent B alone. This relationship is also described by the equation

$$\frac{\text{Dose of A}}{A_e} + \frac{\text{Dose of B}}{B_e} = 1$$

where A_e and B_e are the doses or concentrations of Agent A and Agent B, respectively, needed to produce the selected effect.

Overall, combinations that produce the desired effect that are within the boundaries of Mode I and Mode II are considered additive. Those displaced to the left are greater-than-additive while those displaced to the right are less-than-additive. Combinations that produce effect outside the rectangle defined by the intersections of A_e and B_e are protective. This type of classical isobologram methodology is cumbersome to use experimentally, as each combination must be carefully titrated to produce a constant level of effect. Dewey et al. *(86)* described an analogous form of analysis for the special case in which the dose of one agent was held constant. Using full survival curves of each agent alone, this method produces envelopes of additive effect for different levels of the variable agent. It is conceptually identical to generating a series of isoeffect curves and then plotting the survivals from a series of these at constant dose of Agent A on a log effect by dose of Agent B coordinate system *(87)*. This approach can often be applied to the experimental situation in a more direct and efficient manner, and isobolograms can be derived describing the expected effect (Mode I and Mode II) for any level of the variable agent and constant agent combinations.

It has been recognized that the schedule and sequence of drugs in combination can affect therapeutic outcome. Over the last 15 yr the definition of additivity and therapeutic synergism has evolved with increasing stringency. In the work by Schabel et al. *(88–93)*, Corbett et al. *(94,95)*, and Griswold et al. *(96,97)*, therapeutic synergism between two drugs was defined to mean that "the effect of the two drugs in combination was significantly greater than that which could be obtained when either drug was used alone under identical conditions of treatment." Using this definition, the combination of cyclophosphamide and melphalan administered simultaneously by intraperitoneal injection every 2 wk was reported to be therapeutically synergistic in the Ridgeway osteosarcoma growth delay assay *(88–92)*. Similarly, the combination of cyclophosphamide and melphalan has been reported to be therapeutically synergistic in L1210 and P388 leukemias *(93)*. Cyclophosphamide plus a nitrosourea (BCNU, CCNU, or MeCCNU) have also been reported to be

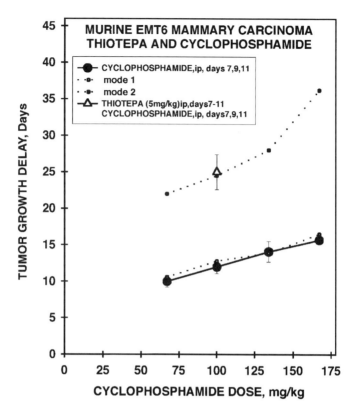

Fig. 1. Isobologram for the growth delay of the EMT6 murine mammary carcinoma treated with combinations of thiotepa and cyclophosphamide. Tumor treatments with cyclophosphamide alone. The dotted area represents the envelope of additivity for treatments with thiotepa and cyclophosphamide. Combination treatment of 5 mg/kg thiotepa × 6 plus 100 mg/kg cyclophosphamide × 3. Points represent three independent experiments (7 animals/group; 21 animals/point); bars represent the SEM (adapted from **ref. 98**).

therapeutically synergistic in increase-in-lifespan and growth delay assays using this definition *(93)*.

In the EMT6 murine mammary carcinoma in vivo, the maximum tolerated combination therapy of thiotepa (5 mg/kg × 6) and cyclophosphamide (100 mg/kg × 3) produced about 25 d of tumor growth delay, which was not significantly different than expected for additivity of the individual drugs *(see* **Fig. 1**) *(98–102)*. The survival of EMT6 tumor cells after treatment of the animals with various single doses of thiotepa and cyclophosphamide was assayed. Tumor cell killing by thiotepa produced a very steep, linear survival curve through 5 logs. The tumor cell-survival curve for cyclophosphamide out

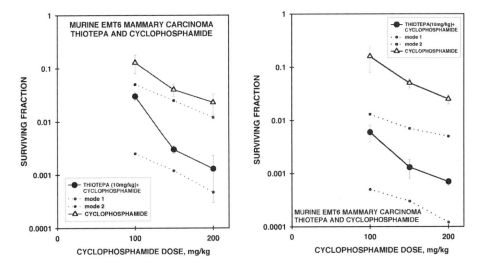

Fig. 2. Isobolograms for the combination treatment of the EMT6 tumor in vivo with 10 or 15 mg/kg thiotepa and various doses of cyclophosphamide. Survival curve for EMT6 tumors exposed to cyclophosphamide only. The dotted area represents the envelope of additivity for the combination treatment. Tumor cell survivals for the combination treatments (adapted from **ref. 98**).

to 500 mg/kg gave linear tumor cell kill through almost 4 logs. In all cases, the combination treatment tumor cell survivals fell well within the envelope of additivity (*see* **Fig. 2**). Both of these drugs are somewhat less toxic toward bone marrow cells by the granulocyte-macrophage colony-forming unit in vitro assay method than to tumor cells. The combination treatments were sub-additive or additive in bone marr ow granulocyte-macrophage colony-forming unit killing. When bone marrow is the dose-limiting tissue, there is a therapeutic advantage to the use of this drug combination *(98–102)*.

The Lewis lung carcinoma arose spontaneously as a carcinoma of the lung of a C57BL mouse in 1951 in the laboratory of Dr. Margaret R. Lewis at the Wistar Institute. The Lewis lung carcinoma was among the earliest transplantable tumors used to identify new anticancer agents. Sugiura and Stock found that the Lewis lung carcinoma produced tumors 100% of the time, producing a very malignant carcinoma. These investigators at the Sloan-Kettering Institute for Cancer Research used the Lewis lung carcinoma along with several other transplantable tumors to determine the antitumor activity of a series of phosphoramides from which the antitumor alkylating agent thiotepa emerged *(103–105)*. Twenty years later, DeWys working at the Strong Memorial Hospital of the University of Rochester School of Medicine, standardized techniques for following primary tumor growth by tumor volume measurements for assessing the response of lung metastases to a therapeutic intervention *(106)*. DeWys observed the Gompertsian pattern of primary tumor growth, effects of tumor burden on therapeutic efficacy, and effects of the presence of the primary tumor on the growth rate of the lung metastases *(107)*. G. Gordon Steel and co-investigators continued working with the Lewis lung carcinoma and in the mid- and late 1970s developed culture colony formation techniques, lung colony formation techniques, and limiting dilution techniques to assess tumor response to new anticancer drugs and radiation therapy *(108,109)*. This syngeneic tumor system mimics the human disease in that from the primary tumor it metastasizes to lungs, bone and liver. It is non-immunogenic and is grown in a host with a fully functional immune system. The rate of tumor growth is relatively rapid with a tumor volume doubling time of 2.5 d and is lethal in 21–25 d. Although this growth rate is rapid, it is in line with the life span of the host, which is about 2 yr.

Vinorelbine (navelbine) is a new, semi-synthetic vinca alkaloid whose antitumor activity is related to its ability to depolymerize microtubules that dissolve the mitotic spindles *(110–115)*. Its activity in cell culture was equal to or greater than other vinca alkaloids *(115)*. Vinorelbine was as effective as vinblastine against the A2780 human ovarian carcinoma cell line and was more cytotoxic than other vinca alkaloids against a human bronchial epidermoid carcinoma *(112)*. In a variety of human tumor cell lines (leukemia, non-small cell lung cancer, small cell lung cancer, colon, breast, melanoma, and brain), vinorelbine was cytostatic at nanomolar concentrations that are significantly below achievable plasma levels *(111,115)*. In a number of in vivo studies exploring activity in rodent tumor models and human tumor xenografts in athymic mice, vinorelbine demonstrated efficacy against P388, L1210, B16, and M5076 in vivo in murine models and in animals with human tumor xenografts. Phase I human trials have shown that in a weekly intravenous administration, the maximum tolerated dose of vinorelbine was 30 mg/m^2; this dose was the recommended dosage to be used in subsequent Phase II human trials employing a weekly schedule *(114,116,117)*. Phase II human trials employing weekly schedules of vinorelbine have demonstrated activity against small cell lung cancer, non-small cell lung cancer, ovarian, and breast cancer *(115)*. Vinorelbine as a single agent was studies in nonrandomized Phase II human trials as first-line therapy in non-small cell lung cancer using a weekly schedule and showed good activity with 23 responders out of 70 evaluable patients producing a response rate of 32.8%. The median duration of response was 34 wk *(115–118)*.

Gemcitabine was an active anticancer agent in animals bearing the Lewis lung carcinoma. Gemcitabine was well tolerated by the animals over the dosage range from 40 mg/kg × 3 to 80 mg/kg × 3 (*see* **Fig. 3**). Navelbine was

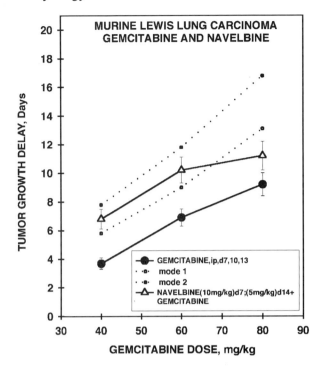

Fig. 3. Growth delay of the Lewis lung carcinoma produced by a range of doses of gemcitabine alone or along with navelbine (15 mg/kg total dose). The dotted area is the envelope of additivity determined by isobologram analysis. The bars are SEM.

administered in three different well-tolerated regimens with total doses of 10, 15, and 22.5 mg/kg. Both gemcitabine and navelbine produced increasing tumor growth delay with increasing dose of the drug. To assess the efficacy of the drug combination, the intermediate dosage regimen of navelbine was combined with each dosage level of gemcitabine. These combination regimens were tolerated and the tumor growth delay increased with increasing dose of gemcitabine. Isobologram methodology *(1,2,13,14)* was used to determine whether the combinations of gemcitabine and navelbine achieved additive antitumor activity (*see* **Fig. 3**). At gemcitabine doses of 40 mg/kg and 60 mg/kg, the combination regimens achieved additivity, with the experimental tumor growth delay falling within the calculated envelope of additivity. At the highest dose of gemcitabine, the combination regimen produced less-than-additive tumor growth delay *(2)*.

The untreated control animals in this study had a mean number of 35 lung metastases on d 20. Gemcitabine was highly effective against disease metastatic to the lungs such that the mean number of lung metastases on d 20 was decreased to 1.0–1.5 or 3–4% of the number found in the untreated controls. Each of the navelbine regimens decreased the number of lung metastases on d 20 to 10 or 11 or to about 30% of the number found in the untreated control animals. The combination regimens were highly effective against Lewis lung carcinoma metastatic to the lungs, with a mean number of <1–0 metastases found on d 20. These results support the notion that gemcitabine and navelbine may be an effective anticancer drug combination against non-small cell lung cancer *(2)*.

The human HCT116 colon carcinoma was selected for the initial study of ALIMTA in combination treatment because the HCT116 tumor is responsive to ALIMTA and because antitumor activity of ALIMTA has been observed in patients with colon cancer *(119–123)*. Treatment of nude mice bearing subcutaneously implanted HCT116 colon tumors with ALIMTA (100 mg/kg) twice daily for 5 d produced a tumor growth delay of 2.7 ± 0.3 d. Irinotecan administered daily for 5 d produced increasing tumor growth delay with increasing dose of the drug (*see* **Fig. 4**) *(124)*. Treatment of HCT116 tumor-bearing animals with ALIMTA and irinotecan resulted in greater-than-additive tumor growth for the two drugs, reaching 27 d when the irinotecan dose was 30 mg/kg. No toxicity was observed when a full standard dose of ALIMTA was administered with a full standard dose of irinotecan.

The combination of ALIMTA and irinotecan can result in synergistic antitumor effect against the human HCT116 colon carcinoma across all the doses of irinotecan examined. In general terms, this may reflect the fixing of the sublethal damage of one of the drugs by the other, or may reflect enhancement of one of the drug targets by the other drug *(125)*. Cell culture studies have shown that combinations of ralittrexed and SN-38, the active metabolite of irinotecan, enhances tumor cell killing *(126)*. Exposure to irinotecan may increase the proportion of tumor cells in S phase, as has been shown on exposure of HL-60 cells to camptothecin in cell culture *(125)*, thus increasing the portion of tumor cells that are susceptible to the cytotoxic action of ALIMTA.

With the availability of computer programs to aid data analysis, several investigators have applied both combination index analysis and isobologram analysis to their data. Satoh et al. *(127)* applied both methods to combinations of TNP-470 and paclitaxel using two human non-small cell lung cancer cell lines in culture. Evaluation of drug interactions with isobologram and combination index values indicated that sequential exposure of the cells to paclitaxel followed by TNP-470 resulted in greater-than-additive growth inhibitory effects. Using an in vitro:in vivo model, murine colon 26 carcinoma cells in culture, the combination of TNP-470 and 5-fluorouracil resulted in greater-than-additive cytotoxicity by isobologram analysis *(128)*. In vivo

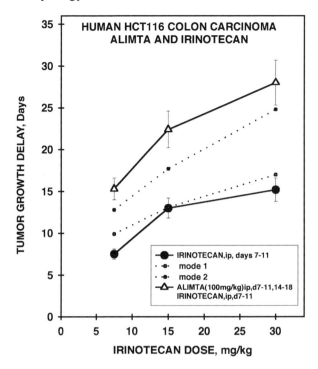

Fig. 4. Growth delay of human HCT116 colon carcinoma growth as a xenograft in nude mice after treatment with irinotecan (7.5, 15, or 30 mg/kg) intraperitoneally on d 7–11 after tumor cell implantation alone or along with ALIMTA (100 mg/kg) intraperitoneally on d 7–11 and d 14–18. The points are the mean values of two experiments with five animals per group per experiment; bars indicate the SEM. The dotted area represents the envelope of additivity by isobologram analysis (adapted from **ref. *124***).

TNP-470 was antiangiogenic in colon 26 tumors and resulted in a greater-than-additive antitumor effect with 5-fluorouracil was inferred, since isobologram analysis was not applied to the in vivo portion of the study. The effects of a recombinant human monoclonal antibody to HER2 simultaneously along with a spectrum of anticancer agents were explored in the SK-BR-3 and MCF-7 human breast cancer cell lines in culture *(129)*. In this paradigm by both isobologram and combination index analyses, greater-than-additive effects were achieved with antitumor alkylating agents, platinum complexes, and topoisomerase II inhibitors, while additivity was seen with taxanes. The combination of cisplatin and radiation therapy was explored using murine EMT6 mammary carcinoma cells and human OV-1063 ovarian cancer cells in culture *(130)*. Scheduling, duration of exposure, and concentration of cisplatin were examined and it was found that these variables had major effects on treatment outcome with exposure to cisplatin shortly after radiation therapy providing greater-than-additive tumor cell killing. A similar study was carried out using human PC-9 and Lu 134A lung cancer cell lines *(131)*. The simultaneous combination of cisplatin and radiation therapy provided primarily additive growth inhibition of the cells as determined by isobologram analysis. In another cell culture study using human LNCaP and DU-145 prostate cancer cells, vitamin D analogs were examined in combination with cisplatin or carboplatin using isobologram analysis. Exposure of the cells to relatively high concentration of the vitamin D analog, 1a,25-dihydroxyvitamin D_3 along with an antitumor platinum complex resulted in greater-than-additive growth inhibition of the cells *(132)*.

4. Conclusion

My doctoral mentor often said that he was interested in biological significance and that he did not care about statistical significance. Indeed, it is often easier to find statistical significance than it is to find biological significance. We are at a point in the science of the study of combinations of treatments that the determination of whether a particular combination regimen in a specific model system produces a greater or lesser effect than expected can readily be assessed by either the median effect/ combination index or the isobologram or other mathematically valid method. We have computers with statistical packages to aid us in these determinations. The challenge remains before us to discern the biologic significance of our findings outside of our model systems. The very useful tools represented by the median effect/combination index and isobologram methodologies supplement scientific intuition. These methods should be applied whenever the experimental system allows.

References

1. Teicher, B. A., Herman, T. S., Holden, S. A., and Eder, J. P. (1991) Chemotherapeutic potentiation through interaction at the level of DNA, in *Synergism and Antagonism in Chemotherapy* (Chou, T.-C. and Rideout, D. C., eds.), Academic Press, Orlando, FL, pp. 541–583.
2. Teicher, B. A. and Frei, E. III. (2000) Laboratory models to evaluate new agents for the systemic treatment of lung cancer, in *Multimodality Treatment of Lung Cancer* (Skarin, A. T, ed.), Marcel Dekker, New York, pp. 301–336.
3. Chou, T. C. and Talalay, P. (1977) A simple generalized equation for the analysis of multiple inhibitions of Michaelis-Menten kinetic systems. *J. Biol. Chem.* **252,** 6438–6442.
4. Chou, T. C. and Talalay, P. (1981) Generalized equations for the analysis of inhibitors of Michaelis-Menten and higher order kinetic systems with two or more mutually exclusive and nonexclusive inihbitors. *Eur. J. Biochem.* **115,** 207–216.

5. Chou, T. C. and Talalay, P. (1983) Analysis of combined drug effects: A new look at a very old problem. *Trends Pharmacol. Sci.* **4,** 450–454.

6. Chou, T. C. and Talalay, P. (1984) Quantitative analysis of dose-effect relationships: The combined effects of multiple drugs or enzyme inhibitors. *Adv. Enzyme Regul.* **22,** 27–55.

7. Chou, T. C. and Talalay, P. (1987) Application of the median-effect principle for the assessment of low-dose risk of carcinogens and for the quantitation of synergism and antagonism of chemotherapeutic agents, in *New Avenues in Developmental Cancer Chemotherapy* (Harrap, K. and Connors, T. A., eds.), Bristol-Myers Symp. vol. 8, Academic Press, Orlando, FL, pp. 37–64.

8. Chou, J. and Chou, T. C. (1985) Dose-effect analysis with microcomputers: Quantitiation of ED_{50}, ID_{50}, synergism, antagonism, low-risk receptor ligand binding and enzyme kinetics. Software for Apple II microcomputers. Elsevier-Biosoft, Cambridge, England.

9. Chou, J. and Chou, T. C. (1987) Dose-effect analysis with microcomputers: Quantitiation of ED_{50}, ID_{50}, synergism, antagonism, low-risk receptor ligand binding and enzyme kinetics. Software for IBM-PC microcomputers. Elsevier-Biosoft, Cambridge, England.

10. Chou, J. and Chou, T. C. (1988) Computerized simulation of dose reduction index (DRI) in synergistic drug combinations. *Pharmacologist* **30,** A231.

11. Chou, T.-C. (1991) The median-effect principle and the combination index for quantiation of synergism and antagonism, in *Synergism and Antagonism in Chemotherapy* (Chou, T.-C. and Rideout, D. C., eds.), Academic Press, Orlando, FL, pp. 61–102.

12. Chou, J. H. (1991) Quantitation of synergism and antagonism of two or more drugs by computerized analysis, in *Synergism and Antagonism in Chemotherapy* (Chou, T.-C. and Rideout, D. C., eds.), Academic Press, Orlando, FL, pp. 223–241.

13. Berenbaum, M. C. (1989) What is synergy? *Pharmacol. Rev.* **41,** 93–141.

14. Berenbaum, M. C. (1977) Synergy, additivism and antagonism in immunosupression. *Clin. Exp. Immunol.* **28,** 1–18.

15. Gemcitabine HCl (LY188011 HCl) clinical investigational brochure. Indianapolis, IN: Eli Lilly and Company, October 1993.

16. Huang, P., Chubb, S., Hertel, L., and Plunkett, W. (1990) Mechanism of action of 2′,2′-difluorodeoxycytidine triphosphate on DNA synthesis (Abstr 2530). *Proc. Amer. Assoc. Cancer. Res.* **31,** 426.

17. Hertel., L., Boder, G. and Kroin, J. (1990) Evaluation of the antitumor activity of gemcitabine 2′,2′- difluoro-2′-deoxycytidine. *Cancer Res.* **50,** 4417–4422.

18. Bouffard, D., Fomparlwer, L., and Momparler, R. (1991) Comparison of the antineoplastic activity of 2′,2′-difluorodeoxycytidine and cytosine arabinoside against human myeloid and lymphoid leukemia cells. *Anticancer Drugs* **2,** 49–55.

19. Heinemann, V., Hertel, L., Grindey, G., and Plunkett, W. (1988) Comparison of the cellular pharmacokinetics and toxicity of 2′,2′-difluorodeoxycytidine and 1-beta-°-arabinofuranosyl cytosine. *Cancer Res.* **48,** 4024–4031.

20. Eckhardt, I. and Von Hoff, D. (1994) New drugs in clinical development in the United States. *Hematol. Oncol. Clin. North Amer.* **8,** 300–332.

21. Anderson, H., Lund, B., and Bach, F. (1994) Single-agent activity of weekly gemcitabine in advanced non-small cell lung cancer: a Phase 2 study. *J. Clin. Oncol.* **12,** 1821–1826.

22. Gatzemeier, U., Shapard, F., LeChevalier, T., et al. (1996) Activity of gemcitabine in patients with non-small cell lung cancer: a multicentre, extended Phase II study. *Eur. J. Cancer* **32A,** 243–248.

23. Verweij, J., Sparreboom, A., and Nooter, K. (1999) Mitomycins. *Cancer Chemother. Biol. Response. Mod.* **18,** 46–58.

24. Yang, X. L. and Wang, A. H. (1999) Structural studies of atom-specific anticancer drugs acting on DNA. *Pharmacol. Therap.* **83,** 181–215.

25. Spanswick, V, J., Cummings, J., and Smyth, J. F. (1998) Current 6 issues in the enzymology of mitomycin C metabolic activation. *Gen. Pharmacol.* **31,** 539–544.

26. Cummings, J., Spanswick, V. J., Tomasz, M., and Smyth, J. F. (1998) Enzymology of mitomycin C metabolic activation in tumor tissue: implications for enzyme-directed bioreductive drug development. *Biochem. Pharm.* **56,** 405–414.

27. Tomasz, M. and Palom, Y. (1997) The mitomycin bioreductive antitumor agents: cross-linking and alkylation of DNA as the molecular basis of their activity. *Pharm. Therap.* **76,** 73–87.

28. Boyer, M. J. (1997) Bioreductive agents: a clinical update. *Oncol. Res.* **9,** 391–395.

29. van Moorse, C. J., Veerman, G., and Bergman, A. M., Guechev, A., Vermorken, J. B., Postmus, P. E., and Peters, G. J. (1997) Combination chemotherapy studies with gemcitabine. *Semin. Oncol.* **24 (Suppl. 7),** 17–23.

30. Aung, T. T., Davis, M. A., Ensminger, W. D., and Lawrence, T. S. (2000) Interaction between gemcitabine and mitomycin C in vitro. *Cancer Chemother. Pharmacol.* **45,** 38–42.

31. Highley, M. S. and Calvert, A. H. (2000) Clinical experience with cisplatin and carboplatin, in *Platinum-Based Drugs in Cancer Therapy* (Kelland, L. R. and Farrell, N. P., eds.), Humana Press, Totowa, NJ, pp. 171–194.

32. Perez, R. P. (1998) Cellular and molecular determinants of cisplatin resistance. *Eur. J. Cancer* **34,** 1535–1542.

33. Eastman, A. (1987) The formation, isolation and characterization of DNA adducts produced by anticancer platinum complexes. *Pharmacol. Ther.* **34,** 155–166.

34. Fink, D. Z. H., Nebel, S., Norris, S., et al. (1997) In vitro and in vivo resistance to cisplatin in cells that have lost DNA mismatch repair. *Cancer Res.* **57,** 1841–1845.

35. van Moorsel, C. J., Veerman, G., Bergman, A. M., et al. (1997) Combination chemotherapy studies with gemcitabine. *Semin. Oncol.* **24,** S717–S723.

36. Peters, G. J., Ruiz van Haperen, V. W., Bergman, A. M., et al. (1996) Preclinical combination therapy with gemcitabine and mechanisms of resistance. *Semin. Oncol.* **23,** 16–24.

37. Braakhuis, B. J., Ruiz van Haperen, V. W., Welters, M. J., and Peters, G. J. (1995) Schedule-dependent therapeutic efficacy of the combination of gemcitabine and cisplatin in head and neck cancer xenografts. *Eur. J. Cancer* **31A,** 2335–2340.
38. Bergman, A. M., Ruiz van Haperen, V. W., Veerman, G., Kuiper, C. M., and Peters, G. J. (1996) Synergistic interaction between cisplatin and gemcitabine in vitro. *Clin. Cancer Res.* **2,** 521–530.
39. Tsai, C. M., Chang, K. T., Chen, J. Y., Chen, Y. M., Chen, M. H., and Perng, R. P. (1996) Cytotoxic effects of gemcitabine-containing regimens against human non-small cell lung cancer cell lines which express different levels of p185neu. *Cancer Res.* **56,** 794–801.
40. Voigt, W., Bulankin, A. Q., Muller, T., et al. (2000) Schedule-dependent antagonism of gemcitabine and cisplatin in human anaplastic thyroid cancer cell lines. *Clin. Cancer Res.* **6,** 2087–2093.
41. Van Moorsel, C. J. A., Pinedo, H. M., Veerman, G., et al. (1999) Mechanisms of synergism between cisplatin and gemcitabine in ovarian and non-small cell lung cancer cell lines. *Br. J. Cancer* **80,** 981–990.
42. Kunimoto, T., Nitta, K., Tanaka, T., et al. (1987) Antitumor activity of 7-ethyl-10-[4-(1-piperidino)-1-piperidino]-caronyloxy-camptothecin, a novel water soluble derivative of camptothecin, against murine tumors. *Cancer Res.* **47,** 5944–5947.
43. Kawato, Y., Aonuma, M., Hirota, Y., Kuga, H., and Sato, K. (1991) Intracellular roles of SN-38, a metabolite of the camptothecin derivative CPT-11, in the antitumor effect of CPT-11. *Cancer Res.* **51,** 4187–4191.
44. Shimada, Y., Rothenberg, M. L., Hilsenbeck, S. G., Burris, H. A., Degen, D., and Von Hoff, D. D. (1994) Activity of CPT-11 (irinotecan hydrochloride), a topoisomerase I inhibitor, against human tumor colony-forming units. *Anticancer Drugs* **5,** 202–206.
45. Kawato, Y., Furuta, T., Aonuma, M., Yasuoka, T., and Matsumotot, K. (1991) Antitumor activity of a camptothecin derivative, CPT-11, against human tumor xenografts in nude mice. *Cancer Chemother. Pharmacol.* **28,** 192–198.
46. Tsuruo, T., Matsuzaki, T., Matsushita, M., Saito, H., and Yokokura, T. (1988) Antitumor effect of CPT-11, a new derivative of camptothecin, against pleiotropic drug-resistant tumors in vitro and in vivo. *Cancer Chemother. Pharmacol.* **21,** 71–74.
47. Bahadori, H. R., Lima, C. M. S. R., Green, M. R., and Safa, A. R. (1999) Synergistic effect of gemcitabine and irinotecan (CPT-11) on breast and small cell lung cancer cell lines. *Anticancer Res.* **19,** 5423–5428.
48. Robinson, M. I. and Osheroff, N. (1990) Stabilization of the topoisomerase II-DNA cleavage complex by antineoplastic drugs: inhibition of enzyme-mediated DNA religation by 4′-(9-acridinylamino)methane-sulfon-*m*-anisidide. *Biochemistry* **29,** 2511–2515.
49. Dombernosky, P. and Nissen, I. (1976) Combination chemotherapy with 4′-demethyl-epipodophyllotoxin 9-(4,6-*O*-ethylidene-β-D-glucopyranoside) VP-16-213 (NCS 141540) in L1210 leukemia. *Eur. J. Cancer* **12,** 181–188.

50. Pommier, Y. (1997) DNA topoisomerase II inhibitors, in *Cancer Therapeutics: Experimental and Clinical Aspects* (Teicher, B. A., ed.), Humana Press, Totowa, NJ, pp. 153–174.

51. van Moorsel, C. J. A., Pinedo, H. M., Veerman, G., et al. (1999) Combination chemotherapy studies with gemcitabine and etoposide in non-small cell lung and ovarian cancer cell lines. *Biochem. Pharmacol.* **57**, 407–415.

52. Rowinsky, E. K. and Donehower, R. C. (1995) Paclitaxel (Taxol). *N. Engl. J. Med.* **332**, 1004–1014.

53. Hortobagyi, G. N., Holmes, F. A., Ibrahim, N., Champlin, R., and Buzdar, A. U. (1997) The University of Texas M. D. Anderson Cancer Center experience with paclitaxel in breast cancer. *Semin. Oncol.* **1 (Suppl. 3)**, S30–S33.

54. McGuire, W. P. and Ozols, R. F. (1998) Chemotherapy of advanced ovarian cancer. *Semin. Oncol.* **3**, 340–348.

55. Schiff, P. B., Fant, J., and Horwitz, S. B. (1979) Promotion of microtubule assembly in vitro by paclitaxel. *Nature* **277**, 665–667.

56. Schiff, P. B. and Horwtiz, S. Paclitaxel stabilizes microtubules in mouse fibroblast cells. *Proc. Natl. Acad. Sci. USA* **77**, 1561–1565.

57. Kumar, N. (1981) Paclitaxel-induced polymerization of purified tubulin. Mechanism of action. *J. Biol. Chem.* **256**, 10,435–10,441.

58. Cos, J., Bellmunt, J., Soler, C., et al. (2000) Comparative study of sequential combinations of paclitaxel and methotrexate on a human bladder cancer cell line. *Cancer Invest.* **18**, 429–435.

59. McDaid, H. M. and Johnston, P. G. (1999) Synergistic interaction between paclitaxel and 8-chloro-adenosine-3′,5′-monophosphate in human ovarian carcinoma cell lines. *Clin. Cancer. Res.* **5**, 215–220.

60. Perez, E. A. and Buckwalter, C. A. (1998) Sequence-dependent cytotoxicity of etoposide and paclitaxel in human breast and lung cancer cell lines. *Cancer Chemother. Pharmacol.* **41**, 448–452.

61. Hamel, E. (1996) Antimitotic natural products and their interactions with tubulin. *Med. Res. Rev.* **16**, 207–231.

62. Sackett, D. I. (1995) Vinca site agents induce structural changes in tubulin different from and antagonistic to changes induced by cholchicine site agents. *Biochemistry* **34**, 7010–7019.

63. Giannakakou, P., Villalba, L., Li, H., Poruchynsky, M., and Fojo, T. (1998) Combinations of paclitaxel and vinblastine and their effects on tubulin polymerization and cellular cytotoxicity: characterization of a synergistic schedule. *Int. J. Cancer* **75**, 57–63.

64. Hoffman, R. M. and Erbe, R. W. (1976) High in vivo rate of methionine biosynthesis in transformed human and malignant rat cells auxotropic for methionine. *Proc. Natl. Acad. Sci. USA* **73**, 1523–1527.

65. Hoffman, R. M. (1984) Altered methionine metabolism, DNA methylation and oncogene expression in carcinogenesis: a review and synthesis. *Biochem. Biophys. Acta* **738**, 49–87.

66. Stern, P. H., Wallace, C. D., and Hoffman, R. M. (1984) Altered methionine metabolism occurs in all members of a set of diverse human tumor cells. *J. Cell Physiol.* **119,** 29–34.
67. Stern, P. H. and Hoffman, R. M. (1984) Elevated overall rates of transmethylation in cell lines from diverse human tumors. *In Vitro* **20,** 663–670.
68. Stern, P. H., Mecham, J. O., Wallace, C. D., and Hoffman, R. M. (1984) Reduced free methionine-dependent SV40 transformed human fibroblasts synthesizing apparently normal of methionine. *J. Cell Physiol.* **117,** 9–14.
69. Breillout, F., Antoine, E., and Poupon, M. F. (1990) Methionine dependency of malignant tumors: a possible approach for therapy. *J. Natl. Cancer Inst.* **82,** 1628–1632.
70. Tanaka, H., Esaki, N., and Soda, K. (1977) Properties of L-methionine-γ-lyase from *Pseudomonas ovalis. Biochemistry* **16,** 100–106.
71. Tan, Y., Xu, M., Tan, X. Z., et al. (1997) Overexpression and large-scale production of recombinant L-methionine-α-deamino-γ-mercaptomethane-lyase for novel anticancer therapy. *Protein Express. Purif.* **9,** 233–245.
72. Miki, K., Al-Refaie, W., Xu, M., et al. (2000) Methioninase gene therapy of human cancer cells is synergistic with recombinant methioninase treatment. *Cancer Res.* **60,** 2696–2702.
73. Tan, Y., Xu, M., Guo, H., Sun, X., Kubota, T., and Hoffman, R. M. (1996) Anticancer efficacy of methioninase in vivo. *Anticancer Res.* **16,** 3931–3936.
74. Yoshioka, T., Wada, T., Uchida, N., et al. (1998) Anticancer efficacy in vivo and in vitro, synergy with 5-fluorouracil and safety of recombinant methionine. *Cancer Res.* **58,** 2583–2587.
75. Tan, Y., Sun, X., Xu, M., et al. (1999) Efficacy of recombinant methioninase in combination with cisplatin on human colon tumors in nude mice. *Clin. Cancer Res.* **5,** 2157–2163.
76. Beran, M., McCredie, K. B., Keating, M. J., and Gutterman, J. U. (1988) Antileukemic effect of recombinant tumor necrosis factor α in vitro and its modulation by α and γ interferons. *Blood* **72,** 728–738.
77. Berenbaum, M. C. (1969) Dose-response curves for agents that impair cell reproductive integrity. A fundamental difference between dose-response curves for antimetabolites and those for radiation and alkylating agents. *Br. J. Cancer* **23,** 426–433.
78. Harsthorn, K. L., Sandstrom, E. G., Neumeyer, D., et al. (1987) Synergistic inhibition of human T-cell lymphotropic virus type III replication in vitro by phosphonoformate and recombinant alpha-A interferon. *Antibiot. Agents Chemother.* **30,** 189–191.
79. Hartshorn, K. L., Vogt, M. W., Chou, T.-C., et al. (1987) Synergistic inhibition of human immunodeficiency virus in vitro by azidothymidine and recombinant alpha A interferon. *Antibiot. Agents Chemother.* **31,** 168–172.
80. Hubbell, H. R. (1988) Synergistic antiproliferative effect of human interferons in combination with mismatched double-stranded RNA on human tumor cells. *Int. J. Cancer* **37,** 359–365.

81. King, T. C. and Krogstad, D. J. (1983) Spectrophotometric assessment of dose-response curves for single antimicrobial agents and antimicrobial combinations. *J. Infect. Dis.* **147,** 758–764.

82. Murohashi, I., Nagata, K., Suzuki, T., Maruyama, Y., and Nara, N. (1988) Effects of recombinant G- CSF and GM-CSF on the growth in methylcellulose and suspension of the blast cells in acute myeloblastic leukemia. *Leuk. Res.* **12,** 433–440.

83. Sobrero, A. F. and Bertino, J. R. (1983) Sequence-dependent synergism between dichloromethotrexate and 5-fluorouracil in a human colon carcinoma line. *Cancer Res.* **43,** 4011–4013.

84. Tallarida, R. J., Stone, D. J., and Raffa, R. B. (1997) Efficient deigns for studying synergistic drug combinations. *Life Sci.* **61,** 417–425.

85. Steel, G. G. and Peckham, M. J. (1979) Exploitable mechanisms in combined radiotherapy-chemotherapy: The concept of additivity. *Ont. J. Radiat. Oncol. Biol. Phys.* **5,** 85–91.

86. Dewey, W. C., Stone, L. E., Miller, H. H., and Giblak, R. E. (1977) Radiosensitization with 5-bromodeoxyuridine of Chinese hamster cells x-irradiated during different phases of the cell cycle. *Radiat. Res.* **47,** 672–688.

87. Deen, D. F. and Williams, M. W. (1979) Isobologram analysis of x-ray-BCNU interactions in vitro. *Radiat. Res.* **79,** 483–491.

88. Schabel, F. M., Trader, M. W., Laster, W. R., Wheeler, G. P., and Witt, M. H. (1978) Patterns of resistance and therapeutic synergism among alkylating agents. *Antibiot. Chemother.* **23,** 200–215.

89. Schabel, F. M., Griswold, D. P., Corbett, T. H., Laster, W. R., Jr., Mayo, J. G., and Lloyd, H. H. (1979) Testing therapeutic hypotheses in mice treated with anticancer drugs that have demonstrated or potential clinical utility for treatment of advanced solid tumors of man. *Meth. Cancer Res.* **17,** 3–51.

90. Schabel, F. M., Jr. (1975) Concepts for systemic treatment of micrometastases. *Cancer* **35,** 15–24.

91. Schabel, F. M., Jr., Griswold, D. P., Jr., Corbett, T. H. and Laster, W. R., Jr. (1984) Increasing the therapeutic response rates to anticancer drugs by applying the basic principles of pharmacology. *Cancer* **54,** 1160–1167.

92. Schabel, F. M., Jr. and Simpson-Herren L. (1978) Some variables in experimental tumor systems which complicate interpretation of data from in vivo kinetic and pharmacologic studies with anticancer drugs. *Antibiotics Chemotherap.* **23,** 113–127.

93. Schabel, F. M., Jr., Griswold, D. P., Jr., Corbett, T. H., and Laster, W. R. (1983) Increasing therapeutic response rates to anticancer drugs by applying the basic principles of pharmacology. *Pharmac. Therap.* **20,** 283–305.

94. Corbett, T. H., Griswold, D. P., Jr., Roberts, B. J., Peckham, J. C., and Schabel, F. M., Jr. (1977) Evaluation of single agents and combinations of chemotherapeutic agents in mouse colon carcinomas. *Cancer* **40,** 2660–2680.

95. Corbett, T. H., Griswold, D. P., Jr., Wolpert, M. K., Venditti, J. M., and Schabel, F. M., Jr. (1979) Design and evaluation of combination chemotherapy trials in experimental animal tumor systems. *Cancer Treat. Rep.* **63,** 799–801.

96. Griswold, D. P., Jr., Corbett, T. H., and Schabel, F. M., Jr. (1980) Cell kinetics and the chemotherapy of murine solid tumors. *Antibiotics Chemother.* **28**, 28–34.

97. Griswold, D. P., Corbett, T. H., and Schabel, F. M., Jr. (1981) Clonogenicity and growth of experimental tumors in relation to developing resistance and therapeutic failure. *Cancer Treat. Rep.* **65 (Suppl. 2)**, 51–54.

98. Teicher, B. A., Herman, T. S., Holden, S. A., et al. (1990) Tumor resistance to alkylating agents conferred by mechanisms operative only in vivo. *Science* **247**, 1457–1461.

99. Teicher, B. A., Holden, S. A, Cucchi, C. A., Cathcart, K. N. S., Korbut, T. T., Flatow, J. L., and Frei, E., III (1988) Combination of N,N′,N″-triethylenethiophosphoramide and cyclophosphamide in vitro and in vivo. *Cancer Res.* **48**, 94–100.

100. Teicher, B. A., Holden, S. A., Eder, J. P., Brann, T. W., Jones, S. M., and Frei, E., III (1990) Preclinical studies relating to the use of thiotepa in the high-dose setting alone and in combination. *Semin. Oncol.* **17**, 18–32.

101. Teicher, B. A., Holden, S. A., Jones, S. M., Eder, J. P., and Herman, T. S. (1989) Influence of scheduling on two-drug combinations of alkylating agents in vivo. *Cancer Chemother. Pharmacol.* **25**, 161–166.

102. Teicher, B. A., Waxman, D. J., Holden, S. A., et al. (1989) Evidence for enzymatic activation and oxygen involvement in cytotoxicity and antitumor activity of N,N′,N″-triethylenethiophosphoramide. *Cancer Res.* **49**, 4996–5001.

103. Sugiura, K. and Stock C. (1955) Studies in a tumor spectrum. III. The effect of phosphoramides on the growth of a variety of mouse and rat tumors. *Cancer Res.* **15**, 38–51.

104. Sugiura, K. and Stock C. (1952) Studies in a tumor spectrum. I. Comparison of the action of methylbis(2-chloroethyl)amine and 3-bis(2-chloroethyl) aqminomethyl-4-methoxymethyl-5-hydroxy-6-methylpyridine on the growth of a variety of mouse and rat tumors. *Cancer* **5**, 282–315.

105. Sugiura, K. and Stock, C. (1952) Studies in a tumor spectrum. II. The effect of 2,4,6-triethyleneimino-S-triazine on the growth of a variety of mouse and rat tumors. *Cancer* **5**, 979–991.

106. DeWys, W. (1972) A quantitative model for the study of the growth and treatment of a tumor and its metastases with correlation between proliferative state and sensitivity to cyclophosphamide. *Cancer Res.* **32**, 367–373.

107. DeWys, W. (1972) Studies correlating the growth rate of a tumor and its metastases and providing evidence for tumor-related systemic growth-retarding factors. *Cancer Res.* **32**, 374–379.

108. Steel, G. G. and Adams, K. (1975) Stem-cell survival and tumor control in the Lewis lung carcinoma. *Cancer Res.* **35**, 1530–1535.

109. Steel, G. G., Nill, R. P., and Peckham, M. J. (1978) Combined radiotherapy-chemotherapy of Lewis lung carcinoma. *Int. J. Radiat. Oncol. Biol. Phys.* **4**, 49–52.

110. Bertelli, P., Mantica, C., Farina, G., et al. (1994) Treatment of non-small cell lung cancer with vinorelbine. *Proc. Amer. Soc. Clin. Oncol.* **13**, 362.

111. Bore, P., Rahmani, R., and VanCamfort, J. (1989) Pharmacokinetics of a new anticancer drug, navelbine, in patients. *Cancer Chemother. Pharmacol.* **23**, 247–251.

112. Cros, S, Wright, M., and Morimoto, M. (1989) Experimental antitumor activity of navelbine. *Semin. Oncol.* **16 (Suppl.)**, 15–20.

113. Cvitkovic, E. (1992) The current and future place of vinorelbine in cancer therapy. *Drugs* **44 (Suppl. 4)**, 36–45.

114. Marquet, P, Lachatre, G., and Debord, J. (1992) Pharmacokinetics of vinorelbine in man. *Eur. J. Clin. Pharmacol.* **42**, 545–547.

115. Navelbine (vinorelbine tartrate) clinical investigational brochure. Burroughs Wellcome Co., October 1995.

116. Fumoleau, P., Delgado, F., Delozier, T., et al. (1993) Phase II trial of weekly intravenous vinorelbine in first line advanced breast cancer chemotherapy. *J. Clin. Oncol.* **11**, 1245–1252.

117. Jehl, F., Quoix, E., and Leveque, D. (1991) Pharmacokinetics and preliminary metabolite fate of vinorelbine in human as determined by high performance liquid chromatography. *Cancer Res.* **51**, 2073–2076.

118. Lepierre, A., Lemarie, E., Dabouis, G., and Garnier, G. (1991) A Phase 2 study of navelbine in the treatment of non-small cell lung cancer. *Amer. J. Clin. Oncol.* **14**, 115–119.

119. Shih, C. and Thornton, D. E. (1998) Preclinical pharmacology studies and the clinical development of a novel multitargeted antifolate, MTA (LY231514), in *Anticancer Drug Development Guide: Antifolate Drugs in Cancer Therapy* (Jackman, A. L., ed.), Totowa, NJ, Humana Press, pp. 183–201.

120. Rinaldi, D. A., Burris, H. A., Dorr, F. A., et al. (1995) Initial Phase I evaluation of the novel thymidylate synthase inhibitor, LY231514, using the modified continual reassessment method for dose escalation. *J. Clin. Oncol.* **13**, 2842–2850.

121. McDonald, A. C., Vasey, P. A., Adams, L., et al. (1998) A phase I and Pharmacokinetic study of LY231514, the multitargeted antifolate. *Clin. Cancer Res.* **4**, 605–610.

122. Takimoto, C. H. (1997) Antifolates in clinical development. *Semin. Oncol.* **24 (Suppl. 18)**, 40–51.

123. Brandt, D. S. and Chu, E. (1997) Future challenges in the clinical development of thymidylate synthase inhibitor compounds. *Oncol. Res.* **9**, 403–410.

124. O'Reilly, S. and Rowinsky, E. C. (1996) The clinical status of irinotecan (CPT-11), a novel water soluble camptothecin analogue. *Crit. Rev. Oncol. Hematol.* **24**, 47–70.

125. Aschele, C., Baldo, C., Sobrero, A. F., et al. (1998) Schedule-dependent synergism between ZD1694 (ralititrexed) and CPT-11 (irinotecan) in human colon cancer in vitro. *Clin. Cancer Res.* **4**, 1323–1330.

126. O'Reilly, S. and Rowinsky, E. C. (1996) The clinical status of irinotecan (CPT-11), a novel water soluble camptothecin analogue. *Crit. Rev. Oncol. Hematol.* **24**, 47–70.

127. Satoh, H., Ishikawa, H., Fujimoto, M., et al. (1998) Combined effects of TNP-470 and taxol in human non-small cell lung cancer cell lines. *Anticancer Res.* **18,** 1027–1030.

128. Ogawa, H., Sato, Y., Kondo, M., et al. (2000) Combined treatment with TNP-470 and 5-fluorouracil effectively inhibits growth of murine colon cancer cells in vitro and liver metastasis in vivo. *Oncol. Rep.* **7,** 467–472.

129. Pegram, M., Hsu, S., Lewis, G., et al. (1999) Inhibitory effects of combinations of HER-2/neu antibody and chemotherapeutic agents used for treatment of human breast cancers. *Oncogene* **18,** 2241–2251.

130. Gorodetsky, R., Levy-Agababa, F., Mou, X., and Vexler, A. M. (1998) Combinations of cisplatin and radiation in cell culture: effect of duration of exposure to drug and timing of irradiation. *Int. J. Cancer* **75,** 635–642.

131. Fujita, M., Fujita, T., Kodama, T., Tsuchida, T., and Higashino, K. (2000) The inhibitory effect of cisplatin in combination with irradiation on lung tumor cell growth is due to induction of tumor cell apoptosis. *Int. J. Oncol.* **17,** 393–397.

132. Moffatt, K. A., Johannes, W. U., and Miller, G. J. (1999) 1a,25-Dihydroxyvitamin D3 and platinum drugs act synergistically to inhibit the growth of prostate cancer cell lines. *Clin. Cancer Res.* **5,** 695–703.

25

Flow Cytometric Methods for Detection and Quantification of Apoptosis

David P. Steensma, Michael Timm, and Thomas E. Witzig

1. Introduction
1.1. Background

The accumulation of cells characteristic of neoplastic disease results from the combination of unrestrained cell growth and diminished cell death. One form of programmed cell death, *apoptosis* (a Greek neologism meaning "dropping off" that conjures images of leaves falling from a tree in autumn), is an important mechanism of normal cellular population control *(1)*. Cells that are physiologically unwanted (e.g., auto-reactive lymphocytes) and cells that have suffered irreversible DNA-damaging injury (e.g., from ultraviolet light or irradiation) may be eliminated via apoptosis. Cytoreductive antineoplastic therapy operates in part by triggering apoptosis of susceptible cells *(2,3)*.

Apoptotic changes are stereotypical, and the process is highly conserved across species *(4)*. Morphologically, apoptosis is characterized by condensation of the cellular nucleus and fragmentation of chromosomal material, followed by the release of membrane-bound apoptotic bodies that are subsequently phagocytized by a wide variety of cells without any release of inflammatory mediators. Biochemically, a family of cysteine proteases called caspases act as the key intracellular effector molecules of apoptosis by cleaving a series of specific cytoskeletal and nuclear proteins at a restricted repertoire of sites resulting in cellular demise *(5)*. Members of the caspase family are activated sequentially following a wide variety of apoptosis-triggering events such as binding of ligand to a cell surface death receptor or the release of cytochrome c from mitochondria. A complex web of pro-apoptotic and anti-apoptotic proteins carefully regulates caspase activity.

From: *Methods in Molecular Medicine, vol. 85: Novel Anticancer Drug Protocols*
Edited by: J. K. Buolamwini and A. A. Adjei © Humana Press Inc., Totowa, NJ

Apoptosis can be detected and quantified by several methods. Apoptosis is a dynamic process, and the diverse methods of apoptosis assessment vary in their sensitivity and specificity for the different stages of apoptosis. As a result, different methods may yield varying results, even when the same specimen is analyzed at the same time.

1.2. Morphologic Assessment of Apoptosis

There are a number of tissue-based assays for detecting apoptosis that are not based on flow cytometric principles. Simple morphologic analysis supplemented by electron microscopy can reveal apoptotic bodies as well as the typical late apoptotic findings of chromatin condensation and nuclear fragmentation. DNA stains such as Hoechst 33258 and 4',6-diamidino-2-phenylindole (DAPI) can facilitate visualization of the condensed nuclear fragments typical of apoptosis. Although morphologic methods are historically important because they were the techniques by which apoptosis was first discovered (the process was originally called "shrinkage necrosis"), they are problematic. Apoptosis is not always easy to recognize in fixed tissue sections, early apoptotic cells have few structural changes and cannot generally be detected, and quantification by such techniques is quite cumbersome *(6)*.

1.3. The DNA Ladder

Agarose gel electrophoresis of cells undergoing apoptosis may reveal the characteristic pattern of a "DNA ladder." The DNA ladder is a bold visual display of DNA fragments of varying lengths, typically multiples of 180–200 base pairs; the rungs are fragments of nuclear DNA that have been degraded by caspases and other endonucleases. Unfortunately, electrophoresis is neither completely sensitive nor totally specific, so the finding of a DNA ladder is not synonymous with apoptosis. DNA ladders, like apoptotic bodies, are a late finding in the apoptosis cascade, if they appear at all. DNA degradation patterns resembling a ladder may be observed in other forms of cell death, and in some forms of apoptosis, DNA cleavage does not proceed all the way to the 180–200 base pair level *(7)*. In addition, the DNA ladder method does not allow spatial localization of the specific cells undergoing apoptosis and is therefore of limited value in tissues with mixed cell populations such as blood and bone marrow.

1.4. ISEL and TUNEL

Other tissue-based methods such as *in situ* end labeling (ISEL) and the related *in situ* terminal deoxynucleotidyl transferase-mediated dUTP nick-end labeling (TUNEL) techniques detect the single- and double-strand DNA breaks that occur during intra-nucleosomal DNA degradation in early apoptosis *(8,9)*.

(The nick-ends can also be detected by flow cytometry, as described below.) These methods can preserve tissue architecture and also allow quantification. However, counting cells in order to obtain an accurate apoptotic index must generally be done manually with ISEL and TUNEL; this is time consuming.

1.5. Flow Cytometry

Flow cytometric methods of apoptosis detection offer several advantages over the above techniques. Flow cytometers make use of a focused beam of laser light to interrogate a single-cell suspension whose laminar flow through a chamber is tightly controlled. The light scattering and fluorescent properties of these cells in fluid suspension and any bound antibodies (which may be labeled with any of several fluorochromes) can be assayed via a series of filters and photomultiplier tubes.

Flow cytometry can rapidly quantify and evaluate the properties of thousands of cells. This is particularly important when the cells of interest are interspersed in a heterogeneous tissue such as bone marrow or blood, as is the case in most hematopoietic malignancies. The flow cytometer can simultaneously assess apoptosis-associated properties as well as the presence of other cell characteristics (e.g., cluster of differentiation markers or other cell surface antigens), allowing isolation and study of specific cellular subspecies ("gating") or correlation of apoptosis with other cellular features.

There are a series of differences between apoptotic cells and normal cells that can be exploited via flow cytometric techniques in order to allow apoptosis detection. These properties were recently reviewed by Darzynkiewicz et al. and include the following *(10)*:

1. *Changes in the plasma membrane:* Assays of plasma membrane alterations are the basis of several of the most useful flow cytometric techniques. One key change in early apoptosis is the translocation of phosphatidylserine from the inner aspect of the plasma membrane phospholipid bilayer to the outer aspect *(11)*. This molecular event can be detected with Annexin V, a calcium-dependent phospholipid binding protein that has a high affinity for negatively charged phospholipids such as phosphatidylserine *(12)*. Annexin V is commercially available conjugated to biotin or directly conjugated to a variety of fluorochromes *(13)*.

   Healthy, living cells with an intact plasma membrane retain the ability to exclude vital dyes such as trypan blue, propidium iodide (PI), 7-amino actinomycin D (7-AAD), ethidium monoazide, and DAPI. During cell death, the cellular plasma membrane becomes progressively altered and degraded and eventually reaches a point where it can no longer prevent the influx of such dyes. This membrane permeability is nonspecific characteristic of both necrosis and of late apoptosis. In apoptosis, the development of membrane permeability occurs subsequent to the phosphatidylserine inversion event labeled by Annexin

V. Because of their particular fluorescent properties, 7-AAD and PI are the most valuable vital dyes for flow cytometry applications *(14)*. Indeed, PI has been called the "flow cytometric equivalent of the trypan blue exclusion assay" *(10)*. This is because most current flow cytometers use a single argon laser that emits monochromatic light at 488 nm, so DNA dyes such as Hoechst 33342 and DAPI which fluoresce primarily under UV light are not useful on such instruments. Dual staining with Annexin V and a DNA-binding dye such as PI can distinguish three cell populations: live cells (Annexin negative and PI negative), early apoptotic cells (Annexin positive and PI negative), and late apoptotic or dead cells (Annexin positive and PI positive) *(13)*.

One final apoptosis-related membrane change is worth mentioning. During apoptosis, specialized plasma membrane structures such as pseudopodia and microvilli are lost and the cell membrane becomes very smooth. F-actin, a component of pseudopodia, can be stained with fluorescein-conjugated phallotoxins, such as phalloidin *(15)*. Phallotoxin staining is progressively lost during apoptosis, and this property can be combined with DNA content analysis to form the basis of a flow cytometric assay. Such assays are not widely used.

2. *Changes in cellular light scattering properties:* Flow cytometers have photometric tubes for detection of laser-generated photons scattered from cells. One key detector is positioned in the axis of the laser beam and another is located at a right angle to the beam. The intensity of laser light that is scattered in a "forward" direction (i.e., along the laser axis) by the cells in suspension is proportional to cell size, while that scattered at more acute angles ("side scatter") correlates with the degree of cell granularity. Side scatter is also dependent on the refractive properties of intracellular substructures. No specific reagents are needed to assess scattering characteristics; these are intrinsic to the cell.

During apoptosis, cells shrink and decrease their forward scatter, but chromatin condensation and other intracellular changes may actually result in increased side scatter early on in the apoptotic cascade *(10)*. In late apoptosis, however, both forward and side scatter decrease as cells continue to shrink and as chromatin and organelles are sloughed off as apoptotic bodies *(16)*. Such properties are unfortunately of limited value for flow cytometric detection of apoptosis because cellular debris (e.g., free nuclei and ruptured cells) and fragments of necrotic cells have similar light scattering properties to that of apoptotic cells.

3. *Changes in cellular DNA content and DNA sensitivity to denaturation:* Cellular DNA content can be quantified by various dyes following cell membrane permeabilization. During the cell permeabilization process, degraded and condensed DNA is poorly preserved. Unlike the case with live, healthy cells, much of the DNA of apoptotic cells is in a degraded and/or condensed form, so apoptotic cells exhibit reduced stainability when probed with DNA staining agents compared with healthy cells. A "sub-G0/G1 peak" (so-called because the DNA content in these cells is less than the normal diploid DNA content of cells in the G0 and G1 phases of the cell cycle) or "A0" peak can then be seen on flow cytometric histograms of DNA content. The utility of this technique varies

with the stage of apoptosis and the specific process of DNA extraction *(17)*. Cellular and nuclear debris also have a sub-G1 DNA content, which can be misleading *(10)*.

Acridine orange (AO) is a fluorochrome that intercalates into double-stranded DNA, preventing renaturation of DNA after partial denaturation of the nucleic acid strands *(10,18)*. Apoptotic cells typically have more DNA in a condensed, denatured form than normal cells. AO staining followed by renaturation of DNA is the basis of one described assay for apoptosis detection *(19)*. It is important to recall that AO also stains lysosomes, and in order for AO to be useful in flow cytometry, cells must be fixed so that lysosomes no longer take up the dye.

4. *Labeling of DNA strand breaks:* Intranucleosomal DNA cleavage by endonucleosomes is characteristic of apoptosis, as described above. DNA strand breaks can be labeled with nucleotides conjugated to biotin or digoxigenin in the TUNEL assay. Once incorporated, these nucleotides can be stained with a variety of fluorochromes. A number of variants of nick-end-labeling techniques have been described. These assays are accurate but technically difficult, so proper controls are essential *(10)*.

5. *Changes in cellular organelles:* Early in apoptosis, the normal mitochondrial transmembrane voltage potential decreases. One method for detecting this alteration uses rhodamine 123, a fluorochrome that normally accumulates in the mitochondria of living, healthy cells. Rhodamine mitochondrial accumulation is dependent on transmembrane potential *(20)*. In early apoptosis, the ability of mitochondria to accumulate rhodamine is lost, a property that can be detected cytometrically.

Another mitochondria-based flow assay takes advantage of the newly described Apo2.7 (7A6) antigen *(21)*. This antigen's expression on the mitochondrial membrane seems to be restricted to cells undergoing apoptosis, but the discrimination between healthy and apoptotic cells appears narrow *(22)*. Apo2.7 based assays may turn out to be useful, but are not currently widely used. Changes in intracellular organelles other than mitochondria have not yet proven to be useful in apoptosis detection.

There are several potential challenges to the investigator using flow cytometric techniques for apoptosis analysis. All of the flow-based techniques described above do not reliably distinguish late apoptosis from necrosis. Apoptotic changes may sometimes be atypical; there is considerable overlap between apoptosis and necrosis *(7,23)*. Analysis of sub-G1 DNA content in particular is susceptible to artifact, as it may be confounded by the presence of cellular debris and nuclear material that escape from non-apoptotic cells during harsh pre-treatments that lyse cells. When in doubt, morphologic correlation can be helpful *(10)*.

Below, we describe the flow cytometric methods we have found most useful in our laboratory: Annexin V staining combined with 7-AAD or PI for assessment of cell permeability, PI or 7-AAD staining alone, sub-G1 DNA population analysis, and TUNEL.

2. Materials

1. Tissue sample of interest.
2. Fine wire mesh for liquefying sample (if tissue is from a solid tumor).
3. Flow cytometer (e.g., FACScan,™ a 3-color flow instrument, or FACScalibur,™ a four-color, dual-laser flow instrument—both available from Becton Dickinson) with computer and software (e.g., CellQuest,™ Becton Dickinson) for data analysis.
3. Fluorochrome-labeled monoclonal antibodies for separating out cell populations of interest—many vendors are available.
4. Streptavidin conjugated to fluorochromes for binding to biotinylated antibodies.
5. A viability staining agent such as 7-amino actinomycin D (7-AAD) or propidium iodide (PI).
6. Phosphate-buffered saline (PBS).
7. Annexin binding buffer with carefully titrated calcium concentration: 10 mM HEPES/NaOH, pH 7.4, 150 mM NaCl, 5 mM KCl, 1.8 mM CaCl$_2$, 1 mM MgCl$_2$.
8. 15-mL conical tubes and 50-mL centrifuge tubes.
9. Ammonium chloride (ACK) erythrocyte lysis buffer.
10. Coulter-style counter or hemocytometer.
11. Ficoll-Hypaque™ solution(s) for cell separation density centrifugation.

For TUNEL, will also need the following:

1. Paraformaldehyde solution: 4% in PBS, pH 7.4.
2. Permeabilization solution: 0.1% Triton X-100 in 0.1% sodium acetate.
3. TdT-mediated dUTP-X nick end labeling (TUNEL) reaction mixture.

3. Methods

3.1. Quantitation of Apoptosis Using Annexin V

1. This method can be used on bone marrow, whole blood, or tissue culture samples.
2. For bone marrow and whole blood samples, pipet 1 mL of sample into a 15-mL conical tube. Add 14 mL of ACK to destroy mature anucleate erythrocytes and incubate at room temperature for 5 min or until the suspension changes its optical properties and becomes transparent (*see* **Note 1**). Centrifuge for 5 min at 300g.
3. Wash pellet twice with PBS and resuspend in cold (4°C) Annexin binding buffer, adjusting cell suspension to a concentration of 1 × 10^6 cells/mL.
4. Add 100 µL of cell suspension and 5 µL of Annexin V to a 12 × 75 Falcon tube. Mix gently and incubate at 4°C for 20 min. If doing three- or four-color flow

cytometry, other antibodies to isolate specific cell populations can also be added at this time. However, it is prudent to avoid spectral overlap with the chosen form of Annexin V as much as possible.

5. Wash cells in 3 mL of cold Annexin binding buffer and centrifuge at 300*g* for 5 min.
6. Resuspend in 500 μL of cold Annexin binding buffer and add 10 μL PI (final concentration of 1 μg/mL, diluted in PBS) or 400 μL of 7-AAD (final concentration of 20 mg/mL in PBS). Incubate for 20 additional min and wash again.
7. Analyze samples on flow cytometer within 30 min. Cytometer will need to be compensated depending on the types and number of flourochromes used in each assay. Control tubes with Annexin only and PI or 7-AAD only are useful for compensation.

3.2. TUNEL Assay

1. Prepare cell suspension as in **steps 1–3** in **Subheading 3.1.**
2. Fix cells in 100 μL of paraformaldehyde solution. Incubate at room temperature for 30 min. Wash in 2 mL of PBS and centrifuge at 300*g* for 10 min. Discard supernatant.
3. Resuspend in permeabilization solution for 2 min on ice. Wash again in 2 mL of PBS and centrifuge at 300*g* for 5 min. Discard the supernatant.
4. Resuspend in 50 μL of TUNEL reaction mixture and incubate for 60 min at 37°C in a humidified atmosphere in the dark. Wash again in 2 mL of PBS and centrifuge at 300*g* for 5 min.
5. Resuspend in 500 μL PBS. Add 10 μL PI (adjust concentration to 1 μg/mL diluted in PBS) and incubate 20 min at 4°C.
6. Analyze.

3.3. Using 7-AAD Penetration (An Assay of Plasma Membrane Permeability) for Detection of Late Apoptosis

1. Prepare cell suspension as in **steps 1–2** in **Subheading 3.1.**
2. Wash cells twice with PBS.
3. Resuspend in PBS; adjust cell concentration to 1×10^6 cells/mL.
4. Add 100 μL of cell suspension and 400 μL of 7AAD (prepare a concentration of 7AAD of 20 μg/mL diluted in PBS) to a 12×75 Falcon tube. Set up another 12×75 Falcon tube without addition of 7-AAD to serve as negative control.
5. Incubate for 20 min at 4°C, wash in 3 mL of PBS and resuspend in 500 μL of PBS.
6. Analyze within 30 min.

3.4. Detection of a Sub-G0/G1 (A0) Population: A DNA Histogram Technique

1. Prepare cell suspension as in **steps 1–2** in **Subheading 3.1.**
2. Wash cell pellet twice in PBS.

3. Add 1×10^6 cells to a 12×75 Falcon tube and incubate pellet in either 2 mL of lysolecithin (final concentration 30 μg/mL) or 0.1% Triton X-100 for 30 min on ice to permeabilize the cells.
4. Wash twice in PBS.
5. Resuspend the cell pellet in 500 mL of PBS and add RNase (30 units/mL) to degrade any double stranded RNA (PI, a double-stranded nucleic acid intercalating agent, can also bind to RNA). Incubate at 37°C for 30 min.
6. Add 50–100 μL of PI (final concentration 1 μg/mL) and incubate at 4°C for 1–2 h before running on the flow cytometer.

4. Notes

1. Ammonium chloride (ACK) and other erythrocyte lysis buffers speed flow cytometry assays by decreasing contamination by red cells, but these agents can increase phosphatidylserine exposure and Annexin V binding on leukocytes up to 300-fold *(24)*. We have observed this phenomenon in our own laboratory in blood and bone marrow preparations; maturing nucleated erythroid precursors seem especially sensitive to ACK, perhaps because normal erythrocyte maturation involves condensation and exclusion of nuclear material—a process very similar to apoptosis, which may already stress the plasma membrane. Even density centrifugation with Ficoll-Hypaque and cell mixing via vigorous use of an agitator/vortex device can artifactually increase Annexin V binding (unpublished observations). If only the relative values of Annexin V binding between samples prepared in similar fashion are to be used, ACK lysis may still be reasonable, but if precise quantitation is important, unprocessed samples must be used. Such samples will naturally take much longer for the flow cytometer to process.
2. Double-density separation using a combination of two different densities of Ficoll-Hypaque (e.g., Histopaque™ 1077 and 1119, whose names indicated their specific gravities) allows separation of mononuclear cells from polymorphonuclear leukocytes in blood and marrow cell preparation. However, late apoptotic cells may preferentially be found in the cell pellet along with dead cells, which may introduce bias in apoptosis measurement.
3. Antibodies to identify specific subpopulations of cells can also be used with the sub G0/G1 method. However, the antibodies used must be tested with the lysolecithin to make sure they still fluoresce after fixation. Other antibodies can be added prior to PI or 7-AAD staining in order to identify specific cell populations *(25,26)*. However, control tubes with those antibodies with and without PI/7-AAD should be set up to serve as a negative control for PI/7-AAD fluorescence, which will also allow adjustment of the flow cytometer for the degree of spectral overlap.
4. One recent study compared morphologic assessment of apoptosis with Annexin V, TUNEL, and Apo2.7 flow-based techniques in samples from patients with B-CLL *(22)*. The Annexin V method consistently stained a higher percentage of cells and achieved a greater separation between positive and negative-staining cell populations.

References

1. Kerr, J. F., Wyllie, A. H., and Currie, A. R. (1972) Apoptosis: a basic biological phenomenon with wide-ranging implications in tissue kinetics. *Br. J. Cancer* **26,** 239–257.
2. Kerr, J. F., Winterford, C. M., and Harmon, B. V. (1994) Apoptosis. Its significance in cancer and cancer therapy. *Cancer* **73,** 2013–2026.
3. Kaufmann, S. H. and Earnshaw, W. C. (2000) Induction of apoptosis by cancer chemotherapy. *Exp. Cell Res.* **256,** 42–59.
4. Yuan, J. (1996) Evolutionary conservation of a genetic pathway of programmed cell death. *J. Cell. Biochem.* **60,** 4–11.
5. Villa, P., Kaufmann, S. H., and Earnshaw, W. C. (1997) Caspases and caspase inhibitors. *Trends Biochem. Sci.* **22,** 388–393.
6. Kerr, J. F. (1971) Shrinkage necrosis: a distinct mode of cellular death. *J. Pathol.* **105,** 13–20.
7. Oberhammer, F., Wilson, J. W., Dive, C., et al. (1993) Apoptotic death in epithelial cells: cleavage of DNA to 300 and/or 50 kb fragments prior to or in the absence of internucleosomal fragmentation. *EMBO J.* **12,** 3679–3684.
8. Wijsman, J. H., Jonker, R. R., Keijzer, R., van de Velde, C. J., Cornelisse, C. J., and van Dierendonck, J. H. (1993) A new method to detect apoptosis in paraffin sections: in situ end- labeling of fragmented DNA. *J. Histochem. Cytochem.* **41,** 7–12.
9. Gavrieli, Y., Sherman, Y., and Ben-Sasson, S. A.(1992) Identification of programmed cell death in situ via specific labeling of nuclear DNA fragmentation. *J. Cell Biol.* **119,** 493–501.
10. Darzynkiewicz, Z., Juan, G., Li, X., Gorczyca, W., Murakami, T., and Traganos F. (1997) Cytometry in cell necrobiology: analysis of apoptosis and accidental cell death (necrosis). *Cytometry* **27,** 1–20.
11. Fadok, V.A., Voelker, D. R., Campbell, P. A., Cohen, J. J., Bratton, D. L., and Henson, P. M. (1992). Exposure of phosphatidylserine on the surface of apoptotic lymphocytes triggers specific recognition and removal by macrophages. *J. Immunol.* **148,** 2207–2216.
12. Koopman, G., Reutelingsperger, C. P., Kuijten, G. A., Keehnen, R. M., Pals, S. T., and van Oers, M. H. (1994) Annexin V for flow cytometric detection of phosphatidylserine expression on B cells undergoing apoptosis. *Blood* **84,** 1415–1420.
13. Vermes, I., Haanen, C., Steffens-Nakken, H., and Reutelingsperger, C. (1995) A novel assay for apoptosis. Flow cytometric detection of phosphatidylserine expression on early apoptotic cells using fluorescein labelled Annexin V. *J. Immunol. Methods* **184,** 39–51.
14. Philpott, N. J., Turner, A. J., Scopes, J., et al. (1996) The use of 7-amino actinomycin D in identifying apoptosis: simplicity of use and broad spectrum of application compared with other techniques. *Blood* **87,** 2244–2251.
15. Endresen, P. C., Prytz, P. S., and Aarbakke, J. (1995) A new flow cytometric method for discrimination of apoptotic cells and detection of their cell cycle specificity through staining of F-actin and DNA. *Cytometry* **20,** 162–171.

16. Ormerod, M. G.. Paul, F., Cheetham, M., and Sun, X. M. (1995) Discrimination of apoptotic thymocytes by forward light scatter. *Cytometry* **21,** 300–304.

17. Gong, J., Traganos, F., and Darzynkiewicz, Z. (1994) A selective procedure for DNA extraction from apoptotic cells applicable for gel electrophoresis and flow cytometry. *Anal. Biochem.* **218,** 314–319.

18. Darzynkiewicz, Z. (1994) Simultaneous analysis of cellular RNA and DNA content. *Methods Cell Biol.* **41,** 401–420.

19. Hotz, M. A., Gong, J., Traganos, F., and Darzynkiewicz, Z. (1994) Flow cytometric detection of apoptosis: comparison of the assays of in situ DNA degradation and chromatin changes. *Cytometry* **15,** 237–244.

20. Johnson, L. V., Walsh, M. L., and Chen, L. B. (1980) Localization of mitochondria in living cells with rhodamine 123. *Proc. Natl. Acad. Sci. USA* **77,** 990–994.

21. Zhang, C., Ao, Z., Seth, A., and Schlossman, S. F. (1996) A mitochondrial membrane protein defined by a novel monoclonal antibody is preferentially detected in apoptotic cells. *J. Immunol.* **157,** 3980–3987.

22. Pepper, C., Thomas, A., Tucker, H., Hoy, T., and Bentley, P. (1998) Flow cytometric assessment of three different methods for the measurement of in vitro apoptosis. *Leuk. Res.* **22,** 439–444.

23. Majno, G. and Joris, I. (1995) Apoptosis, oncosis, and necrosis. An overview of cell death. *Am. J. Pathol.* **146,** 3–15.

24. Tait, J. F., Smith, C., and Wood, B. L. (1999) Measurement of phosphatidylserine exposure in leukocytes and platelets by whole-blood flow cytometry with annexin V. *Blood Cells Mol. Dis.* **25(5–6),** 271–278.

25. Witzig, T. E., Timm, M., Stenson, M., Svingen, P. A., and Kaufmann, S. H. (2000) Induction of apoptosis in malignant B cells by phenylbutyrate or phenylacetate in combination with chemotherapeutic agents. *Clin. Cancer Res.* **6,** 681–692.

26. Witzig, T. E., Timm, M., Larson, D., Therneau, T., and Greipp, P. R. (1999) Measurement of apoptosis and proliferation of bone marrow plasma cells in patients with plasma cell proliferative disorders. *Br. J. Haematol.* **104,** 131–137.

26

Assays for Neoplastic Cell Enrichment in Bone Marrow Samples

Rafael Fonseca and Gregory J. Ahmann

1. Introduction

Most hematological malignancies have clonal cells that reside in the bone marrow environment, and their analysis is critical for diagnosis *(1)*. In the process of procuring a clinical sample, research samples are frequently obtained, and their prompt and appropriate management should allow for their immediate usage or storage for the pertinent research questions. Because of the co-existence of normal cells in that environment, the investigator must decide on the need or appropriateness of selection of the clonal cells. While there will be an initial investment of resources and time, it is our experience that the immediate processing of a sample results in much better material being available for future studies. Furthermore, there is usually a higher yield if the selection process is done immediately as compared to an unsorted sample that is later thawed and selected. Thus, most investigators should seriously consider the possibility of future research in stored samples and decide *a priori* on the best method for enhancing the value of the material.

Given that our laboratory has worked extensively in the plasma cell disorders, we will focus on the processing of samples in this category as an example, but the same procedures could be used for any of the other cell compartments. There are several means by which a selection process can be done. For homogenized solutions (i.e., genomic DNA or mRNA) a sorting process, by flow cytometry or magnetic microbeads, will be mandatory before extraction if subsequent purity is desired. Other chapters deal with the processing of a sample to extract such material. If the experiments are done at the single cell level, it is also possible to use immunofluorescence or other methods for tagging the cells

From: *Methods in Molecular Medicine, vol. 85: Novel Anticancer Drug Protocols*
Edited by: J. K. Buolamwini and A. A. Adjei © Humana Press Inc., Totowa, NJ

of interest. In selected cases, an investigator may wish to use both methods simultaneously to improve on the ease of scoring without losing specificity. This is especially important for those situations with a low percentage involvement of the bone marrow, such as the monoclonal gammopathy of undetermined significance. So for samples of patients with the monoclonal gammopathy of undetermined significance and primary systemic amyloidosis, we first perform bead selection followed by interphase fluorescent *in situ* hybridization (FISH) analysis *(2)*.

In this chapter we will explore some of the techniques that we currently use for the optimal processing of the samples. The reader is referred to other chapters of this book to obtain details about the sample processing specific for the different applications.

2. Materials

1. Cytospin machine.
2. Blood tubes containing ethylenediamine tetraacetic acid (EDTA) or heparin.
3. RPMI 1640 cell culture medium.
4. Ficoll-hypaque.
5. Fetal calf serum (FCS).
6. Cytospin machine (Thermo Shandon, Pittsburgh, PA).
7. Magnetic micro-bead selection system.
8. Ethidium bromide solution: (2 g/200 mL H_2O).
9. Colcemid.
10. DNAse.
11. Phosphate buffered saline (PBS).
12. Hypotonic solution: (KCl:citrate, 50:50).
13. KCl.
14. Carnoy's fixative (methanol:acetic acid, 3:1 v/v).

3. Methods

3.1. Preparation and Enrichment of Bone Marrow Aspirates for Mononuclear Cells

3.1.1. Procurement of Sample

There are several methods to obtain a bone marrow sample, but most rely on the use of posterior iliac crest aspiration. Because the bone marrow is quickly diluted with blood if more than 3 mL is aspirated at the same site, it is important to perform small aspirates (<3 mL) and inserting the needle at a separate site (P.R. Greipp, personal communication). Thus, it is important to redirect the aspirate needle if a research sample is to be obtained. We have an IRB-approved protocol for such purpose. Patients provide informed consent

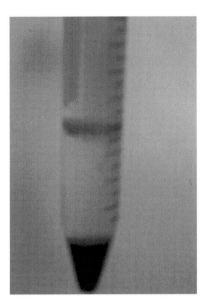

Fig. 1. Ficol tube showing the sediment layers.

after discussion of participation, subsequent to which bone marrow is aspirated and placed into a tube containing EDTA or heparin. EDTA is preferred as it is less likely to interfere with subsequent molecular biology assays.

3.1.2. Ficoll Separation of the Mononuclear Cells

By simple gradient centrifugation, it is possible to separate the mononuclear cell such that the bulk of neutrophilic series cells and red blood cells can be separated. In addition, a red blood cell lysis buffer can be utilized to further remove unwanted red blood cells. What follows is the standard Ficoll method for separation of the mononuclear cells. We normally use a density of 1.076 for this purpose.

1. Mix the sample one to one with RPMI 1640 cell culture medium.
2. Layer this mixture over 5 mL of Ficoll-hypaque and centrifuged for 25 min at 400g.
3. Remove the supernatant up to the mononuclear cell (MNC) interface (*see* **Fig. 1**).
4. Remove the MNCs and place into a 15-mL conical tube and fill tube with RPMI 1640 medium.
5. Centrifuge the cells again for 5 min at 300g.
6. Decant the supernatant and resuspend the cells in 15 mL of new medium and again centrifuge for 5 min at 300g.

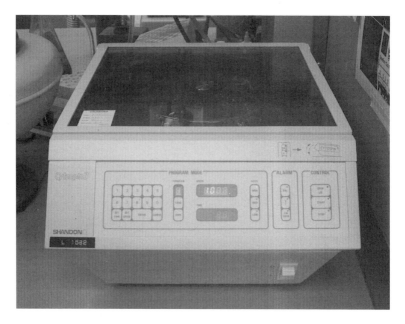

Fig. 2. Cytospin machine.

7. Decant the supernatant and resuspend the cells in 1 mL of RPMI medium
   containing 10% fetal calf serum (FCS). Then, count the MNCs either manually
   with a hemacytometer or automatically with a Coulter counter.

3.1.3. Cytospin Slide Preparation

In order to perform assays that involve the preservation of the cell morphology, we have found that the use of the Cytospin machine (Thermo Shandon,
Pittsburgh, PA) significantly helps to achieve this (*see* **Fig. 2**). This low-speed
centrifuge allows cells in suspension to be attached to slides in a discrete spot
area. The low-speed centrifugation preserves the cytoplasm. A filter-paper
interphase between the loading cartridge and the slide absorbs the suspending
medium, allowing immediate drying of the cells. This prevents the changes
in osmotic pressure involved in the air drying of a cell suspension drop, and
thus prevents the formation of crenocytes. If the preservation of nuclei is not
important, then the cytospin machine is not needed but can still be used.
New cartridges allow for the simultaneous deposition of several spots in a
single slide (2–8), and allow for multiple experiments to be carried out on a single
slide (*see* **Fig. 3**). The slides can be immediately fixed or left unfixed for future
usage. We normally use positively-charged slides, but others can be used as
needed according to the desired assays. If *in situ* RNA work is desired, the

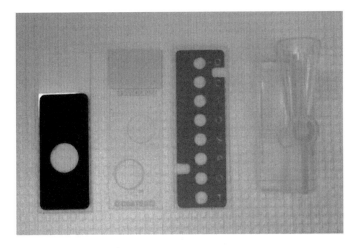

Fig. 3. Cytospin slides showing the capacity of 1 (left) to 8 spots (right) being analyzed simultaneously.

slides must be autoclaved and treated with a diethyl pyrocarbonate (DEPC) solution.

3.1.4. Magnetic Micro-Bead Selection

To further enrich a sample, our preferred method is the magnetic micro-bead selection. While multiple providers are available, we have used the one from Miltenyi (Auburn, CA) with great success. Overall, this results in a 20-fold enrichment of the sample. In the processing of the plasma cells, we have about a 50% yield. What follows is the description of the positive selection method we use to enrich for the monoclonal plasma cells. We find this method to be more affordable than to perform flow cytometric cell sorting and less dependent on the availability of equipment. In addition, multiple samples can be processed at once. The availability of an automated system makes the process even easier. While multiple antibodies bound to the micro-beads are available, essentially any cluster-of-differentiation (CD) marker can be used, since an anti-IgG magnetic micro-bead is available. Furthermore, the bound antibody can be removed after the cell selection so that processing of the sample can be performed after the sample is bead selected, including flow cytometric analysis.

1. Transfer a total of 2.0×10^7 MNCs into a 1-mL conical micro-centrifuge tube and add 0.5 mL of bead buffer, composed of phosphate buffered saline (PBS), pH 7.4, 5 mM EDTA, and 0.5% bovine serum albumin (BSA).

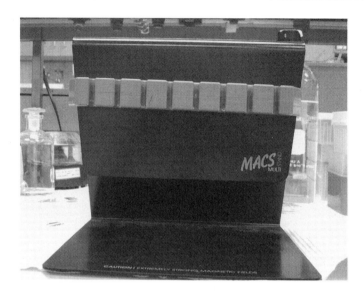

Fig. 4. Magnet stand used for the micro-bead selection.

2. Centrifuge the sample for 5 min at 300g and remove the supernatant.
3. Resuspend the cells in 180 μL of bead buffer and 20 μL of microbeads conjugated to an anti-human antigen is added (CD138 in the case of the plasma cell disorders).
4. Incubate the cells for 15 min at 8°C.
5. Centrifuge at 300g for 5 min at 4°C. While the cells are in the centrifuge, a Miltenyi microbead MS column is placed into a magnet, 0.5 mL of bead buffer is added to the column, and the flowthrough is collected into a clean 12 × 75-mm tube (*see* **Fig. 4**).
6. After centrifugation, resuspend the cell pellet in 0.5 mL of bead buffer.
7. Add the suspension to the column and allow it to flow through.
8. After the fluid has gone through, add 0.5 mL of bead buffer to the column and allow to flow through.
9. Repeated this washing step two more times. After the last wash, add 1.0 mL of bead buffer to the column and remove the column from the magnet.
10. Place the column onto a new 12 × 75 tube and push the plunger into the column. This forces the "bound" cells out of the column and may be repeated to increase cell recovery.
11. Count the sample. Depending on the number of plasma cells recovered, cytospin slides are made and cells are frozen for later retrieval of DNA, RNA, or more cytospin slides.

3.1.5. Thawing Bone Marrow for Bead Separation

It is sometimes necessary to thaw stored samples for enrichment and this section deals with the necessary steps to achieve this. It should be mentioned that the yield of this process is much lower than that of processing samples before freezing.

1. Retrieve a vial of bone marrow from liquid nitrogen and place it on ice.
2. Thaw the vial of bone marrow in a 37°C water bath just until it gets "slushy." Rinse vial with 70% ethanol and place on ice.
3. Transfer to a 15-mL conical tube and dilute one drop at a time at room temperature up to 10 mL over 12 min using room temperature RPMI containing 20% FCS, 2 mM EDTA and 10 units/mL DNAse (For 50 mL: 10 mL FCS, 200 µL 0.5 M EDTA, and 1 mg DNase, depending upon the activity of the DNase). Let the sample sit at room temperature for 30 min.
4. Centrifuge in Ficoll (density 1.076, Amersham Pharmacia, Uppsala Sweden) at room temperature for 15 min with the brake function of the centrifuge off. While centrifuging, prepare buffer for bead separation. Use PBS containing 0.5% FCS and 2 mM EDTA (Macs Buffer).
5. Collect interface of cells after Ficol centrifugation, count and wash with micro-bead buffer in 15-mL conical tube.
6. Spin for 10 min at room temperature at 300g.
7. Add 60 µL of bead buffer per 1×10^6 cells and subsequently add 40 µL of CD138 microbeads per 1×10^6 cells.
8. Incubate the sample in the cold room for 15 min and wash once with bead buffer and spin for 10 min at room temperature at 300g.
9. Resuspend the cells in 1 mL of bead buffer and count. Some of the automated machinery can process samples twice to increase the yield. A test of purity such as a Wright stain, immunofluorescence, or flow cytometric counting is highly recommended to assess for purity. Magnetic micro-beads can also be used to deplete the sample of an unwanted population of cells (i.e., T-cell depletion).

3.1.6. Colcemid Pulsing of Cultured Cells

In order to obtain cells arrested in metaphase for cytogenetic analysis a standard procedure is to incubate cells with a tubulin-disrupting agent such as Colcemid. Through this procedure, one can produce mitotic arrest and can observe condensed chromosomes. This will result in the direct evaluation of metaphases, and in the possibility of their use for the more sophisticated molecular cytogenetic analysis, such as spectral kerotyping (SKY).

1. To 10 mL of culture medium add 50 µL of ethidium bromide (2 g/200 mL H_2O) and 100 µL of Colcemid (0.001%) and incubate for 2 h at 37°C.

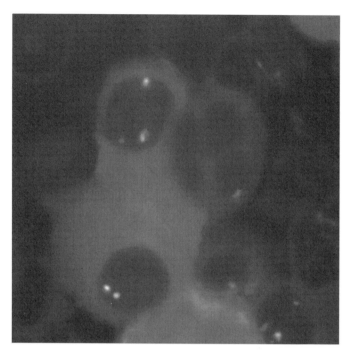

Fig. 5. cIg-FISH technique. The intense blue fluorescence of the cytoplasm also for the detection of the clonal plasma cells. The cells are also subjected to FISH and display discrete signals.

2. Spin down and resuspend in 10 mL of hypotonic solution (KCl : citrate, 50 : 50) or just KCl (0.075 *M*) and incubate for 20 min at room temperature or 37°C.
3. Add 5 mL of 3 : 1 Carnoy's fixative (methanol : acetic acid), mix gently and spin for 5 min.
4. Resuspend in 3 : 1 fixative and drop on slides. If there are not enough metaphase cells present try an overnight Colcemid pulsing. Add 10 µL of colcemid with no ethidium bromide to 10 mL of media and follow the rest of the procedure.

3.2. Immunofluorescence

It is also possible to select cells of interest in an unsorted cytospin preparation through the use of immunodetection. We have performed this best using immunofluorescent-labeled antibodies directed against the cytoplasmic light chain, in the case of the plasma cells, or against other cell surface markers *(3)*. By using a light-chain restricted antibody, we can limit the analysis to the cells forming part of the clones (*see* **Fig. 5**). It is important to perform the immunodetection of the antigen of interest before proceeding with other experimental steps that might disrupt the recognition sites and prevent success-

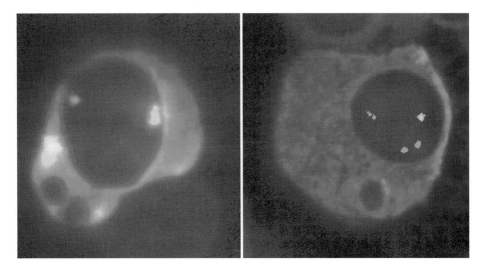

Fig. 6. Multicolor immunofluorescence detection of various cell populations. The green cell is detected with an anti-IgG antibody while the red one is detected with an anti-IgA antibody. Cell specific FISH analysis can be performed.

ful binding. We have found that paraformaldehyde fixation performed after the binding of the antibody permits subsequent steps (i.e., high temperature, 80°C, denaturation) that would normally preclude immunodetection, with no discernible loss of the signal. The antibody concentration has to be experimentally determined for the individual assays. We like to use direct antibody detection with a second step amplification. Antibodies are normally diluted in a protein-containing solution at 1:10 to 1:1000 concentrations. The use of a blue fluorophore allows for two-color fluorescent *in situ* hybridization experiments to be performed on the same cell. We have successfully used this technique to detect cytogenetic abnormalities in the myeloid cells and not in the cells of the clone *(4)*.

3.2.1. Multiple Color Immunofluorescence

We have also explored the use of a combination of antibodies for the selection of cells that require further selection. This can be performed with two different antibodies that allow for the separation of two populations under study to detect co-existence of the same marker in a single cell (*see* **Fig. 6**). For instance, with combinatorial immunofluorescence, one can positively select only plasma cells that are IgA kappa with an anti-A and anti-kappa antibodies bound to different fluorophores. Only those cells with positive staining for both markers are considered positive.

3.3. Flow Cytometry

Flow cytometry allows for the selection of samples and subpopulations of cells contained within the sample. While the technique has some advantages such as immediate double gating, it is more expensive, time consuming and dependent on equipment availability, compared to the magnetic micro-bead selection process.

4. Notes

1. Multiple mechanisms are available for the sorting of samples obtained from the bone marrow. The selection of a sample prior to freezing is technically simpler and with much higher yields. Investigators should seriously consider processing of the samples at this time.
2. The use of direct cell detection can further enhance the assay specificity.

References

1. Kyle, R. A. (1992) Diagnostic criteria of multiple myeloma. *Hematol. Oncol. Clin. North Am.* **6,** 347–358,
2. Fonseca, R., Ahmann, G. J., Jalal, S. M., et al. (1998) Chromosomal abnormalities in systemic amyloidosis. *Br. J. Haematol.* **103,** 704–710.
3. Ahmann, G. J., Jalal, S. M., Juneau, A. L., et al. (1998) A novel three-color, clone-specific fluorescence in situ hybridization procedure for monoclonal gammopathies. *Cancer Genet. Cytogenet.* **101,** 7–11.
4. Fonseca, R., Rajkumar, S. V., Ahmann, G. J., et al. (2000) FISH demonstrates treatment related chromosome damage in myeloid cells but not plasma cells in primary systemic amyloidosis. *Leuk. Lymphoma* **39,** 391–395.

Index

343